D1571126

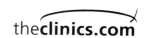

MEDICAL CLINICS
OF NORTH AMERICA

Antimicrobial Therapy

GUEST EDITOR
Burke A. Cunha, MD, MACP

November 2006 • Volume 90 • Number 6

SAUNDERS

An Imprint of Elsevier, Inc.
PHILADELPHIA LONDON TORONTO MONTREAL SYDNEY TOKYO

W.B. SAUNDERS COMPANY
A Division of Elsevier Inc.

1600 John F. Kennedy Boulevard • Suite 1800 • Philadelphia, Pennsylvania 19103-2899

http://www.theclinics.com

MEDICAL CLINICS OF NORTH AMERICA	**Volume 90, Number 6**
November 2006	**ISSN 0025-7125**
Editor: Rachel Glover	**ISBN 1-4160-3889-2**

The ideas and opinions expressed in *Medical Clinics of North America* do not necessarily reflect those of the Publisher. The Publisher does not assume any responsibility for any injury and/or damage to persons or property arising out of or related to any use of the material contained in this periodical. The reader is advised to check the appropriate medical literature and the product information currently provided by the manufacturer of each drug to be administered to verify the dosage, the method and duration of administration, or contraindications. It is the responsibility of the treating physician or other health care professional, relying on independent experience and knowledge of the patient, to determine drug dosages and the best treatment for the patient. Mention of any product in this issue should not be construed as endorsement by the contributors, editors, or the Publisher of the product or manufacturers' claims.

Medical Clinics of North America (ISSN 0025-7125) is published bimonthly by W.B. Saunders, 360 Park Avenue South, New York, NY 10010-1710. Business and editorial offices: 1600 John F. Kennedy Boulevard, Suite 1800, Philadelphia, PA 19103-2899. Accounting and circulation offices: 6277 Sea Harbor Drive, Orlando, FL 32887-4800. Periodicals postage paid at New York, NY, and additional mailing offices. Subscription prices are USD 157 per year for US individuals, USD 273 per year for US institutions, USD 81 per year for US students, USD 200 per year for Canadian individuals, USD 347 per year for Canadian institutions, USD 119 per year for Canadian students, USD 227 per year for international individuals, USD 347 per year for international institutions and USD 119 per year for international students. To receive student/resident rate, orders must be accompanied by name of affiliated institution, date of term, and the *signature* of program/residency coordinator on institution letterhead. Orders will be billed at individual rate until proof of status is received. Foreign air speed delivery is included in all *Clinics* subscription prices. All prices are subject to change without notice. POSTMASTER: Send address changes to *Medical Clinics of North America*, Elsevier Periodicals Customer Service, 6277 Sea Harbor Drive, Orlando, FL 32887-4800. **Customer Service: 1-800-654-2452 (US). From outside of the USA, call (+1) 407-345-1000. E-mail: hhspcs@harcourt.com.**

Reprints. For copies of 100 or more, of articles in this publication, please contact the Commercial Reprints Department, Elsevier Inc., 360 Park Avenue South, New York, New York 10010-1710. Tel.: (+1) (212) 633-3813; Fax: (+1) (212) 462-1935; E-mail: reprints@elsevier.com.

Medical Clinics of North America is also published in Spanish by McGraw-Hill Interamericana Editores S. A., P.O. Box 5-237, 06500 Mexico, D.F., Mexico.

Medical Clinics of North America is covered in *Index Medicus, Current Contents, ASCA, Excerpta Medica, Science Citation Index,* and *ISI/BIOMED.*

Printed in the United States of America.

GOAL STATEMENT

The goal of *Medical Clinics of North America* is to keep practicing physicians up to date with current clinical practice by providing timely articles reviewing the state of the art in patient care.

ACCREDITATION

The *Medical Clinics of North America* is planned and implemented in accordance with the Essential Areas and Policies of the Accreditation Council for Continuing Medical Education (ACCME) through the joint sponsorship of the University of Virginia School of Medicine and Elsevier. The University of Virginia School of Medicine is accredited by the ACCME to provide continuing medical education for physicians.

The University of Virginia School of Medicine designates this educational activity for a maximum of 90 *AMA PRA Category 1 Credits*™. Physicians should only claim credit commensurate with the extent of their participation in the activity.

The American Medical Association has determined that physicians not licensed in the US who participate in this CME activity are eligible for *AMA PRA Category 1 Credits*™.

Credit can be earned by reading the text material, taking the CME examination online at http://www.theclinics.com/home/cme, and completing the evaluation. After taking the test, you will be required to review any and all incorrect answers. Following completion of the test and evaluation, your credit will be awarded and you may print your certificate.

FACULTY DISCLOSURE/CONFLICT OF INTEREST

The University of Virginia School of Medicine, as an ACCME accredited provider, endorses and strives to comply with the Accreditation Council for Continuing Medical Education (ACCME) Standards of Commercial Support, Commonwealth of Virginia statutes, University of Virginia policies and procedures, and associated federal and private regulations and guidelines on the need for disclosure and monitoring of proprietary and financial interests that may affect the scientific integrity and balance of content delivered in continuing medical education activities under our auspices.

The University of Virginia School of Medicine requires that all CME activities accredited through this institution be developed independently and be scientifically rigorous, balanced and objective in the presentation/discussion of its content, theories and practices.

All authors/editors participating in an accredited CME activity are expected to disclose to the readers relevant financial relationships with commercial entities occurring within the past 12 months (such as grants or research support, employee, consultant, stock holder, member of speakers bureau, etc.). The University of Virginia School of Medicine will employ appropriate mechanisms to resolve potential conflicts of interest to maintain the standards of fair and balanced education to the reader. Questions about specific strategies can be directed to the Office of Continuing Medical Education, University of Virginia School of Medicine, Charlottesville, Virginia.

The authors/editors listed below have identified no professional or financial affiliations for themselves or their spouse/partner:
Amira Ali-Ibrahim, MD; Emilio Bouza, MD, PhD; Almudena Burillo, MD, PhD; Jason Collins, MD; Burke A. Cunha, MD (Guest Editor); Rachel Glover (Acquisitions Editor); Kathryn Momary, Pharm.D.; Patricia Munoz, MD, PhD; Shilpa M. Patel, MD; David Schlossberg, MD, FACP; and Duane T. Smoot, MD, FACP, FACG.

The authors/editors listed below identified the following professional or financial affiliations for themselves or their spouse/partner:
Gary Doern, MD is on the speakers' bureau for Abbott, Bayer, Astra-Zeneca, Pfizer, Roche and Aventis; is an independent consultant to Abbott, Bayer, and AstraZeneca.
Nancy Khardori, MD is on the speakers' bureau for GSK, Merck, Ortho, Pfizer, Roche, and Schering; serves as a consultant for GSK, Ortho, Pfizer, and Wyeth; and, owns stock in Merck.
Manjunath (Amit) P. Pai, Pharm.D is an independent contractor conducting research for Pfizer, Astellas Pharma, Inc., and Cubist Pharmaceuticals, Inc..
Keith A. Rodvold, Pharm.D is on the speakers' bureau for Ortho-McNeil Pharmaceutical, Wyeth Research, Abbott Laboratories, Astra-Zeneca and Daiichi; is on the advisory board for Ortho-McNeil, Abbott Laboratories, Astra-Zeneca, Glaxo-SmithKline, Ortho Biotech, Baxter and Elan; and, is an independent contractor for Wyeth Reseach and Sanofi-Aventis.
Louis Saravolatz, MD is an independent contractor for Pfizer and Theravance; is on the advisory committee for Pfizer; and, is a consultant and on the speakers' bureau for Schering.
Charles W. Stratton, MD is on the speakers' bureau for Aventis.

Disclosure of Discussion of non-FDA approved uses for pharmaceutical products and/or medical devices:
The University of Virginia School of Medicine, as an ACCME provider, requires that all faculty presenters identify and disclose any "off label" uses for pharmaceutical and medical device products. The University of Virginia School of Medicine recommends that each physician fully review all the available data on new products or procedures prior to instituting them with patients.

TO ENROLL

To enroll in the Medical Clinics of North America Continuing Medical Education program, call customer service at 1-800-654-2452 or visit us online at http://www.theclinics.com/home/cme. The CME program is available to subscribers for an additional fee of USD 205.

FORTHCOMING ISSUES

RECENT ISSUES

GUEST EDITOR

BURKE A. CUNHA, MD, Professor of Medicine, State University of New York School of Medicine, Stony Brook; Chief, Infectious Disease Division, Winthrop-University Hospital, Mineola, New York

CONTRIBUTORS

AMIRA ALI-IBRAHIM, MD, Gastroenterology Section, Department of Medicine, Howard University College of Medicine, Washington, District of Columbia

EMILIO BOUZA, MD, PhD, Department of Clinical Microbiology and Infectious Diseases, Hospital General Universitario Gregorio Marañón, Universidad Complutense, Madrid, Spain

ALMUDENA BURILLO, MD, PhD, Servicio de Microbiología Clínica, Hospital de Madrid-Monteprincipe, Madrid, Spain

JASON COLLINS, MD, Gastroenterology Section, Department of Medicine, Howard University College of Medicine, Washington, District of Columbia

BURKE A. CUNHA, MD, Professor of Medicine, State University of New York School of Medicine, Stony Brook; Chief, Infectious Disease Division, Winthrop-University Hospital, Mineola, New York

GARY V. DOERN, PhD, Director, Clinical Microbiology Laboratories, University of Iowa Hospital; and Clinics Professor of Pathology, University of Iowa College of Medicine, Iowa City, Iowa

NANCY KHARDORI, MD, PhD, Professor of Medicine and Microbiology/Immunology and Chief, Division of Infectious Diseases, Department of Internal Medicine, Southern Illinois University School of Medicine, Springfield, Illinois

KATHRYN M. MOMARY, PharmD, Research Fellow, College of Pharmacy, University of Illinois at Chicago, Chicago, Illinois

PATRICIA MUÑOZ, MD, PhD, Department of Clinical Microbiology and Infectious Diseases, Hospital General Universitario Gregorio Marañón, Universidad Complutense, Madrid, Spain

MANJUNATH P. PAI, PharmD, Assistant Professor, College of Pharmacy, University of New Mexico, Albuquerque, New Mexico

SHILPA M. PATEL, MD, Division of Infectious Diseases, Department of Internal Medicine, St. John Hospital and Medical Center, Grosse Pointe Woods, Michigan; Assistant Professor of Internal Medicine, Wayne State University, Detroit, Michigan

KEITH A. RODVOLD, PharmD, Professor of Pharmacy Practice, Associate Professor of Medicine in Pharmacy, Colleges of Pharmacy and Medicine, University of Illinois at Chicago, Chicago, Illinois

LOUIS D. SARAVOLATZ , MD, MACP, Professor and Chairman, Department of Medicine, St. John Hospital and Medical Center, Grosse Pointe Woods, Michigan

DAVID SCHLOSSBERG, MD, FACP, Medical Director, Tuberculosis Control Program, Department of Health, Philadelphia; Professor of Medicine, Temple University School of Medicine, Philadelphia, Pennsylvania

DUANE T. SMOOT, MD, FACP, FACG, Professor and Chair, Department of Medicine, Howard University College of Medicine, Washington, District of Columbia

CHARLES W. STRATTON, MD, Associate Professor of Pathology and Medicine, Vanderbilt University School of Medicine, Nashville, Tennessee

CONTENTS

Caused by the toxins of certain strains of *C difficile*, CDAD represents a growing concern, with epidemic outbreaks in some hospitals where very aggressive and difficult-to-treat strains have recently been found. Incidence of CDAD varies ordinarily between 1 to 10 in every 1,000 admissions. Evidence shows that CDAD increases morbidity, lengths of stay, and costs. This article describes the clinical manifestations of CDAD, related risk factors, considerations for confirming CDAD, antimicrobial and nonantimicrobial treatment of CDAD, and issues related to relapses. The article concludes with a discussion of recent epidemic outbreaks involving CDAD.

Antibiotic resistance among pneumococci, enterococci, and staphylococci has become increasingly important in recent decades. Clinicians should be familiar with the nuances of antibiotic susceptibility testing and interpretation in selecting antibiotics for these infections. The clinical significance of penicillin-resistant *Streptococcus pneumoniae*, macrolide-resistant *S pneumoniae*, and multidrug-resistant *S pneumoniae* is discussed. The clinical spectrum and therapeutic approach to *Enterococcus faecalis* (ie, vancomycin-sensitive enterococci) and *E faecium* (ie, vancomycin-resistant enterococci) are discussed. Differences in therapeutic approach between methicillin-sensitive *Staphylococcus aureus* and methicillin-resistant *S aureus* (MRSA) infections are reviewed. Differences between in vitro susceptibility testing and in vivo effectiveness of antibiotics for hospital-acquired MRSA (HA-MRSA) are described. Lastly, the clinical features of infection and therapy of HA-MRSA and community-acquired MRSA (CA-MRSA) infections are compared.

The science of antibiotic therapy for infectious diseases continues to evolve. In many instances where empiric coverage is necessary, treatment with more than one agent is considered prudent. If an etiology is identified, antibiotics are modified based on culture and susceptibility data. Even when the organism is known, more than one antibiotic may be needed. Decisions about antibiotics should be made after assessments of pertinent clinical information, laboratory and microbiology information, ease of administration, patient compliance, potential adverse effects, cost, and available evidence supporting various treatment options. Clinicians also need to consider synergy and local resistance patterns in selecting therapeutic options. In this article, the authors outline monotherapy and combination therapy options for several common infectious diseases.

THE MEDICAL
CLINICS
OF NORTH AMERICA

Med Clin N Am 90 (2006) xiii–xiv

Preface

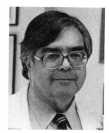

Burke A. Cunha, MD, MACP
Guest Editor

Since the author first edited a volume of the *Medical Clinics of North America* on Antimicrobial Therapy in 1982, the ensuing decades have witnessed a conceptual evolution in antimicrobial therapy. Emerging pathogens and antibiotic resistance have fueled the search for new antibiotics to cope with these ongoing challenges. Over the years, additional antimicrobial agents have been introduced to clinical use. Because the number of newly introduced antibiotics has been limited, clinicians have re-evaluated older agents with activity against newly resistant organisms. Recent decades have also witnessed an increase in the appreciation of the pharmacokinetic aspects of antimicrobials, which has led to an increase in the use of oral antibiotics to treat more and more infectious diseases. This volume of the *Medical Clinics of North America* on Antimicrobial Therapy builds on the previous volumes of 1995 and 2001, edited by the author, and focuses on the currently most relevant topics relating to antimicrobial therapy.

This issue contains articles written by recognized authorities on antibiotics from the United States and Europe. The contributors have been selected on the basis of their clinical experiences and expertise. The issue consists of 12 articles covering the most important aspects of antimicrobial therapy at the present time. It begins with an overview by Dr. Nancy Khardori of antimicrobial therapy past, present, and future, which places today's antimicrobial therapy in perspective. Dr. Charles Stratton contributes an article reviewing in vitro susceptibility testing versus in vivo clinical effectiveness of antibiotics. Other antibiotic concepts that are problematic for many physicians include the relative merits of monotherapy and

doi:10.1016/j.mcna.2006.07.001

combination therapy for various infectious diseases, which are ably reviewed by Dr. Louis Saravoltaz. Older antibiotics are being "rediscovered" for new uses against resistant organisms. An article by the author focusing on new uses for older antibiotics is also included in this issue.

Antibiotic resistance among gram-positive cocci is a problem worldwide. Multidrug-resistant *Streptococcus pneumonia*, vancomycin-resistant enterococci, and methicillin-resistant *Staphylcoccus aureus* are the most frequently encountered gram-positive therapeutic challenges for physicians. Nationally, there is an underrecognized and underappreciated epidemic of macrolide-resistant *S pneumoniae*, and this important topic is well reviewed by Dr. Gary Doern.

The antimicrobial therapies for *Helicobacter pylori* and *Clostridium difficile* diarrhea/colitis remain thorny therapeutic problems. Key components of this issue are articles reviewing the current state of the art for the antimicrobial therapy of *H pylori,* by Dr. Duane Smoot, and for that of *C difficile* diarrhea/colitis, by Dr. Emilio Bouza.

The remaining articles are devoted to potential problems related to antimicrobial prescription. The common dilemma of selecting an antibiotic in the penicillin-allergic patient is reviewed by the author. The important topic of antibiotic drug interactions is carefully covered by Dr. Keith Rodvold. The issue concludes with the important subject of apparent antibiotic failure, covered by Dr. David Schlossberg.

This issue of the *Medical Clinics of North America* on Antimicrobial Therapy is an up-to-date desk reference source dealing with the most important clinical problems related to antimicrobial therapy that are currently faced by physicians.

Burke A. Cunha, MD, MACP
Chief, Infectious Disease Division
Winthrop-University Hospital
Minneola, NY 11501

THE MEDICAL
CLINICS
OF NORTH AMERICA

Med Clin N Am 90 (2006) 1049–1076

Antibiotics—Past, Present, and Future

Nancy Khardori, MD, PhD*

*Department of Internal Medicine, Southern Illinois University School of Medicine,
PO Box 19636, Springfield, IL 62794-9636, USA*

The drug therapy for diseases other than those caused by microbial agents involves treating the host. In infectious diseases therapy, the goal is to rid the host of the pathogen. Hence, drug therapy is aimed at the pathogen. Because a second living agent is involved in the triangle, drug therapy is affected by the pathogen's nature, its tissue specificity, and, most importantly, the changes it undergoes to survive. The history of antimicrobial therapy has clearly demonstrated that the drugs that are used to treat infections are also responsible for making them more difficult to treat in the future. The only way to keep antimicrobial agents useful is to use them appropriately and judiciously.

The slow but glorious beginning

The "Ice Man," whose mummified body was retrieved from underneath a receded glacier in northern Italy in 1991, had lived about 5310 years ago [1]. The dead body had been dried quickly by alpine winds, then frozen and enclosed in the perennial ice—explaining its extraordinarily well-preserved state. The study of this mummy has produced important archaeologic and medical findings. Among them are the presence of *Trichuris trichura* eggs in his rectum and his probable use of a fungus, *Piptoporus betulinus,* for these intestinal parasites. The toxic oils in the fungus were probably the only remedy available in Europe until the introduction of more toxic chenopod oil from the Americas. The efficacy of chenopod oil was increased by a strong laxative, resulting in expulsion of the dead and dying worms and eggs. *Piptoporus betulinus* contains oils that are toxic against metazoans and have known antimicrobial properties against mycobacteria. The fungus also contains toxic resins and agaric acid, which are powerful laxatives. For

---

* Infectious Disease Division, PO Box 19636, 701 North First Street, Room A-478, Springfield, IL 62794-9636.
E-mail address: nkhardori@siumed.edu

doi:10.1016/j.mcna.2006.06.007

more than five millennia, human beings have treated their ailments with extraordinary creativity. For example, in 2000 BC, Assyrian and Babylonian doctors used a salve made of frog bile and sour milk for treating infected eyes, but this concoction was considered effective only after the patient took a swig of beer and a sliced onion [2].

It was in the mid-nineteenth century that Louis Pasteur observed that some micro-organisms destroy others—the phenomenon that later came to be known as antibiosis or "against life." The search for antimicrobial chemical agents revealed that antiseptics were too toxic for anything but surface use on wounds. German bacteriologist Paul Ehrlich systematically tested chemical agents, searching for the "magic bullet" that could be taken internally, but he ended up with only a high-risk arsenic-based treatment for syphilis. Alexander Fleming in London had been looking for antibacterial agents in human secretions. The discovery of the antibacterial activity of the enzyme lysozyme was made because of an accidental sneeze on a petri dish [3]. Fleming observed that, when bacteria later formed colonies on the plate, none developed in the spots occupied by mucus. Further tests showed that lysozyme acted mostly against harmless organisms. In 1928, serendipity made another notable visit to Fleming's laboratory at St. Mary's Hospital in London. He had left a culture plate of *Staphylococci* uncovered in his laboratory while on a vacation. On his return, he noticed mold in the petri dish along with a clear space between the *Staphylococci* and the blue-green spotted mold. It was the classic example of what Pasteur had referred to as fortune's accommodating a willing mind.

Fleming identified the mold as *Penicillium natatum*, a culture filtrate of which was able to kill bacteria. He named the agent in the filtrate penicillin. Because of a paucity of financial resources and Fleming's modest ambitions (according to some historians), it took another 12 years for penicillin to emerge as the greatest medical advance of the twentieth (or any other) century. But the golden age of anti-infective medicine actually began in 1934. Gerhard Domagk, a German pharmacologist, discovered that a dye used to tint cloth cured streptococcal infections in mice. His own dying daughter survived a streptococcal infection after he injected her with the dye. Daniel Bovert, a Swiss-born scientist, identified the active compound as sulfanilamide. Domagk was awarded the Nobel Prize in Medicine in 1939.

Florey and Chain, working at Oxford University, were interested to note that staphylococci, though resistant to sulfanamides and lysozyme, were apparently sensitive to the penicillium mold [4]. World War II provided a crucial spur to and much-needed resources for research on antimicrobial agents. Staphylococcal infections and gas gangrene were killing more men than the immediate organ damage caused by shell and bullet wounds. In the spring of 1940, Florey and Chain were able to make a small amount of yellowish-brown powder from Fleming's mold. This first sample of "penicillin powder" was a million times more potent than Fleming's original filtrate. In 1941, the Fermentation Division of the newly created Northern

Regional Research Laboratory in Peoria, Illinois became the first site for commercial production of penicillin [5]. By mid-1944, when the Allies invaded France, large supplies of the yellow liquid were available. When treated with penicillin, 95% of the wounded lived. The Nobel Prize in Medicine was awarded to Fleming, Florey, and Chain in 1945.

Selman A. Waksman, a Russian immigrant to the United States, gave the name "antibiotics" to chemicals (produced by soil-borne fungi and micro-organisms) that destroy or slow the growth of other microbes. Waksman spent his lifetime hunting for "antibiotic"-producing micro-organisms and in 1943 found a mold that was able to kill *Tubercle* bacilli. He called this aminoglycoside streptomycin. On November 20, 1944, streptomycin was administered to a young woman who had advanced pulmonary tuberculosis at the Mayo Clinic in Rochester, Minnesota. Her life was saved by streptomycin. Dr. Waksman received the Nobel Prize in 1952 for its discovery.

The rest is history: awakening to the possibilities and confronting the challenges

Subsequently, more broad-spectrum penicillins and other aminoglycosides were developed, followed by more antibiotic classes. More than 5000 antibiotics are now known. Approximately a thousand of these have been carefully investigated, and about 100 are currently used to treat infections. Most are produced by actinomycetes and bacteria, many of which are then chemically modified (semisynthetic). Others are completely synthetic.

The β-lactams

Penicillin, the prototype β-lactam, is a 6-aminopenicillanic acid consisting of a thiazolidine ring, an attached β-lactam ring, and a side chain [6]. Manipulations of the side chain have altered β-lactamase susceptibility, antibacterial spectrum, and pharmacokinetic properties. Other groups of antibacterial agents that contain the β-lactam ring include cephalosporins, carbapenems, and monobactams. In actively dividing bacteria, the β-lactams inhibit enzymes (transpeptidase, carboxypeptidase, and endopeptidase) located beneath the cell wall that are termed the "penicillin-binding proteins." This inhibition prevents the development of normal peptidoglycan structure, because these enzymes are involved in creating the cross-linkage between the peptide chains. Various bacteria differ in the permeability of their cell walls to antibiotics and the type and concentration of penicillin-binding proteins. Subsequent activation of the endogenous autolytic system of bacteria by β-lactams initiates cell lysis and death [7].

Penicillins

The penicillin family of antibiotics remains an important part of today's antimicrobial armamentarium. Penicillins are bactericidal against most susceptible bacteria (an important exception is *Enterococcus* spp) and have an excellent safety profile. The initial introduction of aqueous penicillin G for treatment of streptococcal and staphylococcal infections in 1941 to 1944 was followed by the emergence of penicillinase-producing *Staphylococcus aureus*. This finding prompted the development of penicillinase-resistant penicillins (methicillin, oxacillin, and nafcillin), in which an acyl side chain prevents disruption of the β-lactam ring by penicillinase. The aminopenicillins (ampicillin, amoxicillin, and bacampicillin) were developed because of the need for antibiotics with activity against gram-negative bacteria. Aminopenicillins initially were effective against *Escherichia coli*, *Proteus mirabilis*, *Shigella* spp, *Salmonella* spp, *Hemophilus* spp, and *Neisseria* spp. Carboxypenicillins (carbenicillin and ticarcillin) and ureidopenicillins (mezlocillin, azlocillin, and piperacillin) offer additional activity that includes Enterobacteriaceae, such as *Klebsiella* spp and *Enterobacter* spp, and *Pseudomonas aeruginosa*. Many gram-negative bacteria, including Enterobacteriaceae and *Hemophilus influenzae*, are now resistant to penicillins because of β-lactamase production. β-lactamase inhibitors (clavulanic acid, sulbactam, and tazobactam) inhibit the non–group 1 β-lactamases of resistant bacteria. They are available as combinations of amoxicillin-clavulanate, ampicillin-sulbactam, ticarcillin-clavulanate, and piperacillin-tazobactam. The current penicillin group of drugs is ineffective against gram-negative bacteria that produce other types of β-lactamases, including extended-spectrum β-lactamases.

Cephalosporins

This large family of broad-spectrum β-lactam agents was introduced for clinical use in the 1960s [8]. They are bactericidal, with favorable pharmacokinetic profiles and low rates of drug-associated toxicity. In general, first-generation cephalosporins (cefazolin, cephalexin) are most active against aerobic, gram-positive cocci, including methicillin-susceptible *S aureus*. Second-generation cephalosporins are more active against selected gram-negative organisms, such as *Klebsiella* spp, *E coli*, and *Proteus* spp. Cefoxitin and cefotetan (technically cephamycins) are active against anaerobic bacteria as well. Third-generation cephalosporins are the most active against gram-negative aerobic organisms. From this group, ceftazidime and, to a lesser extent, cefoperazone are active against *P aeruginosa*. Cefepime, classified as a fourth-generation cephalosporin, has an extended spectrum of activity against both gram-positive and gram-negative organisms, including *P aeruginosa*.

Carbapenems

Carbapenems are a class of β-lactam antibiotics with a broad spectrum of activity against aerobic and anaerobic gram-positive and gram-negative organisms [9]. Imipenem in combination with cilastatin became available in 1985 and meropenem in 1996. With the exception of enterococci, carbapenems are bactericidal against susceptible bacteria. The spectrum of activity of carbapenems includes streptococci, methicillin-susceptible staphylococci, *Neisseria* spp, *Haemophilus* spp, anaerobes, and aerobic gram-negative pathogens, including *P aeruginosa*. *Stenotrophonomas maltophilia* is typically resistant to carbapenems. Imipenem is more active against gram-positive cocci in vitro, and meropenem has better in vitro activity against gram-negative bacilli. A third carbopenem, ertapenem, has become available recently; however, it does not have activity against *P aeruginosa* or enterococci.

Monobactams

The only available monobactam, aztreonam, is a synthetic compound with a β-lactam ring that is activated by its sulfonic acid group [9]. Because of the lack of affinity for the penicillin-binding proteins of gram-positive and anaerobic bacteria, the antibacterial spectrum of aztreonam is limited to aerobic gram-negative bacilli, similar to that of aminoglycosides. However, it is not nephrotoxic and is only weakly immunogenic. Therefore, aztreonam, in susceptible bacteria, is a useful nonnephrotoxic alternative to the aminoglycosides and may be used with caution in patients with significant penicillin hypersensitivity reactions.

The aminoglycosides

The first aminoglycoside, streptomycin, was introduced in 1942 for treatment of tuberculosis [10]. It was followed by the availability of neomycin, which has formidable toxicity and is not useful for systemic therapy. Kanamycin, isolated in 1957, was the aminoglycoside of choice until gentamicin became available in 1963. Gentamicin provided a breakthrough in the therapy for infections caused by aerobic gram-negative bacilli, including *P aeruginosa*. Tobramycin, amikacin, and netilmicin became available in 1968, 1972, and 1975, respectively. Dibekacin, sisomicin, and isepamicin are not available in the United States.

The aminoglycosides bind irreversibly to the 30S bacterial ribosomes and inhibit protein synthesis. The irreversible binding may explain the bactericidal effect of aminoglycosides as compared with other inhibitors of protein synthesis. Low pH and anaerobic conditions inhibit an energy- and oxygen-dependent transport mechanism, which is an essential prelude to the binding of aminoglycosides to ribosomes. When such conditions exist within a focus of infection (such as purulence, abscess formation), the activity of aminoglycosides is limited. The uptake of aminoglycosides is facilitated in the presence of inhibitors of cell-wall synthesis (ie, β-lactams and glycopeptides). Aminoglycosides demonstrate concentration-dependent killing and a prolonged postantibiotic effect. The postantibiotic effect leads to continued bacterial killing even after serum concentrations fall below the minimum inhibitory concentrations. Aminoglycosides are useful in the treatment of infections caused by aerobic gram-negative bacilli (including *P aeruginosa*), particularly in combination with β-lactams. Most institutions have noted little change in the patterns of aminoglycoside resistance among gram-negative bacilli, despite alarming increases in aminoglycoside-resistant enterococci. Amikacin may be active against gentamicin-resistant gram-negative bacilli and is useful in the treatment of infections caused by *Nocardia* and nontuberculous mycobacteria. Streptomycin is an important agent for the treatment of infections due to multidrug-resistant *Mycobacterium tuberculosis* and may be useful in the treatment of some gentamicin-resistant enterococccal infections.

The macrolides and ketolides

The prototype macrolide, erythromycin derived from *Streptomyces erythrus*, became available in the 1950s [11]. Macrolides inhibit RNA-dependent protein synthesis by reversibly binding to the 50S ribosomal subunit of susceptible organisms. They inhibit bacterial growth by inducing dissociation of peptidyl transfer RNA from the ribosome during the elongation phase. In general macrolides are bacteriostatic, although bactericidal activity may occur under certain conditions or against specific micro-organisms. Erythromycin is active against streptococci, including group A β-hemolytic streptococci and *Streptococcus pneumoniae*, methicillin-susceptible staphylococci, *Treponema pallidum*, *Ureaplasma urealyticum*, *Mycoplasma pneumoniae*, *Legionella pneumophila*, *Chlamydia* spp, some strains of *Rickettsia*, *Neisseria meningitidis*, *Neisseria gonorrhoeae*, *Bordetella pertussis*, and *Campylobacter jejuni*. The two new macrolides, clarithromycin and azithromycin, are more stable, have a longer half-life, and are better tolerated than erythromycin. The new macrolides have a broader antimicrobial spectrum than erythromycin against *Mycobacterium avium complex*, other nontuberculous mycobacteria, *H influenzae*, and *Chlamydia trachomatis*.

Ketolides are a new class of macrolides with activity against gram-positive organisms (*S pneumoniae* and *Streptococcus pyogenes*) that are resistant to macrolides [12]. The ketolides have a higher (10- to 100-fold) affinity for the ribosome binding site (domain V) than does erythromycin. In addition, they bind to domain II of the $23S_rRNA$, do not induce methylase production, and resist active drug efflux. Because of these attributes, the ketolides are able to overcome both low-level and high-level resistance to macrolides. Telithromycin, a ketolide and a semisynthetic derivative of erythromycin, became available in 2005 for treatment of community-aquired pneumonia, acute exacerbation of chronic bronchitis, and acute sinusitis.

The tetracyclines

Aureomycin, the first tetracycline, was discovered by Duggar in 1948 [13]. After amoxicillin and erythromycins, tetracyclines remain the most widely prescribed antibiotic class in the world. Tetracycline, oxytetracycline, doxycycline, minocycline, and demeclocycline are available in the United States. The low cost, reduced toxicity, and superior pharmacokinetic properties of doxycycline make it the agent of choice among tetracyclines. Tetracyclines inhibit protein synthesis by reversible binding to the 30S ribosome and by blocking the attachment of transfer RNA to an acceptor site on the messenger RNA ribosomal complex. These agents are generally bacteriostatic against a wide array of aerobic and anaerobic bacteria, including many *Rickettsiae, Chlamydiae*, mycoplasmas, spirochetes, mycobacteria, and some protozoa. Minocycline and doxycycline have excellent in vitro inhibitory activity against staphylococci, including methicillin-resistant *S aureus, Staphylococcus epidermidis,* and *Mycobacterium* spp, including *M marinum, M fortuitum,* and *M chelonei.* In contrast to other tetracyclines, the dose of doxycycline and minocycline does not need to be adjusted in patients who have renal dysfunction. Both are eliminated through the hepatobiliary and gastrointestinal tracts.

The lincosamides

Lincomycin was first isolated from *Streptomyces lincolnesis* in 1962. Clindamycin, a derivative of lincomycin with better absorption and improved antibacterial activity, was introduced in 1966 [14]. The lincosamides inhibit bacterial protein synthesis by reversible binding to the 50S ribosomal subunit. The macrolides and chloramphenicol also act at this site and can be antagonistic to each other and to lincosamides. Clindamycin facilitates opsonization, phagocytosis, and intracellular killing of bacteria. It has also been found to interfere with biofilm formation associated with device-related infection and chronic infections like osteomyelitis. Clindamycin is active against anaerobic gram-positive and gram-negative organisms, with the exception of *Clostridium difficile* and *Fusobacterium varium.* Aerobic gram-positive organisms except enterococci are also susceptible to clindamycin. All aerobic gram-negative organisms should be considered resistant to clindamycin. Clindamycin-susceptible organisms that are resistant to erythromycin can rapidly become resistant to clindamycin because of the macrolide-lincosamide-streptogramin cross-resistance mechanism.

Trimethoprim-sulfamethoxazole

The combination of trimethoprim (TMP) with sulfamethoxazole (SMX) was widely used before it became available in the United States in 1974 [15]. SMX, like all sulfonamides, is a structural analogue of ρ-aminobenzoic acid (PABA), which bacteria use to initiate the synthesis of folic acid. Bacterial dihydropteroate synthetase is the enzyme involved in incorporating PABA into dihydrofolic acid and is competitively inhibited by SMX. Dihydrofolate reductase then converts dihydrofolic acid to tetrahydrofolic acid, the metabolically active cofactor for synthesis of purines, thymidine, and DNA. TMP competitively binds to dihydrofolate reductase. By virtue of sequential inhibition of two enzymes in the synthesis of folic acid, TMP-SMX acts synergistically and has bactericidal activity against many aerobic gram-positive and gram-negative bacteria involved in community-acquired infections. Some nosocomial pathogens, such as *Stenotrophomonas maltophilia*, *Burkholderia cepacia*, and *Serratia marcescens*, are also susceptible to TMP-SMX. It is active against *Nocardia asteroides*, *Listeria monocytogenes*, *Pneumocystis jirovecii*, *Isospora belli*, and cyclospora. TMP-SMX is one of the most widely used antimicrobial agents in the world. However, increasing bacterial resistance and occasional severe adverse effects are diminishing the usefulness of this cost-effective antimicrobial agent combination.

The glycopeptides

Vancomycin, the first glycopeptide antibiotic, was isolated from *Streptomyces orientalis* in the mid-1950s and introduced for clinical use in 1958 [16]. It became an important agent for treatment of infections caused by penicillin-resistant staphylococci and other gram-positive bacteria, which were becoming increasingly prevalent. Early impure preparations of vancomycin were associated with significant nephrotoxicity and ototoxicity. With the availability of β-lactamase–stable penicillins like oxacillin and naficillin, the need for vancomycin use decreased dramatically until the emergence of methicillin-resistant staphylococci in the early 1980s. Vancomycin demonstrated constant activity against all common gram-positive bacteria for more than 3 decades of clinical use. The gradually increasing prevalence of vancomycin resistance in enterococci and the recent emergence of vancomycin–intermediately susceptible *S aureus* and vancomycin-resistant *S aureus* have created a need for alternatives to vancomycin in the management of serious infections caused by resistant gram-positive organisms [17].

Vancomycin is a bactericidal agent (except against enterococci) that complexes with the D-alanyl D-alanine portion of peptide precursor units at the crucial site of attachment and inhibits peptidoglycan polymerase and transpeptidation reactions. Because vancomycin inhibits the stage of peptidoglycan synthesis at a site earlier than the site of action of β-lactams, no cross-resistance with β-lactams occurs. Vancomycin also affects the permeability of cytoplasmic membranes and may impair RNA synthesis. The combination of vancomycin and gentamicin is synergistic against *S aureus* and enterococci. The spectrum of activity of vancomycin is limited to gram-positive organisms, including *Staphylococci, Streptococci, Enterococci, Corynebacteria, Bacillus* spp, *Listeria monocytogenes*, anaerobic cocci, *Actinomyces*, and *Clostridia*. Infrequently encountered gram-positive organisms that are resistant to vancomycin include leuconostoc, *Pediococcus*, *Lactobacillus*, and *Erysipelothrix*.

Teicoplanin, a glycopeptide derived from the fermentation products of *Actinoplanes teicnomyceticus*, is chemically similar to vancomycin [18]. Teicoplanin is more lipophilic than vancomycin, a property that results in rapid and excellent tissue penetration and intracellular concentration. It is water soluble at physiologic pH, releases slowly from tissues, and has a long elimination half-life. It may be given once a day intramuscularly or intravenously. Although widely used in Europe and Asia for treatment of gram-positive infections, teicoplanin is still investigational in the United States.

The fluoroquinolones

Fluoroquinolones are synthetic compounds that first became available in the mid-1980s. They have been developed extensively to optimize antibacterial activity against gram-negative and gram-positive bacteria as well to improve pharmacokinetic properties and safety [19]. Topoisomerase (I, II, III, and IV) maintains cellular DNA in an appropriate state of supercoiling in both replicating and nonreplicating regions of the bacterial chromosome. The fluoroquinolones target topoisomerase type II (DNA gyrase) and topoisomerase type IV. The activity of the quinolones against gram-positive bacteria may primarily be the result of targeting topoisomerase IV and topoisomerase II, whereas DNA gyrase may be the primary target in gram-negative bacteria. The complexity of the interaction of various fluoroquinolones with different topoisomerases is the basis of differences in the antibacterial spectrum and resistance patterns among fluoroquinolones. The prototype quinolone, nalidixic acid, is considered a first-generation fluoroquinolone. The second-generation fluoroquinolones, such as norfloxacin, ciprofloxacin, and ofloxacin, have predominantly gram-negative activity. Ciprofloxacin remains the most active fluoroquinolone against *P aeruginosa*. In contrast, the third- and fourth-generation fluoroquinolones, like levofloxacin, gatifloxacin, and moxifloxacin, have better activity against gram-positive organisms, particularly *S pneumoniae*, including penicillin-resistant strains.

The streptogramins

The first streptogramin antibiotic, pristinamycin, produced by *Streptomyces pristinaespiralis,* was developed in France more than 35 years ago. It has been used primarily for the treatment of respiratory and skin structure infections [20]. Quinupristin/dalfopristin (30:70) is a water-soluble derivative of pristinamycin with a selective spectrum of activity against gram-positive organisms. It became available in the United States in 1999 for the treatment of infections caused by vancomycin-resistant *Enterococcus faecium* and those caused by other gram-positive organisms for which the other available agents are ineffective or not tolerated. The target of quinupristin (streptogramin A) and dalfopristin (streptogramin B) is the bacterial ribosome. Dalfopristin blocks an early step of protein synthesis (elongation) and causes a conformational change leading to increased affinity of ribosomes for quinupristin. Quinupristin blocks a subsequent step by inhibiting peptide bond formation, resulting in the release of incomplete protein chains. This sequential dual mechanism of action results in synergy and bactericidal activity against most susceptible organisms except enterococci. The combination is active against *E faecium*, including Vancomycin resistant *Enterococcus faecalis* (VREF), but not against *Enterococcus faecalis*, against staphylococci, including methicillin-resistant and vancomycin-resistant strains, against streptococci, including penicillin-resistant *S pneumoniae*, and against *Corynebacteria* and *Clostridrium perfringens*. Other susceptible organisms include *Neisseria meningitidis*, *Moraxella catarrhalis*, *Legionella pneumophilia*, and *Mycoplasma pneumoniae* [21].

The oxazolidinones

The first oxazolidinone was developed in the late 1970s for control of bacterial and fungal foliage diseases of tomatoes and other plants [22]. A number of the oxazolidinones studied in the 1980s showed an in vitro spectrum of activity against staphylococci, streptococci, enterococci, anaerobes, and *M tuberculosis*. Because of adverse effects, particularly monomine oxidase inhibition and bone marrow toxicity, they were not further developed for human use. Some also showed acute (lethal) animal toxicity. Further chemical modifications have resulted in safer agents with superior pharmacokinetic properties. Linezolid first became available in the United States in 2000 for treatment of infections caused by vancomycin-resistant enterococci and respiratory and skin structure infections caused by gram-positive bacteria [23]. Linezolid is bacteriostatic against enterococci as well as staphylococci. It inhibits ribosomal protein synthesis by interfering with initiation complex formation. Linezolid is active against most gram-positive cocci, including those resistant to methicillin and vancomycin. It is also active against *Legionella* spp, *Chlamydia pneumoniae*, and *H influenzae*.

The lipopeptides

Daptomycin, a fermentation byproduct of *Streptomyces roseosporus*, is a naturally occurring cyclic lipopeptide antibiotic [24]. It exhibits a rapid bactericidal activity in a concentration-dependent manner. The spectrum of activity involves a broad range of gram-positive pathogens, including those that are resistant to methicillin, vancomycin, and other currently available agents [25]. The mechanism of action is binding to the cell membrane in a calcium-dependent manner, leading to depolarization of the bacterial membrane potential, which results in termination of bacterial DNA, RNA, and protein synthesis, release of intracellular potassium, and cell death. Daptomycin first became available in the United States in 2004 for the treatment of complicated skin and soft tissue infections [26].

The glycylcyclines

Tigecycline, a derivative of the tetracycline minocycline, is a broad-spectrum glycylcycline antibiotic [27]. It is a bacteriostatic agent, acts by binding to the 30s ribosomal subunit of bacteria, and prevents elongation of peptide chains, which leads to inhibition of protein synthesis. Tigecycline is not affected by the known mechanisms of resistance (efflux and ribosomal) to tetracyclines and has activity against bacterial isolates that are resistant to other antibiotic classes such as β-lactams and fluoroquinolones. These attributes give tigecycline a broad spectrum of activity against vancomycin-resistant enterococci, methicillin-resistant *S aureus*, and many species of multiresistant aerobic and anaerobic gram-negative bacteria. Its activity against *P aeruginosa* and *Proteus* spp is very limited. Tigecycline first became available in the United States in 2005 for the treatment of complicated intra-abdominal infections and complicated skin and skin structure infections [28–30].

Many battles won but the war goes on—the evolution of antimicrobial resistance

More than 6 decades following the availability of penicillin, and in the wake of the eradication of naturally occurring smallpox by global vaccination and dramatic decreases in infections like diphtheria, tetanus, and poliomyelitis by their respective vaccines, infectious diseases remain a major cause of morbidity and mortality in the world. Although many new drugs have been discovered, so have many new infectious agents. However, the biggest hurdle in the path to victory has been the development of resistance to antibiotics by most types of bacteria [31]. Given that antibiotics are mediating a war between the human species and thousands of bacterial species, the counterstrike was expected and anticipated at a pace determined by the genetic constitution of various bacteria. What was not a part of the long-range plan was the widespread use, abuse, and misuse of antibiotics prevalent in various forms in different parts of the world.

To quote Frank L. Meleney from 1947, "We have to get experience all over again on the behavior of infection under treatment with these new drugs. There is a temptation to use them promiscuously and yet certainly if we are to improve our results we must use them with discrimination" [32]. The indiscriminate use of antibiotics significantly enhances the natural occurrence of bacterial resistance by exerting selective pressure. Although time to clinically relevant resistance varies, no class of antimicrobial agents is exempt from bacterial resistance [33–37]. Resistance to antimicrobial agents in bacteria can be intrinsic or acquired. Naturally occurring intrinsic resistance determines the spectrum of activity of an antimicrobial agent at the time it becomes available, for example, resistance of *P aeruginosa* to vancomycin and that of anaerobic bacteria to aminoglycosides. Acquired resistance occurs when bacteria that have been susceptible to an antimicrobial agent develop resistance. This process can occur by mutation or by acquisition of new DNA. Mutation leading to chromosomal resistance is an event that occurs whether the organism is exposed to antimicrobial agents or not. However, the presence of an antimicrobial agent results in rapid killing of the susceptible populations, including the normal flora at various sites, and offers the resistant ones a selective survival advantage. If the antimicrobial use happens to be inappropriate or unnecessary, the net health outcome is negative. Transferable resistance was first recognized in 1959, when plasmids were shown to transfer resistance genes from *Shigella* to *E coli*. Plasmids and other genetic material may be transferred between bacteria by a number of mechanisms [34]:

> Transduction—Plasmid DNA is enclosed in bacteriophages (viruses with bacteria as the host) and transferred to another organism of the same species. An example of this mechanism is the transfer of β-lactamase production from a penicillin-resistant to a penicillin-susceptible staphylococcus.
> Transformation—Naked DNA from dead bacteria can be taken up by certain bacterial species (eg, *S pneumoniae*), resulting in an altered genotype including antibiotic resistance. In the laboratory, this is the principle behind DNA recombinant technology, in which this process is facilitated by various experimental steps. This process is increasingly being recognized as an important means of genetic transfer between bacteria in the environment. It is also probably the main route for the spread of penicillin resistance in *S pneumoniae* by creation of a "mosaic penicillin-binding protein gene."
> Conjugation—Bacterial conjugation refers to a unilateral transfer of genetic material between bacteria of the same or different genera. Resistance (R) factors are a class of plasmids that carry genes for resistance to antimicrobial agents and heavy metals. The transfer occurs through a process of mating (conjugation) mediated by a fertility (F) factor. This results from the extension of sex pili (fimbriae) from the donor (F+) cell to the recipient. Plasmids or other extrachromosomal DNA particles are transferred to the recipient cell through these protein tubules. A series of closely linked genes may then transfer resistance to multiple antimicrobial agents. Such resistance transfer factors (RTFs) are the most common method of spread for multidrug resistance among gram-negative bacteria. Plasmids transfer resistance to penicillins and cephalosporins by carrying genes for formation of β-lactamases. They also code for acetyltransference that destroys chloramphenicol and for enzymes that acetylate, adenylate, or phosphorylate various aminoglycosides. Plasmids also determine the active transport of tetracyclines across the cell membrane and code for many other enzymes that destroy antimicrobial agents.
> Transposition—Transposons (transposable elements or "jumping genes") transfer short DNA sequences between plasmids or between

a plasmid and a portion of the bacterial chromosome. This process extends the range of bacteria to which plasmids spread. The mecA gene found in methicillin resistant *Staphylococcus aureus* (MRSA) may have been acquired by transposition.

The major mechanisms of resistance to various antibiotic classes and their genetic basis are listed in Table 1 [36].

Origin of resistance genes

At the time antibiotics were first introduced, the biochemical and molecular basis of resistance was not known. Bacteria collected between 1914 and 1950 (the Murray Collection) were found to be completely sensitive to antimicrobial agents, including sulfanamides that had been introduced in the mid-1930s [38]. However, they contained a large number of plasmids capable of conjugative transfer. Antimicrobial resistance was reported in the early 1940s in streptococci, gonococci, and staphylococci. Recognition of the mutation of the target genes for streptomycin in *M tuberculosis* soon after its introduction led to the concept of multidrug therapy for tuberculosis.

To understand the evolution and dissemination of antimicrobial resistance genes, it is important to appreciate the rapidity of bacterial multiplication and the constant exchange of bacteria among human, environmental, animal, and agricultural sources throughout the world. Evidence supports the notion that the antimicrobial resistance determinants were not derived from the currently observed bacterial hosts of the resistance plasmids [39–41]. Because the evolutionary time-frame is only 60 years, it is difficult to create a model in which mutations from common ancestral genes alone would have led to the current level of antimicrobial resistance. It is more likely that they were derived from a large and diverse gene pool, presumably already present in environmental bacteria. Many fungi and bacteria that produce antibiotics possess determinants of resistance that are similar to those found in pathogenic bacteria. Could this be nature's way of putting us in our place? It has been reported that commercial antibiotic preparations contain DNA including antibiotic resistance gene sequences from the producing bacteria [42]. Gene exchange occurs in soil or, more likely, in the gastrointestinal tract of humans and animals. This is where the selection pressure by antimicrobial agents is the heaviest. The injudicious use of antimicrobial agents in medical practice is certainly responsible for that selection pressure. However, agricultural, veterinary, and lately household use of antibacterial agents contributes significantly to resistance in human pathogens. The search for newer antimicrobial agents with different mechanisms of action is ongoing and most likely will only result in temporary improvement in the antimicrobial resistance scenario, as has been seen in the past 6 decades.

Table 1
Common mechanisms of resistance among bacteria and genetic basis

Mechanisms of resistance	Antibiotic class	Genetics	Example micro-organisms
Enzymatic inhibition			
β-lactamases			
Group 1 — cephalosporin hydrolyzing not inhibited by CA	β-lactam	Chromosomal, produce β-lactamases constitutively	*Enterobacter*, *Klebsiella*, and *Citrobacter* spp resistant to third-generation cephalosporins
Group 2a — penicillinases inhibited by CA	β-lactam	Plasmid mediated	*Staphylococcus aureus* resistant to penicillin but sensitive to amoxicillin CA
Group 2bN — broad spectrum not inhibited by CA	β-lactam	Plasmid, chromosomal	*Escherichia coli* resistant to amoxicillin CA
Group 2b — extended broad spectrum	β-lactam	Plasmid mediated	*Plasmodium aeruginosa* and *Klebsiella* spp resistant to ceftazidime and other third-generation cephalosporins
Group 2c — carbenicillinases, oxacillinases	β-lactam	Plasmid, chromosomal	*P aeruginosa* resistant to carbenicillin and piperacillin
	β-lactam	Plasmid, chromosomal	*Nocardia*, *Actinomadura*, *Bacillus*, and *Mycobacterium* spp
Group 2e — cephalosporins inhibited by CA	β-lactam	Plasmid, chromosomal	*Stenotrophomonas maltophilia* susceptible to ticarcillin-CA; bacteroides spp resistant to β-lactams
Group 3 — metalloenzymes	β-lactam	Plasmid, chromosomal	*S maltophilia* resistant to carbapenems
Group 4 — penicillinases not inhibited by CA	β-lactam	Plasmid, chromosomal	*Ralstonia* (*Burkholderia*) *cepacia* resistant to β-lactams
Acetyltransferases, adenyltransferases, phosphotransferases	Aminoglycosides	Plasmid mediated except *Enterococcus faecium* (chromosomal)	Enterococci and gram-negative bacilli highly resistant to β-lactams
Chloramphenicol acetyltransferases	Chloramphenicol	Plasmid, chromosomal	

Mechanism	Antibiotic class	Genetic basis	Examples
Esterases, phosphotransferases	Macrolides, streptogramins (dalfopristin)	Plasmid	Enterobacteriaceae highly resistant
Permeability-uptake	β-lactam, aminoglycosides, and macrolides	Chromosomal	P aeruginosa resistant to β-lactams; gram-negative bacteria, enterococci, and staphylococci resistant to aminoglycosides
Porin channels	β-lactam and carbapenems	Chromosomal	P aeruginosa, S maltophilia, and Aeromonas spp
Drug efflux	Quinolones, tetracycline, chloramphenicol, and β-lactam	Tet gene for tetracycline resistance—plasmid or chromosomal	P aeruginosa and S aureus
Target site alteration			
Altered penicillin-binding protein	β-lactam	Plasmid mediated in S aureus; mosaic genes in penicillin-resistant Streptococcus pnumoniae	S aureus resistant to methicillin; S pneumoniae resistant to penicillin
Altered cell wall oligopeptide	Glycopeptide	vanA and vanB-transferable plasmid; vanC-contitutive plasmid	Enterococci resistant to vancomycin and teicoplanin
Altered ribosomal target	Tetracycline, macrolides and aminoglycosides, streptogramins (quinupristin), oxazolidinone		Enterococci, E coli, and Neisseria gonorrhoeae resistant to streptomycin; S aureus, streptococci, and enterococci spp resistant to macrolides
Competitive inhibition by overproduction of P-aminobenzoic acid or altered dihydropteroate synthetase	Sulfonamides	Plasmid mediated; cross-resistance common	E coli, S aureus, and Neisseria spp
Auxotrophs—utilization of alternative growth requirements	Trimethoprim		Enterococci

Abbreviation: CA, Clavulanic acid.
Adapted from Virk A, Steckelberg JM. Symposium on antimicrobial agents. Part XVII. Clinical aspects of antimicrobial resistance. Mayo Clin Proc 2000;75(2):200; with permission.

The future of antibiotic therapy

The strategies for developing new antibacterial agents will continue to involve inhibition of bacterial growth and multiplication, bacterial death, and interference with cellular attachment. In addition, improving drug delivery systems, reducing side effect profiles, improving antimicrobial susceptibility testing and reporting, and improving antibiotic use in the clinical setting will all play important roles in determining the future of antibacterial therapy [43].

Antibiotics with novel modes of action

No novel antibiotic classes were licensed in the 1970s, 1980s, or 1990s [44]. Since 2000, oxazolidinones (linezolid) and the cyclic lipopeptides (doplomycin) with novel modes of action have been approved for the treatment of infections caused by gram-positive bacteria. Molecular biology and genomics have not yet proved useful in the discovery of new antimicrobial agents. Researchers are now focusing in part on virulence factors rather than on the organisms directly. One of the fascinating potential targets is the quorum-sensing mechanism. After a threshold of high cell density or "quorum" is reached, bacteria sense one another's presence. This process results in the production of a protective biofilm or an orchestrated production of virulence factors. Early studies suggest a promising role for anti–quorum-sensing agents as adjuncts to standard antimicrobial therapy.

A group of enzymes capable of duplicating damaged DNA and creating new mutations was reported by Livneh [45]. Suppression of the activity of these enzymes could potentially slow the spread of antibiotic-resistant bacteria. Vancomycin-resistant and multiresistant pathogenic strains of *E faecalis* differ from nonpathogenic strains in that their genomes contain a 150-kb–long "pathogenicity island" [46]. The virulence factors encoded by these genes include the enterococcal toxin cytolysin (a surface protein that aids colonization) and factors that contribute to bacterial clumping, adherence to host tissues, and resistance to phagocytosis. The function of many of the genes in the pathogenicity island is unknown, and none of them is known to code for antibiotic resistance. They may represent putative targets for novel antimicrobial drugs, and it may be possible to design a prophylactic agent that prevents colonization with these virulent strains. Hung and colleagues [47] have described a small molecule, virstatin, which inhibits the activation of cholera toxin genes and abolishes the production of both cholera toxin and toxin coregulated pilus. It did not interfere with the growth of the organism in laboratory media but was a highly potent inhibitor of intestinal colonization by the bacteria. In an infant mouse model, virstatin was shown significantly to reduce colonization of the small bowel and reduce the numbers of *Vibrio cholerae* from already colonized mice. Combination of antivirulence drugs with conventional antibiotics may prove to be the safest and most efficacious approach, with the potential to extend the useful life of both types of agents [48]. Antivirulence drugs may facilitate an active immune response in the host, because they will not inhibit the growth of the pathogen.

Chemical modification of known agents

Addition of β-lactamase inhibitors to current β-lactam agents continues to be explored. This approach may reach a saturation point because of the emergence of extended-spectrum β-lactamases. LY333328 is a glycopeptide in which the vancosamine sugar has been derivitized, resulting in activity against vancomycin (glycopeptide)–resistant gram-positive bacteria, including enterococci. This compound possesses bactericidal activity against enterococci [49]. L786392 is a carbapenem in which the side chain at the 2 position has been modified to improve affinity of penicillin-binding protein 2a of methicillin-resistant staphylococci and penicillin-binding protein 5 of penicillin-resistant *E faecium* [22].

Antibiotic hybrids

It is now possible to synthesize a single molecule composed of two antibiotics [50]. This development could overcome the obstacles to the use of combinations as two separate drugs, which may preclude simultaneous effective concentrations at the target site. Hybrids have been produced mostly between β-lactam antibiotics (cephalosporins and carbapenems) and fluoroquinolones, including ciprofloxacin. Some of the hybrids have shown antibacterial effects attributable to both types. Others may be able to use bacterial enzymes (such as β-lactamases) to produce two separate antibacterials from a prodrug. Some hybrids have already been administered safely to humans in clinical trials, but none have become available for clinical use.

Antimicrobial peptides

Ubiquitous natural antibiotics

Peptides with antibacterial activity, such as β-defensins and cathelicidius, are expressed on epithelial surfaces and in neutrophils in mammals [51,52]. They have been proposed to provide a first line of defense against infection by acting as "natural antibiotics." The naturally occurring peptides demonstrate a broad spectrum of activity against bacteria, fungi, viruses, and cancer cells. Insects do not possess lymphocytes, immunoglobulins, or any of the complex components of an acquired immune system, yet they have existed and thrived on this planet for millions of years. They rely on the transient synthesis of potent antimicrobial peptides to combat microbial invasion and subsequent infections. Thus these peptides are a part of innate defense ("natural immunity") and may be found in all multicellular organisms, including humans. The antimicrobial peptides are typically found at sites that come in direct contact with the environment, such as eyes, ears, oral cavity, lungs, and gastrointestinal tract. The process of bacterial lysis by antimicrobial peptides starts with the lipid–peptide interaction between the bacterial membrane and the peptide, followed by binding and insertion of the peptide molecules into the cytoplasmic membrane. This process leads to disruption of the cytoplasmic membrane and lysis. Defensins have also been reported to damage bacterial DNA by inducing single-strand breaks. The naturally occurring peptides are gene coded and are produced by all species, including bacteria. Some of the larger families of these ribosomally synthesized peptides include the cecropins, defensins, magainins, and protegrins.

Non–ribosomally synthesized, high-molecular-weight peptide antibiotics are produced by bacteria, fungi, and streptomyces. Of these, gramicidin S, polymixin B, polymixin E, and bacitracin have been in clinical use. These are made of multienzyme complexes rather than being synthesized on ribases. This class of peptide antibiotics must be drastically modified to reduce toxicity. Gramicidin, derived from *Bacillus brevis*, was the first antibiotic to be used commercially to treat bacterial infection, a few years before the introduction of penicillin. The availability of safer agents for systemic use relegated these agents to topical use. As resistance develops to all currently available agents, the need to develop more active, stable, and nontoxic variants of naturally occurring peptides has led to the synthesis of "new and improved" peptides. *Streptococcus macedonicus* (ACA-DC198), isolated from Greek cheese, has been shown to produce an antimicrobial peptide that could prevent food spoilage and the growth of pathogenic micro-organisms [53]. This new food-grade bacteriocin has been named "macedocin," and its safety, stability, and effectiveness in food products is being assessed. At present, the only bacteriocin approved as a food additive is nisin.

Designed antimicrobial peptides

Designed antimicrobial peptides (DAPs) are laboratory-synthesized peptides based on novel designs or modifications of existing natural peptides. Many DAPs have been designed using natural peptides as templates. They include D2A21 and D4E1, which are currently under investigation. It remains to be seen whether they will become effective and safe systemic antimicrobial agents in the future.

Bacterial attachment inhibitors

For pathogens, including bacteria, a prelude to initiating invasive disease is recognizing and attaching themselves to epithelial/mucosal cells. This process involves the binding of specific bacterial receptors to oligosaccharide complexes expressed on mucosal cells. When these oligosaccharides can be competitively replaced by noncellular oligosaccharides to saturate the bacterial receptors, the attachment or subsequent invasion may be prevented [43]. Mucosal surfaces do produce free oligosaccharides, but these may not be produced in quantities sufficient to alter the course of microbial invasion. The protection afforded by breast milk against neonatal infections may be related to large amounts of oligosaccharides present in the breast milk. Administration of large amounts of oligosaccharides specific for the bacterial receptors may dissociate bound bacteria from their target cells, preventing further invasion. This concept has been used with some success in preventing *E coli* infections in newborn calves and monkeys. The only selective pressure applied by this strategy is nonlethal and so is not likely to lead to resistance. If and when such agents become available, we may finally have the "good" in antimicrobial therapy without the "bad."

Bacteriophages as antimicrobial agents

Bacteriophages, the viruses with bacteria as their hosts, are among the most common organisms on earth. Bacteriophage-induced lysis (killing) of bacteria is highly efficient and specific for different types of bacteria. In the war of species between phages and bacteria, humans are bystanders. Bacteriophages were discovered during World War I by Twort and d'Herelle at the Pasteur Institute [54]. They were named in 1917 by d'Herelle, who predicted that these biologic agents would produce a revolution in the treatment of infectious diseases. He believed that nature had provided us with a living weapon against bacteria. However, their role as therapeutic agents has not shown much promise.

Hundreds of types of phages exist; each kills only one type of bacteria, and contaminants of bacterial lysis left in phage preparations are toxic to humans. Although Eli Lilly manufactured therapeutic phages for the United States market in the 1930s, they were quickly outpaced by penicillin. However, their simple molecular structure made them an ideal tool for DNA research and molecular biology. In 1934, d'Herelle joined the Institute of Bacteriology in Tubilis, which was founded by a young Georgian microbiologist named George Eliava. Eliava Institute became the world's leading center for therapeutic phage research, with a library of more than 300 phage clones. During World War II, it supplied a powerful dysentery phage to the Red Army, and it subsequently provided precisely targeted phages to hospitals all over the Soviet bloc.

Bacteriophage research has continued for more than 80 years. The creation of an intravenous phage preparation for *S aureus* has been the most remarkable contribution of Eliava Institute. In the past 15 years, lack of financial resources and difficult working conditions have decreased the production of phage sprays, salves, ointments, and tablets. A significant part of the phage library has been lost. With the need for and the interest in antibiotic alternatives, bacteriophage therapy is suddenly looking "very promising." Three start-up companies in the United States and others in Europe are once again exploring the broad therapeutic potential of bacteriophages. Although wild phages are expelled quickly by the body's filtering system, engineered mutant phages have been shown to remain in experimental animals for much longer. A single phage can produce 400,000 daughter cells in an hour, with subsequent exponential increase in numbers. If they do become available for commercial therapeutic use, they will be the only drugs that make more of themselves in the hosts they are treating.

Societal issues outside the medical world

It is time for global society to accept bacteria as normal, generally useful components of the living world and to refrain from trying to eliminate them except when they give rise to disease. To prevent or reverse the problem of antibiotic resistance, society must recognize that most bacteria are a natural and needed part of life on this planet. The antimicrobial agents affect the "good" as well as the "bad" bacteria [55]. In addition to physician education and other interventions to promote appropriate use of antimicrobial agents, consumers need to be educated [56]. They must stop demanding antibiotics for themselves and their children based on self-diagnosis and previous experiences. They should use antibiotics for the intended purpose only and complete a full course in spite of improvement in their symptoms. When members of the public save antibiotics from a current prescription for later use, disastrous outcomes can result. Meats and eggs should be well cooked and fresh vegetables thoroughly washed. Antibacterials in soaps and other products at home are unnecessary. They should only be used in consultation with health care providers by people who are highly susceptible to infection because of an immunocompromised state. Hand washing with soap and water leads to physical removal of bacteria that are not normal inhabitants of the skin and is the most effective day-to-day means of preventing transmission of bacteria, including those that are resistant to antibiotics.

It is also time for global society to acknowledge that the use of an antimicrobial anywhere can increase resistance to antimicrobial agents anywhere else [57]. Antibiotic resistance certainly crosses all barriers. The use of antimicrobials in animals, agriculture, and humans contributes to the global pool of resistance genes in the environment. Common bacteria, including normal flora in humans and animals, contribute to antimicrobial resistance by serving as reservoirs of resistance genes transferable to pathogenic organisms. In the United States, the amount of antimicrobials administered to animals is comparable to that used in humans [58,59]. Much of this use is nontherapeutic, for purposes of growth promotion and disease prevention. Such use selects for resistant strains and is followed by dissemination in the environment and transmission to other animals and humans. Transfer of bacteria from food animals to humans is common through direct contact and undercooked meats. Use of fecal waste from food animals as a fertilizer is also implicated in contamination of the environment with resistant bacteria. The net result is a significant contribution to the growing problem of antibiotic ineffectiveness in animal and human infections.

The effect of antimicrobial use in plant agriculture on antimicrobial resistance is largely unknown [60]. In the United States, only streptomycin and oxytetracycline are currently approved for treatment of bacterial diseases in plants. Most applications are by spray treatments in orchards and are primarily prophylactic.

Antibiotic use in developing countries

Because the world is a "global village" when it comes to antibiotic resistance, any efforts toward prevention in the developed world will be less than successful unless and until the issue is addressed on a global level [61]. It is estimated that 4123 million (78%) of the world's population of 5267 million lived in the developing countries in 1990. Infectious diseases were estimated to have caused 9.2 million of the 39.5 million deaths. Infections are the most common cause of death in children, and 98% of these occur in the developing world.

The four major issues regarding the use of antibiotics in developing countries are

The unavailability of health care facilities and appropriate management of infections to the large majority of the population. In developing countries, antibiotic use is confined to those who have resources to afford them.

The unregulated use of antimicrobial agents for treating people and animals. Antibiotics may be purchased with or without a prescription from drug stores, general stores, and even roadside market stalls. A survey of rural medical practitioners with an average of 11 years' experience in the Rajbari district of Bangladesh showed that they each saw an average of 380 patients per month and prescribed antibiotics to 60% of them based on symptoms alone. Antibiotics were prescribed to 14,950 patients in a month—a total of 291,500 doses. Of these, only 109,500 doses had been dispensed by pharmacies, and 100,000 doses a month were dispensed without a prescription. This widespread and uncontrolled use of antibiotics unfortunately is more prevalent among the educated and the affluent than among those who cannot afford health care. The misplaced notion among the public's higher socioeconomic classes that they can diagnose and treat infectious diseases themselves is a societal menace of tremendous magnitude. It is understandable that people unable to afford a full course of antibiotics might not complete the accepted duration of treatment for an infectious disease. What is not understandable is the erratic and incomplete use of antibiotic courses by those who can afford both health care and a full course of antibiotics.

The quality and efficacy of locally manufactured antimicrobial drugs are also largely unregulated in the developing countries. Often multiple brands of the same agent are available, and potency equivalents of the active antibiotic may be a fraction of the appropriate dose.

In most developing countries, there is no effective surveillance of antibiotic use or antibiotic resistance patterns. The infrastructure for laboratory diagnosis of infectious diseases is nonexistent in most areas and largely "academic" in major institutions. A lack of resources for these purposes is understandable, but what is not is the use of available resources for diseases that are not transmissible and that affect smaller segments of the population.

In summary, the antibiotic use—more aptly antibiotic abuse—that occurs in the developing countries involves much more complex issues than just that of affordability. Worst of all, the issue is largely ignored by all concerned.

In case of the status quo, prospects for the future

The antimicrobial resistance that emerged in the last century will continue into the current one. The number of multiresistant bacteria for which no effective antibiotics exist at this point will expand. Breeding grounds of resistance in communities, hospitals, nursing homes, and ultimately homes will make both the current and future treatment of infectious diseases ineffective. The patients in hospitals who cannot be treated will become reservoirs of resistant bacteria, leading to further spread unless drastic isolation precautions and quarantines are instituted. Along with resistance genes, bacteria will acquire critical virulence genes that lead to more serious infections. International travel and economic globalization will hasten the exchange of resistant bacteria between countries and continents. A gloomy picture at best.

The hope of altering these gloomy prospects

For any hope to materialize, there is an absolute need for cooperation between health administrations, health care agencies, scientists, practicing physicians, the public, and the industry, particularly the agricultural and pharmaceutical industries. What medical science has to offer is summarized in the section on "The Future of Antibiotic Therapy." Molecular genetics and drug modeling may help produce engineered drugs designed to inhibit new bacterial targets. Bacteria-carrying engineered antiresistance genes may be used as colonizers and may be able to compete with invading pathogens. Although possible, these futuristic approaches are not predictable. What is predictable is that, through extensive and intensive interventions at multiple levels, the life-span of the existing and currently experimental antibiotics can be extended.

The role of community physicians lies in educating local communities and learning the most appropriate use of antimicrobial agents. The use of antibacterial agents for noninfectious illnesses and nonbacterial infections can only have harmful effects, eradicating the normal flora that are part of natural host defenses. Some of the measures to deal with antimicrobial resistance are listed in Box 1. Changes seen in antimicrobial prescribing for children after a community-wide campaign in Knox County (United States) certainly offer hope [62]. McCaig and colleagues [63] studied the impact of various national campaigns and interventions on the antimicrobial prescription rate for children and adolescents. The rate of antimicrobial prescribing in general and for respiratory tract infections in particular by office-based physicians for children and adolescents younger than 15 years differed significantly between 1989 to 1990 and 1990 to 2000. However, we must maintain reminders if these changes are to progress and spread.

The Alliance for Prudent Use of Antibiotics (APUA), founded by Dr. Stuart B. Levy in 1981, has provided a model that may be used to improve antimicrobial use at all levels and in all countries [64]. The group shares information with members in more than 90 countries. APUA, the Centers for Disease Control and Prevention, and many other public health agencies have published educational brochures for the public and for health professionals. APUA has published the findings and the recommendations of a 2-year project called "Facts About Antimicrobials in Animals and the Impact on Resistance" [65]. This report is expected to help United States officials determine how much of total antimicrobial use is directed toward food animals and what proportion is used for treatment and prevention of infections in animals as opposed to nontherapeutic uses. The panel concluded that the elimination of nontherapeutic use of antimicrobials in food animals and in agriculture, with the exception of inophores and coccidiostats, will lower the burden of antimicrobial resistance in the environment with consequent benefits to human and animal health. Restrictions on the agricultural uses of antimicrobials have been put in place by regulatory agencies in the European Union, Australia, New Zealand, Japan, and other nations. United States officials are in the process of considering the facts.

Medical schools all over the world need to extend and improve the curriculum for microbiology and infectious disease. The emphasis should be on understanding the fundamentals of host defenses, bacteriology, bacterial genetics, antibiotic chemistry, and pharmacokinetics. The disease-based study of infectious diseases is a suboptimal and dangerous approach. This is an area of medicine where new diseases are constantly discovered along with new organisms. The behavior of existing diseases and organisms changes because of the changing host susceptibilities and antibiotic resistance. "Empiric antibiotic" therapy is justified when it is properly controlled and based on host- as well as pathogen-related factors. This principle would help change empiric into "presumptive antibiotic" therapy and give a method to the madness.

Box 1. If and when we must use antibiotics

- Have a working knowledge of the spectrum of pathogens involved in common infections and the spectrum of activity of commonly used antibiotics.
- Treat early and treat aggressively.
- In the absence of a microbiologic diagnosis, treat the most resistant of possible pathogens. This is particularly important in patients with serious, life-threatening infection.
- If and when the infection is microbiologically documented, use the most narrow-spectrum agent possible.
- Use combination antibiotic therapy with agents known to have synergistic activity against the infecting organism.
- Use bactericidal agents whenever possible. Bacteriostatic agents, particularly in the absence of normal host-defense mechanisms, contribute to suboptimal therapy.
- Understand the role of pharmacokinetics of antimicrobial agents. Among the appropriate agents available for the infecting organisms, use those with high bioavailability, higher volume of distribution, and better tissue/phagocyte penetration.
- Use the optimal dose for appropriate duration. Subinhibitory concentration of antibiotics for even a short period is highly likely to induce resistance in the pathogens as well as normal flora.
- Use local resistance surveillance data to guide initial antibiotic selection and to decide on the most appropriate choices for presumptive therapy when cultures are not available or helpful.
- Follow infection control practices for designated organisms stringently and consistently. When in doubt, consult local infection control practitioners. The least that should be done for all patients is to wash hands between patient contacts.
- Use all available vaccines for children and adults optimally, with initial immunization and periodic boosters as needed. Vaccines not only offer protection against infection, they also reduce the need for antibiotic use and thereby prevent antibiotic resistance.

Information about resistance is needed at local, national, and international levels. Strong national surveillance systems are necessary for international surveillance of antimicrobial resistance. In many developing countries, organized networks of laboratory facilities and information networks will need to be established and strengthened. This process will entail redirection of the nations' resources, as well as intellectual and financial support from international agencies. The World Health Organization (WHO) is assisting member countries in strengthening their surveillance capacity through support for training, education, and quality assurance [66]. In addition, WHO is working with its partners to achieve international consensus on standards for surveillance of antimicrobial resistance and to create a repository of information about resistance in key pathogens worldwide. This resource could provide an official mechanism, currently lacking, for international alert when new phenotypes (such as vancomycin-resistant *S aureus*) are identified.

In developing countries, it is time for the mass media to educate the public and demand that governmental and nongovernmental organizations pay serious attention to the growing and largely hidden problem of antibiotic resistance. Among other things, these countries need to develop infectious diseases as a specialty, teach applied microbiology and infectious diseases in the undergraduate medical curriculum, and start postgraduate training programs in infectious diseases. The models for such training programs are already existent in a number of countries. Such programs exist in some developing countries for cardiology, nephrology, endocrinology, and many other specialties. Evidence indicates that specialists trained in infectious diseases, working with multidisciplinary teams, have a significant impact on improving the quality of antibiotic prescribing and costs [67]. Any team providing advice on antibiotic prescribing must include an infection specialist (preferably both an infectious disease physician and a microbiologist) and a pharmacist. Somehow, the fact that infectious diseases are the major cause of morbidity and mortality in developing countries has been largely ignored, and the weapons against "germs" continue to be in untrained hands, including those of the public at large.

References

[1] Capasso L. 5300 years ago, the Ice Man used natural laxatives and antibiotics. Lancet 1998; 352(9143):1864.
[2] Hoel D, Williams DN. Antibiotics: past, present, and future. Unearthing nature's magic bullets. Postgrad Med 1997;101(1):114–8, 121–2.
[3] Alexander Fleming—medicine's accidental hero. US News World Rep 1998:58–63.
[4] Goldsworthy PD, McFarlane AC. Howard Florey, Alexander Fleming and the fairy tale of penicillin. Med J Aust 2002;176(4):176–8.
[5] Raper K. The penicillin saga remembered. ASM News 1978;44:645–53.
[6] Wright AJ. Symposium on antimicrobial agents. Part VI. The penicillins. Mayo Clin Proc 1999;74(3):290–307.
[7] Tomasz A. From penicillin-binding proteins to the lysis and death of bacteria: a 1979 view. Rev Infect Dis 1979;1(3):434–67.
[8] Marshall WF, Blair JE. Symposium on antimicrobial agents. Part V. The cephalosporins. Mayo Clin Proc 1999;74(2):187–95.
[9] Hellinger WC, Brewer NS. Symposium on antimicrobial agents. Part VII. Carbapenems and monobactams: imipenem, meropenem, and aztreonam. Mayo Clin Proc 1999;74(4):420–34.
[10] Edson RS, Terrell CL. Symposium on antimicrobial agents. Part VIII. The aminoglycosides. Mayo Clin Proc 1999;74(5):519–28.

[11] Alvarez-Elcoro S, Enzler MJ. Symposium on antimicrobial agents. Part IX. The macrolides: erythromycin, clarithromycin, and azithromycin. Mayo Clin Proc 1999;74(6):613–34.

[12] Zuckerman JM. Macrolides and ketolides: azithromycin, clarithromycin, telithromycin. Infect Dis Clin North Am 2004;18(3):621–49.

[13] Smilack JD. Symposium on antimicrobial agents. Part X. The tetracyclines. Mayo Clin Proc 1999;74(7):727–9.

[14] Kasten MJ. Symposium on antimicrobial agents. Part XI. Clindamycin, metronidazole, and chloramphenicol. Mayo Clin Proc 1999;74(8):825–33.

[15] Smilack JD. Symposium on antimicrobial agents. Part VI. Trimethoprim-sulfamethoxazole. Mayo Clin Proc 1999;74(7):730–4.

[16] Wilhelm MP, Estes L. Symposium on antimicrobial agents. Part XII. Vancomycin. Mayo Clin Proc 1999;74(9):928–35.

[17] Centers for Disease Control and Prevention. Staphylococcus aureus resistant to vancomycin—United States, 2002. MMWR Morb Mortal Wkly Rep 2002;51(26):565–7.

[18] Murray B, Nannini EC. Glycopeptides (vancomycin and teicoplanin), streptogramins (quinupristin-dalfopristin), and lipopeptides (daptomycine). In: Mandell GBJ, Raphael D, Mandell D, editors. Bennett's principles and practice of infectious diseases. 6th edition. Philadelphia: Elsevier; 2005. p. 417–34.

[19] Walker RC. Symposium on antimicrobial agents. Part XIII. The fluoroquinolones. Mayo Clin Proc 1999;74(10):1030–7.

[20] Nadler H, Dowzicky M, Feger C, et al. Quinupristin/dalfopristin: a novel selective-spectrum antibiotic for the treatment of multi-resistant and other gram-positive pathogens. Clin Microbiol Newsl 1999;21:103–12.

[21] Quinupristin/dalfopristin. Med Lett Drugs Ther 1999;41(1066):109–10.

[22] Moellering RC Jr. A novel antimicrobial agent joins the battle against resistant bacteria. Ann Intern Med 1999;130(2):155–7.

[23] Linezolid (Zyvox). Med Lett Drugs Ther 2000;42(1079):45–6.

[24] Lundstrom TS, Sobel JD. Antibiotics for gram-positive bacterial infections: vancomycin, quinupristin-dalfopristin, linezolid, and daptomycin. Infect Dis Clin North Am 2004; 18(3):651–68, x.

[25] Arbeit RD, Maki D, Tally FP, et al. The safety and efficacy of daptomycin for the treatment of complicated skin and skin-structure infections. Clin Infect Dis 2004;38(12): 1673–81.

[26] Daptomycin (Cubicin) for skin and soft tissue infections. Med Lett Drugs Ther 2004; 46(1175):11–2.

[27] Noskin GA. Tigecycline: a new glycylcycline for treatment of serious infections. Clin Infect Dis 2005;41(Suppl 5):S303–14.

[28] Babinchak T, Ellis-Grosse E, Dartois N, et al. The efficacy and safety of tigecycline for the treatment of complicated intra-abdominal infections: analysis of pooled clinical trial data. Clin Infect Dis 2005;41(Suppl 5):S354–67.

[29] Ellis-Grosse EJ, Babinchak T, Dartois N, et al. The efficacy and safety of tigecycline in the treatment of skin and skin-structure infections: results of 2 double-blind phase 3 comparison studies with vancomycin-aztreonam. Clin Infect Dis 2005;41(Suppl 5):S341–53.

[30] Tigecycline (tygacil). Med Lett Drugs Ther 2005;47(1217):73–4.

[31] Wise R, Hart T, Cars O, et al. Antimicrobial resistance. Is a major threat to public health. BMJ 1998;317(7159):609–10.

[32] Meleney F. Treatment of surgical infections by chemical and antibiotic agents. Postgrad Med 1947;1:87–96.

[33] Jacoby GA, Archer GL. New mechanisms of bacterial resistance to antimicrobial agents. N Engl J Med 1991;324(9):601–12.

[34] Brooks GF, Butel JS, Morse A. Microbial genetics. In: Brooks GF, Butel JS, Morse A, editors. Jawetz, Melnick, and Adelberg's review of medical microbiology. 23rd edition. New York: McGraw-Hill; 2004. p. 96–118.

[35] Gold HS, Moellering RC Jr. Antimicrobial-drug resistance. N Engl J Med 1996;335(19): 1445–53.

[36] Virk A, Steckelberg JM. Symposium on antimicrobial agents. Part XVII. Clinical aspects of antimicrobial resistance. Mayo Clin Proc 2000;75(2):200–14.

[37] Davies J. Inactivation of antibiotics and the dissemination of resistance genes. Science 1994; 264(5157):375–82.

[38] Hawkey PM. The origins and molecular basis of antibiotic resistance. BMJ 1998;317(7159): 657–60.

[39] Pillay D, Zambon M. Antiviral drug resistance. BMJ 1998;317(7159):660–2.

[40] Hughes VM, Datta N. Conjugative plasmids in bacteria of the 'pre-antibiotic' era. Nature 1983;302(5910):725–6.

[41] Davies J. Origins, acquisition and dissemination of antibiotic resistance determinants. In: Chadwick D, Goode J, editors. Antibiotic resistance: origins, evolution, selection and spread. Chicester (UK): Wiley; 1997. p. 15–35.

[42] Webb V, Davies J. Antibiotic preparations contain DNA: a source of drug resistance genes? Antimicrob Agents Chemother 1993;37(11):2379–84.

[43] Ellis R, Pillay D. Antimicrobial therapy: toward the future. Br J Hosp Med 1996;56(4): 145–50.

[44] Wenzel RP. The antibiotic pipeline—challenges, costs, and values. N Engl J Med 2004; 351(6):523–6.

[45] Goldsmith M, Sarov-Blat L, Livneh Z. Plasmid-encoded MucB protein is a DNA polymerase (pol RI) specialized for lesion bypass in the presence of MucA', RecA, and SSB. Proc Natl Acad Sci USA 2000;97(21):11227–31.

[46] Shankar N, Baghdayan AS, Gilmore MS. Modulation of virulence within a pathogenicity island in vancomycin-resistant *Enterococcus faecalis*. Nature 2002;417(6890):746–50.

[47] Hung DT, Shakhnovich EA, Pierson E, et al. Small-molecule inhibitor of *Vibrio cholerae* virulence and intestinal colonization. Science 2005;310(5748):670–4.

[48] Waldor MK. Disarming pathogens—a new approach for antibiotic development. N Engl J Med 2006;354(3):296–7.

[49] Jones RN, Barrett MS, Erwin ME. In vitro activity and spectrum of LY333328, a novel glycopeptide derivative. Antimicrob Agents Chemother 1997;41(2):488–93.

[50] Hamilton-Miller JM. Dual-action antibiotic hybrids. J Antimicrob Chemother 1994;33(2): 197–200.

[51] Nizet V, Ohtake T, Lauth X, et al. Innate antimicrobial peptide protects the skin from invasive bacterial infection. Nature 2001;414(6862):454–7.

[52] Gabay JE. Ubiquitous natural antibiotics. Science 1994;264(5157):373–4.

[53] Georgalaki MD, Van Den Berghe E, Kritikos D, et al. Macedocin, a food-grade antibiotic produced by *Streptococcus macedonicus* ACA-DC 198. Appl Environ Microbiol 2002; 68(12):5891–903.

[54] Stone R. Bacteriophage therapy. Stalin's forgotten cure. Science 2002;298(5594):728–31.

[55] Levy SB. The challenge of antibiotic resistance. Sci Am 1998;278(3):46–53.

[56] Turnidge J. What can be done about resistance to antibiotics? BMJ 1998;317(7159):645–7.

[57] O'Brien TF. Emergence, spread, and environmental effect of antimicrobial resistance: how use of an antimicrobial anywhere can increase resistance to any antimicrobial anywhere else. Clin Infect Dis 2002;34(Suppl 3):S78–84.

[58] McEwen SA, Fedorka-Cray PJ. Antimicrobial use and resistance in animals. Clin Infect Dis 2002;34(Suppl 3):S93–106.

[59] Gorbach SL. Antimicrobial use in animal feed—time to stop. N Engl J Med 2001;345(16): 1202–3.

[60] Vidaver AK. Uses of antimicrobials in plant agriculture. Clin Infect Dis 2002;34(Suppl 3): S107–10.

[61] Hart CA, Kariuki S. Antimicrobial resistance in developing countries. BMJ 1998;317(7159): 647–50.

[62] Perz JF, Craig AS, Coffey CS, et al. Changes in antibiotic prescribing for children after a community-wide campaign. JAMA 2002;287(23):3103–9.

[63] McCaig LF, Besser RE, Hughes JM. Trends in antimicrobial prescribing rates for children and adolescents. JAMA 2002;287(23):3096–102.

[64] Barza M, Gorbach S, DeVincent SJ. Introduction. Clin Infect Dis 2002;34(Suppl 3):S71–2.

[65] Select findings and conclusions. Clin Infect Dis 2002;34(Suppl 3):S73–5.

[66] Williams RJ, Ryan MJ. Surveillance of antimicrobial resistance—an international perspective. BMJ 1998;317(7159):651.

[67] Nathwani D, Davey P. Antibiotic prescribing—are there lessons for physicians? QJM 1999; 92(5):287–92.

THE MEDICAL
CLINICS
OF NORTH AMERICA

Med Clin N Am 90 (2006) 1077–1088

In Vitro Susceptibility Testing Versus In Vivo Effectiveness

Charles W. Stratton, MD

Room 4525-TVC, 21st and Edgehill Road, Vanderbilt University School of Medicine
Nashville, TN 37232, USA

In vitro susceptibility testing is widely done and relied on for the antimicrobial therapy of infectious diseases. Yet the clinical relevance of such testing has been questioned partly because of the difficulty of correlating in vitro susceptibility testing with in vivo clinical effectiveness. It is useful to review this issue periodically and update the clinical relevance of susceptibility testing with new information. When this is done carefully, it becomes clear that the correlation of in vitro susceptibility testing with clinical outcome is actually improving because of the impact of newer approaches, methods, and breakpoints combined with the teamwork of clinical microbiologists, clinical pharmacologists, and infectious diseases practitioners. There are still host/pathogen factors that influence the clinical outcome that cannot be predicted by the results of susceptibility testing. A better understanding of the science behind these factors now allows many of them to be recognized and appropriate therapy to be given. Improved understanding of pharmacodynamic and pharmacokinetic parameters has greatly improved the use of antimicrobial agents. Most importantly, the integration of these pharmacodynamic and pharmacokinetic indices has greatly improved the correlation between in vitro susceptibility testing and in vivo clinical effectiveness and allows more realistic breakpoints. Finally, the clinical microbiology laboratory has advanced with improved methods to detect resistance as well as the adaptation of breakpoints that are more realistic. Examples of these factors and their science, the pharmacokinetic/pharmacodyamic indices and their integration as well as advances in breakpoint determination and detection of resistance are discussed in this review.

E-mail address: Charles.Stratton@Vanderbilt.edu

0025-7125/06/$ - see front matter © 2006 Elsevier Inc. All rights reserved.
doi:10.1016/j.mcna.2006.07.003

Introduction

A British microbiologist, Sir Alexander Fleming, was among the first to perform an in vitro susceptibility test [1]. The introduction of sulfonamides in 1935 and penicillin in 1942 initiated the antimicrobial era. Within a decade of antimicrobial therapy, the correlation of clinical results with laboratory susceptibility tests was first questioned [2]. Others have continued to ask this question. Another British microbiologist, David Greenwood, perhaps framed this important question the best when he asked, "In vitro veritas?" in regards to antimicrobial susceptibility tests and their clinical relevance [3]. This author also has addressed this important topic in the past [4–6] and will do so again for this issue of *The Medical Clinics of North America*. Factors that influence the effectiveness of antimicrobial therapy will be reviewed with attention to newer concepts and information. Host/pathogen factors will be updated to include new scientific information that explains why the results of susceptibility testing cannot predict the clinical response for all infections and all patients. New information on the effects of antimicrobial agents on microorganisms will be addressed. For example, the differentiation between concentration-dependent killing versus time-dependent killing is very important in terms of the antimicrobial dosing needed to achieve optimal killing and thus improve clinical efficacy. Indeed, the impact of the integration of pharmacokinetics with pharmacodynamics will be discussed in detail as this integration has greatly improved the correlation of in vitro susceptibility testing with in vivo clinical effectiveness. Finally, the impact of newer susceptibility testing methods designed to detect specific resistant phenotypes as well as the impact of redefined breakpoints for existing methods based on the integration of pharmacodynamics and pharmacokinetics will be addressed as will the impact of the teamwork of clinical microbiologists, clinical pharmacologists, and infectious disease practitioners who have made this happen. Because of space limitations, this review will not be exhaustive, but instead will focus on what is new. For those wishing more detail on older concepts, the author refers them to reference 6.

Host/pathogen factors that influence the effectiveness of antimicrobial therapy

There are many host/pathogen factors that influence the effectiveness of antimicrobial therapy. Many of these factors are well known [7–7b], but some are worth reviewing in brief. The first and most important of these host/pathogen factors is the host immune system [7–7b,8]. The immune system today is recognized as a complex collection of defenses that include the innate immune system and the adaptive immune system [8]. The innate immune system uses multiple families of pattern-recognition receptors that trigger a variety of antimicrobial defense mechanisms [9] while the adaptive immune encompasses T- and B-cell responses to somatically recombined antigen receptor genes to recognize virtually any antigen [10].

It is widely appreciated that the host immune system may result in clinical cure despite the use of an antimicrobial agent to which the microorganism is resistant. After all, the mortality of bacteremic pneumococcal pneumonia in the pre-antibiotic era was not 100%. Using an antimicrobial agent that has no activity against the pneumococcus is no different than using no antimicrobial agent at all. What is less appreciated is that the host immune system may result in clinical failure despite the use of an antimicrobial agent to which the microorganism is susceptible. This is because virulence factors produced by the microorganism may accelerate or retard the immune response and contribute to poor clinical outcomes.

A recent example is toxic shock syndrome (TSS) caused by staphylococcal and streptococcal superantigens [11]. Penicillin-susceptible stains of group A streptococci can cause TSS, an acute onset illness characterized by fever, rash formation, and hypotension that can lead to multiple organ failure and lethal shock despite penicillin therapy. TSS is caused by bacterial superantigens that bypass normal antigen presentation by binding to class II major histocompatibility complex molecules on antigen-presenting cells and to specific variable regions on the beta-chain of the T-cell antigen receptor. This interaction allows more rapid and intense activation of T cells, resulting in massive Th1 cytokine storm that includes an early tumor necrosis factor alpha (TNF-alpha) burst from splenic T cells during the acute cytokine response. It is this early TNF-alpha response from the cytokine storm that can lead to sepsis syndrome, disseminated intravascular coagulation, multiple organ failure, and death [12]. Fortunately, most persons have antibodies to superantigens produced by streptococci and staphylococci and thus don't suffer TSS [13]. The results of in vitro susceptibility testing cannot be expected to predict the clinical response to penicillin therapy in patients with group A streptococcal infection when the clinical outcome may be greatly influenced by TSS. Necrotizing fasciitis and other severe tissue infections caused by group A streptopcocci also involve superantigens [14]. Of clinical interest is that severe group A streptococcal soft tissue infections can be managed with antimicrobial therapy combined with intravenous polyspecific immunoglobulin together with a conservative surgical approach [15].

A similar disconnect between the results of in vitro susceptibility testing and in vivo clinical effectiveness can be seen with necrotizing pneumonia caused by community-acquired methicillin-resistant *Staphylococcus aureus* having the Panton-Valentine leukocidin (PVL) gene [16]. PVL is an exotoxin produced by some, but not all, strains of *S aureus*; this exotoxin kills human granulocytes and monocytes. The effects of this exotoxin, if present in a patient with pneumonia, would not be predicted by the results of in vitro susceptibility testing, and patients may die of necrotizing pneumonitis despite receiving appropriate antimicrobial therapy. Thus, it is clear that the immune response may be accelerated as seen with superantigens or may be suppressed at the site of infection as seen with exotoxins such as PVL. In either case, the result may be a poor clinical outcome that would not be predicted by the results of in vitro susceptibility testing.

Other recognized host factors include the site of infection. Site-specific effectiveness of the host immune response and penetration of antimicrobial agents into the site are two factors related to the site of infection. These factors are nicely illustrated by pneumococcal meningitis [17]. Pneumococcal meningitis, unlike pneumococcal pneumonia, has a mortality approaching 100% if untreated. Antimicrobial therapy of pneumococcal meningitis has reduced the mortality to 30% [18]. Early in the antimicrobial era, the necessity of using a bactericidal agent such as penicillin versus a bacteristatic agent such as tetracycline for the therapy of pneumococcal meningitis readily became apparent. In addition, the problem of antimicrobial penetration into the central nervous system (CNS) was appreciated. Specifically, this was and remains an issue of the concentration of antibiotic in the CNS being sufficient to kill the pneumococcus. Newer cephalosporins were more active against pneumococci and were able to achieve killing at CNS concentrations until beta-lactam resistance became a problem. The addition of vancomycin or rifampin to a third-generation cephalosporin became necessary for pneumococcal isolates that were resistant to beta-lactam agents [19]. The immune response in the CNS remains a problem; the use of intravenous dexamethasone before or with the first dose of antibiotic is able to cut the mortality in half (15% rather than 30%), but is not yet widely done [17]. Finally, there are experimental models of pneumococcal meningitis studying the antioxidant N-acetylcysteine that suggest that the current mortality and morbidity rates may be lowered yet further with this kind of adjunctive treatment [20]. There are several important lessons here. The first is that the site of infection is an important factor in the pathogenesis of an infection. The immune response in the CNS is not sufficient to deal with pneumococcal meningitis, yet contributes greatly to the morbidity and mortality. The second is that the site of infection also is an important factor in the clinical effectiveness of antimicrobial agents. The concentrations in the cerebrospinal fluid achieved by a third-generation cephalosporin are not sufficient to provide killing of the penicillin-intermediate or penicillin-resistant pneumococci at that site [21].

In vitro susceptibility testing can be directly influenced by the pathogen such that the results of susceptibility testing would predict clinical effectiveness, but the actual result would be clinical failure. A recent example of this is the staphylococcal small colony variants [22]. Staphylococci are well-recognized pathogens because of their ability to cause overwhelming sepsis and death; the emergence of staphylococci resistant to multiple antimicrobial agents has created great concern. Staphylococcal small colony variants (SCVs) are slow-growing subpopulations with altered metabolism and reduced antimicrobial susceptibility that can cause persistent and recurrent intracellular infections [22,23]. Persistent recurrent infections caused by *S aureus* small colony variants typically include chronic osteomyelitis and cyctic fibrosis. The slow growth of *S aureus* small colony variants often makes susceptibility testing by disk diffusion or by automated methods invalid [24]. Methicillin resistance, for example, is best detected by detection of the mecA gene by polymerase chain reaction (PCR). Even when staphylococcal SCVs are susceptible to beta-lactam agents, antimicrobial therapy must be prolonged, and complete eradication of the microorganism is not guaranteed [22]. SCVs have novel mechanisms for antimicrobial resistance, which involve alterations in electron transport [25]. These strains appear to be defective for the biosynthesis of one or more of the following compounds: menadione, heme, or thiamine. These compounds are required for biosynthesis of electron transport chain component; hence, staphylococcal SCVs are deficient in electron transport. SCVs may represent a stringent response in which a spore-like form allows this pathogen to survive within the host when the conditions are unfavorable. The clinical importance of SCV isolates is that they may appear susceptible, yet clinical therapy may fail. Of interest is that supplying either menadione or hemin in vitro reverses the resistance to antimicrobial agents. This suggests that vitamin K (isoprenylated menadione) therapy might be a useful adjunct.

Intrinsic factors that influence the effectiveness of antimicrobial therapy

There are many factors that are intrinsic to the antimicrobial agents themselves that determine their therapeutic effectiveness [6]. The understanding of these factors continues to evolve in line with new scientific information and collectively can be viewed as the standards of antibacterial performance [26]. These factors include the effect of the agent on the microorganism, which is what most clinicians think of when considering the results of in vitro susceptibility testing. Actually, it is recognized today that this concept is a bit more complicated, and these effects are now more broadly defined as pharmacodynamics [27].

Pharmacodynamics is the effect of the antimicrobial agent on the microorganism; in other words, the effect of the drug on the bug [28]. There are a number of effects of the drug on the bug [6,26–28]: these include whether the drug is bacteristatic or bactericidal; the actual susceptibility of the pathogen to the drug (ie, potency or minimal inhibitory concentration); the relationship between the concentration of the drug and its antimicrobial effects; the postantibiotic effect, if any; and the concentration required to prevent the emergence of resistance. Of course, these effects are dependent on the antimicrobial agent reaching the microorganism. With in vitro susceptibility testing, this is not a major issue, but in vivo effectiveness of antimicrobial agents in the infected human greatly depends on the antibiotic reaching the pathogen.

The ability of the agent to reach the infected tissue site is determined by pharmacokinetics; in other words, the effect of the drug on the patient. Pharmacokinetics, then, describes the basic processes of absorption, distribution, metabolism, and elimination of the antimicrobial agent administered to an infected patient and is usually described by a concentration-versus-time profile of the agent at the site of infection [29]. Pharmacokinetic parameters are determined with free drug concentrations as only free drug has an effect on microorganisms; these parameters include peak concentration (C_{max}), the serum half-life ($t_{1/2}$), and cumulative exposure to an antibiotic (area-under-the-concentration-time curve [AUC]).

After 60 years of antimicrobial therapy, the single most important advance in the ability of in vitro susceptibility testing results to correlate with in vivo clinical effectiveness has been the integration of pharmacodynamic and pharmacokinetic parameters [30,31]. This integration has been termed pharmacological indices [32] and offers a more scientific approach to determining breakpoints for susceptibility testing [33,34] as well as allowing optimal and rational antimicrobial therapy. A historical perspective of these pharmacological indices is provided by the review by Barger and colleagues [32]. These pharmacodynamic/pharmacokinetic parameters and their integration have been defined [35] and updated [36] to facilitate their usage.

A brief review of the pharmacological indices and their integration follows. The goal of antimicrobial therapy is bacterial eradication, whereas the goal of susceptibility testing is to predict bacterial eradication [37]. Eradication can be achieved by the antimicrobial agent killing the microorganisms (bactericidal activity) or by holding their replication in check (bacteristatic activity) until the host immune system can eradicate the microorganisms. The most common method for determining the susceptibility of a microorganism to an antimicrobial agent is the minimal inhibitory concentration (MIC). This per se only measures the inhibitory concentration, yet eradication (ie, killing in the absence of an effective host immune response) of the microorganism is the desired endpoint. Therefore, assessment of the in vitro killing ability of an antimicrobial agent is a basic step necessary for understanding the antimicrobial activity of an agent. Some antimicrobial agents, such as macrolides and tetracyclines, are considered bacteristatic; yet both can be bactericidal under certain conditions against certain microorganisms, particularly with prolonged exposure of the microorganism to the agent. Generally, antimicrobial agents that rapidly kill microorganisms after a relatively short exposure are considered to be bactericidal, and this killing effect is further defined as being either concentration dependent (eg, aminoglycosides) or time dependent (eg, cephalosporins). A more detailed review of bacteristatic versus bactericidal activity will be provided in the article by Dr Khardori elsewhere in this issue. A brief review of how bactericidal activity relates to clinical effectiveness follows.

For antimicrobial agents with concentration-dependent bactericidal effects, these effects may depend on the Cmax:MIC ratio (eg, aminoglycosides) or the AUC:MIC ratio (eg, fluoroquinolones). The goal of antimicrobial therapy with an aminioglycoside is to achieve a very high peak concentration, while that for a fluoroquinolone is to maximize drug exposure by achieving both a high peak and trough concentration. Remember, this concentration is calculated on free drug. Other antimicrobial agents that characteristically exhibit concentration-dependent killing include azolides (ie, azithromycin), ketolides (ie, telithromycin), and vancomycin. Therefore, dosing becomes a critical factor in achieving the proper concentration-dependent bactericidal effect. Another pharmacodynamic parameter that influences dosing is the postantibiotic effect (PAE). PAE is defined as persistent suppression of microbial growth following exposure of the microorganism to an antimicrobial agent. Prolonged in vivo PAEs are usually seen with antimicrobial agents that inhibit protein and nucleic acid synthesis. Both aminoglycosides and fluoroquinolones have significant PAEs and thus may be administered less frequently than would be predicted based on elimination half-life. Related to the PAE is the postantibiotic sub-MIC effect (PAE-SME) in which a long period of growth suppression may be obtained when a low concentration is added to microorganisms previously exposed to a supra-inhibitory concentration. The PAE-SME probably more accurately reflects the clinical situation more closely than does PAE because there usually is a period with sub-inhibitory concentrations between the doses when intermittent dosing of antimicrobial agents is used. Both PAE and PAE-SME influence dosing. A recently proposed pharmacodynamic parameter that also influences dosing is the mutant prevention concentration (MPC). The MPC is defined as the lowest concentration of an antimicrobial agent that prevents microbial colony formation from a culture containing more that 10^{10} microorganisms. This deals with the observation that at the site of infection, therapeutic concentrations of antimicrobial agents that are able to kill the majority of susceptible microorganisms may allow the selective emergence of those strains with resistant mutations. A similar term is the mutant selection window, which is defined as the antimicrobial concentration range in which the resistant mutants are able to selectively emerge during antimicrobial therapy.

For antimicrobial agents with time-dependent bactericidal effects, the killing depends on the duration of time that the microorganism is exposed to the antimicrobial agent. Antimicrobial agents with time-dependent killing include beta-lactam agents (ie, penicillins, cephalosporins, carbapenems, and monobactams), macrolides, clindamycin, and oxazolidinones (ie, linazolid). Because agents that exhibit time-dependent killing generally have minimal PAE or PAE-SME, the goal of a dosing regimen for these agents is to optimize the duration of exposure of the microorganism to antimicrobial concentrations above its MIC. As with concentration-dependent killing, this effect is calculated with free drug. The necessary time required above the MIC varies depending on the pathogen, infection site, and drug, but is usually thought to be 40% to 50% of the dosing interval. Concentrations need to be above the MIC, but concentrations greater than four to five times the MIC do not offer any advantage. Again, there can be some variations based on the microorganism or the antimicrobial agent. For example, staphylococci exhibit PAE for all antimicrobial agents, while there is some evidence that carbapenems require a shorter time above the MIC (20% to 30%). There are some antimicrobial agents that appear to exhibit both concentration-dependent killing and time-dependent killing and have PAE/PAE-SME; these include azithromycin, tetracyclines, vancomycin, and linezolid. For these agents, the AUC/MIC seems to be the primary parameter that correlates with clinical efficacy.

This integration of pharmacokinetic and pharmacodynamic parameters is being used to define pharmacokinetic/pharmacodynamic breakpoints that are based on the dosing regimen and the site of infection. It will take time to apply these more relevant breakpoints to all antimicrobial agents, but the potential is there to do so. The Clinical and Laboratory Standards Institute (CLSI) (formerly the National Committee for Clinical Laboratory Standards [NCCLS]) is engaged in this process currently and for the foreseeable future.

Susceptibility testing and the clinical microbiology laboratory

Susceptibility testing remains one of the principal functions of the clinical microbiology laboratory. If the results of in vitro susceptibility testing did not correlate with in vivo clinical effectiveness, clinicians would have no use for this information. In fact, today the clinician considers the results of susceptibility testing as being of utmost importance in directing proper antimicrobial therapy, particularly in the current era of increasing resistance. Indeed, detection of resistance has become more important as well as more difficult because of the development and spread of bacterial resistance to antimicrobial agents [38]. Unfortunately, many of these resistant phenotypes have proven difficult to detect by routine susceptibility test methods [39]. For example, proficiency-testing surveys have demonstrated that decreased susceptibility to beta-lactam agents in pneumococci and decreased susceptibility to vancomycin in staphylococci are difficult to detect [40]. In the past, resistant bacteria were easy to detect in the laboratory because the concentration of drug needed to inhibit their growth was quite high in comparison to that needed to inhibit susceptible strains. This means that today the clinical microbiology laboratory must use a variety of susceptibility test methods, each tailored specifically to a particular pathogen or group of pathogens [39]. Previously, clinical microbiology laboratories attempted to use one method for susceptibility testing, choosing from the broth microdilution, disk diffusion, antibiotic gradient (E-test), and automated instrument methods. However, clinical microbiologists have now recognized that a single method, whether conventional or automatic, is not capable of testing all antimicrobial agents against all microorganisms and detecting all resistance mechanisms. Moreover, any susceptibility testing method used must be accurate, reliable, and provide clinically relevant results. A number of important examples of these varied methods are as follows. Glycopeptide-intermediate S aureus can be detected by a screening method using vancomycin-containing brain-heart infusion agar followed by confirmation by broth microdilution testing [40]. Similar screening methods have been developed to detect vancomycin resistance in enterococci [41] and such active surveillance has been shown to reduce the incidence of vancomycin-resistant enterococcal bacteremia [42]. The susceptibility testing of Streptococcus pneumoniae has similarly evolved in the past 2 decades from no susceptibility testing at all to a screening process that only looked for penicillin resistance [43] to susceptibility testing of multiple antimicrobial agents [44] that uses specific penicillin breakpoints for pneumococcal isolates from cerebral spinal fluid [45]. Pneumococcal resistance in vitro to macrolides and fluoroquinolones has been associated with clinical failures [46,47], whereas in vitro penicillin resistance is important for meningitis, but not for other pneumococcal infections [48]. Other techniques have evolved for screening for extended-spectrum beta-lactamases [49], which continue to become more prevalent and treatment of such isolates that may appear susceptible to some extended spectrum cephalosporins has been associated with high failure rates [50]. Most clinical microbiology laboratories now use the erythromycin-induction test (D test) to detect the presence of in vitro inducible macrolide-lincosamide-streptogramin B resistance in clindamycin-susceptible, erythromycin-resistant methicillin-resistant S aureus (MRSA) [51]. Each of these methods has been shown to be accurate and reliable and is included in the CLSI (formerly NCCLS) M100 Performance Standards for Antimicrobial Susceptibility Testing [44]. This approach using multiple susceptibility testing methods continues to evolve. A current issue is the susceptibility testing of the polymyxin class of antimicrobial agents (colistin or polymyxin B and polymyxin B) for the therapy of infections caused by multidrug-resistant isolates of Pseudomonas aeruginosa and Acinetobacter species [52]. Quality control guidelines for testing gram-negative control strains with polymyxin B and colistin have been established for the broth microdilution method [53] and are included in the CLSI M100 document [44]. However, there currently are no recommendations for disk diffusion testing of polymyxins. It is important to appreciate that this shift in the manner in which clinical microbiology laboratories approach susceptibility testing has been driven, in part, by the requirement that in vitro susceptibility test results correlate with in vivo clinical effectiveness.

Summary

Thirty years of experience as both an infectious diseases specialist and the director of a clinical microbiology laboratory with a primary research interest in susceptibility testing, antimicrobial mechanisms of action, and microbial resistance mechanisms allows me a somewhat unique perspective on in vitro susceptibility testing versus in vivo effectiveness. I began as a skeptic based on the current status of susceptibility testing and pointed out specific problems related to susceptibility testing and suggested future directions that susceptibility testing needed to take [4]. Others were voicing the same message [3]. The message was heard and things began to change [5]. By 15 years, the advances had reached the point where I was able state that "There is need to improve the correlation of susceptibility with clinical outcome. Fortunately these newer methods combined with the teamwork of clinical microbiologists, clinical pharmacologists, and infectious diseases practitioners is already impacting on this need" [6]. In the past 15 years, the advances have been staggering, to say the least. Although there remains work to be done, I can confidently say that we are moving rapidly in the right direction. For reasons described in this review, there will always be instances where in vitro susceptibility testing will not predict in vivo effectiveness. The use of the improved tools of the trade, to include the pharmacological indices and their integration as well as improved methods of detecting microbial resistance, now allows more clinically relevant breakpoints as well as the foundation for proper dosing of existing or new antimicrobial agents. This has been a job well done.

References

[1] Fleming A. On the antibacterial action of cultures of a penicillium with special reference to their use in the isolation of *B influenzae*. Br J Exp Pathol 1929;10:226–36.
[2] Rodger KC, Branch A, Power EE. Antibiotic therapy: correlation of clinical results with laboratory susceptibility tests. Can Med Assoc J 1956;74:605–12.
[3] Greenwood D. In vitro veritas? Antimicrobial susceptibility tests and their clinical relevance. J Infect Dis 1981;144(4):380–5.
[4] Stratton CW. Susceptibility testing revisited. In: Stafenini M, Gorstein F, Fink LM, editors. Progress in clinical pathology, vol IX. New York: Grune & Stratton; 1983. p. 65–100.
[5] Stratton CW. Susceptibility testing today. Myth, reality, and new direction. Infect Control Hosp Epidemiol 1988;9(6):264–7.
[6] Stratton CW. In vitro testing: correlations between bacterial susceptibility, body fluid levels and effectiveness of antibacterial therapy. In: Lorian V, editor. Antibiotics in laboratory medicine. 3rd edition. Baltimore, MD: The Williams & Wilkins Company; 1991. p. 849–79.
[7] Weinstein L, Dalton AC. Host determinants of response to antimicrobial agents. N Engl J Med 1968;279(9):467–73.
[7a] Weinstein L, Dalton AC. Host determinants of response to antimicrobial agents. N Engl J Med 1968;279(10):524–31.
[7b] Weinstein L, Dalton AC. Host determinants of response to antimicrobial agents. N Engl J Med 1968;279(11):580–8.
[8] Clark R, Rupper T. Old meets new: the interaction between innate and adaptive immunity. J Invest Dermatol 2005;125(4):629–37.
[9] Hargreaves DC, Medzhitov R. Innate sensors of microbial infections. J Clin Immunol 2005;25(6):503–10.
[10] Pancer Z, Cooper MD. The evolution of adaptive immunity. Annu Rev Immunol 2006;24:497–518.

[11] McCormick JK, Yarwood JM, Schlievert PM. Toxic shock syndrome and bacterial super-antigens: an update. Annu Rev Microbiol 2001;55:77–104.
[12] Faulkner L, Cooper A, Fantino C, et al. The mechanism of superantigen-mediated toxic shock: not a simple Th1 cytokine storm. J Immunol 2005;175(10):6870–7.
[13] Parsosnnet J, Hansmann MA, Delaney ML, et al. Prevalence of toxic shock syndrome toxin 1-producing *Staphylococcus aureus* and the presence of antibodies to superantigen in men-struating women. J Clin Microbiol 2005;43(9):4628–34.
[14] Norrby-Teglund A, Thulin P, Gan BS, et al. Evidence for superantigen involvement in severe group A streptococcal tissue infections. J Infect Dis 2001;184(7):853–60.
[15] Norrby-Teglund A, Muller MP, Mcgeer A, et al. Successful management of severe group A streptococcal soft tissue infections using an aggressive medical regimen including intrave-nous polyspecific immunoglobulin together with a conservative surgical approach. Scand J Infect Dis 2005;37(3):166–72.
[16] Tseng MH, Wei BH, Lin WJ, et al. Fatal sepsis and necrotizing pneumonia in a child due to community-acquired methicillin-resistant *Staphylococcus aureus*: case report and literature review. Scand J Infect Dis 2005;37(6–7):504–7.
[17] Kastenbauer S. Pneumococcal meningitis: a 21st century perspective. Lancet Neurol 2006;5(2):104–5.
[18] Weisfelt M, van de Beek D, Spanjaar L, et al. Clinical features, complications, and outcome in adults with peumococcal meningitis: a prospective case series. Lancet Neruol 2006;5(2):123–9.
[19] John CC. Treatment failure with use of a third-generation cephalosporin for penicillin-resistant pneumococcal meningitis: case report and review. Clin Infect Dis 1994;18(2):188–93.
[20] Koedel U, Pfister HW. Protective effect of the antioxidant N-acetyl-L-cysteine in pneumo-coccal meningitis in the rat. Neurosci Lett 1997;225(1):33–6.
[21] Stratton CW, Aldridge KE, Gelfand MS. In vitro killing of penicillin-susceptible, -interme-diate, and -resistant strains of *Streptococcus pneumoniae* by cefotaxime, ceftriaxone, and cef-tizoxime: a comparison of bactericidal and inhibitory activity with achievable CSF levels. Diagn Microbiol Infect Dis 1995;22(2):35–42.
[22] Proctor RA, Peters G. Small colony variants in staphylococcal infections: diagnostic and therapeutic implications. Clin Infect Dis 1998;27(3):419–22.
[23] Baumert N, von Eiff C, Schaaff F, et al. Physiologic and antibiotic susceptibility of *Staphy-lococcus aureus* small colony variants. Microb Drug Resist 2002;8(4):253–60.
[24] Kipp F, Becker K, Peters G, et al. Evaluation of different methods to detect methicillin re-sistance in small-colony variants of *Staphylococcus aureus*. J Clin Microbiol 2004;42(3):1277–9.
[25] Proctor RA, Kahl B, von Eiff C, et al. Staphylococcal small colony variants have novel mech-anisms for antibiotic resistance. Clin Infect Dis 1998;27(Suppl 1):S68–74.
[26] Finch RG. Introduction: standards of antibacterial performance. Clin Microbiol Infect 2004;10(Suppl 2):S1–5.
[27] Craig WA. Basic pharmacodynamics of antibacterials with clinical applications to the use of beta-lactams, gycopeptides, and linezolid. Infect Dis Clin North Am 2003;17:479–501.
[28] Drusano GL. Antimicrobial pharmacodynamics: critical interactions of "bug and drug." Nat Rev Microbiol 2004;2(4):289–300.
[29] McKinnon PS, Davis SL. Pharmacokinetic and pharmacodynamic issues in the treatment of bacterial infectious diseases. Eur J Clin Microbiol Infect Dis 2004;23(4):271–88.
[30] Jacobs MR. Optimisation of antimicrobial therapy using pharmacokinetic and pharmaco-dynamic parameters. Clin Microbiol Infect 2001;7(11):589–96.
[31] Schentag JJ, Gilliland KK, Paladino JA. What have we learned from pharmacokinetic phar-macodynamic theories? Clin Infect Dis 2001;32(Suppl 1):S39–46.
[32] Barger A, Fuhst C, Wiedemann B. Pharmacologic indices in antibiotic therapy. J Antimi-crob Chemother 2003;52(6):893–8.

[33] Mouton JW. Breakpoints: current practice and future perspectives. Int J Antimicrob Agents 2002;19(4):323–31.

[34] Mouton JW. Impact of pharmacodynamics on breakpoint selection for susceptibility testing. Infect Dis Clin North Am 2003;17(3):579–98.

[35] Mouton JW, Dudley MN, Cars O, et al. Standardization of pharmakinetic/pharmacodynamic (PK/PD) terminology for anti-infective drugs. Int J Antimicrob Agents 2002;19(4): 355–8.

[36] Mouton JW, Dudley MN, Cars O, et al. Standardization of pharmakinetic/pharmacodynamic (PK/PD) terminology for anti-infective drugs: an update. Int J Antimicrob Agents 2005;55(5):601–7.

[37] Jacobs MR. How can we predict bacterial eradication? Int J Infect Dis 2003;7(Suppl 1): S13–20.

[38] Tenover FC. Development and spread of bacterial resistance to antimicrobial agents: and overview. Clin Infect Dis 2001;33(Suppl 3):S108–15.

[39] Turnidge JD, Ferraro MJ, Jorgensen JH. Susceptibility test methods: general considerations. In: Murray PR, Baron EJ, Jorgensen JH, et al, editors. Manual of clinical microbiology. 8th edition. Washington, DC: ASM Press; 2003. p. 1102–7.

[40] Hubert SK, Mohammed JM, Fridkin SK, et al. Glycopeptide-intermediate *Staphylococcus aureus*: evaluation of a novel screening method and results of a survey of selected US hospitals. J Clin Microbiol 1999;37(11):3590–3.

[41] Endtz HP, Van Den Braak N, Ban Belkum A, et al. Comparison of eight methods to detect vancomycin resistance in enterococci. J Clin Microbiol 1998;36(2):592–4.

[42] Price CS, Paule S, Noskin GA, et al. Active surveillance reduces the incidence of vancomycin-resistant enterococcal bacteremia. Clin Infect Dis 2003;37(7):921–8.

[43] Decker MD, Gregory DW, Boldt J, et al. The detection of penicillin-resistant pneumococci. The compliance of hospital laboratories with recommended methods. Am J Clin Pathol 1985;84(3):357–60.

[44] Clinical and Laboratory Standards Institute. Performance standards for antimicrobial susceptibility testing. 16th informational supplement. CLSI document M100–S16. Wayne, PA: Clinical and Laboratory Standards Institute; 2006.

[45] Tan TQ, Schutze GE, Mason EO Jr, et al. Antibiotic therapy and acute outcome of meningitis due to *Streptococcus pneumoniae* considered intermediately susceptible to broad-spectrum cephalosporins. Antimicrob Agents Chemother 1994;38(5):918–23.

[46] Empey PE, Jennings HR, Thornton AC, et al. Levofloxacin failure in a patient with pneumococcal pneumonia. Ann Pharmacother 2001;35(6):687–90.

[47] Dylewski J, Davidson R. Bacteremic pneumococcal pneumonia associated with macrolide failure. Eur J Clin Microbiol Infect Dis 2006;25(1):39–42.

[48] Peterson LR. Penicillins for treatment of pneumococcal pneumonia: does in vitro resistance really matter? Clin Infect Dis 2006;42(2):224–33.

[49] Dunne WM Jr, Hardin DJ. Use of several inducer and substrate antibiotic combinations in a disk approximation assay format to screen for AmpC induction in patient isolates of *Pseudomonas aeruginosa*, *Enterobacter* spp, *Citrobacter* spp, and *Serratia* spp. J Clin Microbiol 2005;43(12):5945–9.

[50] Paterson DL, Bonomo RA. Extended-spectrum beta-lactamases: a clinical update. Clin Microbiol Rev 2005;18(4):657–86.

[51] Siberry GK, Tekle T, Carroll K, et al. Failure of clindamycin treatment of methicillin-resistant *Staphylococcus aureus* expressing inducible clindamycin resistance *in vitro*. Clin Infect Dis 2003;37(9):1257–60.

[52] Stein A, Raoult D. Colistin: an antimicrobial for the 21st century. Clin Infect Dis 2002;35(7): 901–2.

[53] Jones RN, Anderegg TR, Swenson JM. Quality control guidelines for testing Gram-negative control strains with polymyxin B and colistin (polymyxin E) by standardized methods. J Clin Microbiol 2005;43(2):925–7.

ELSEVIER
SAUNDERS

THE MEDICAL
CLINICS
OF NORTH AMERICA

Med Clin N Am 90 (2006) 1089–1107

New Uses for Older Antibiotics: Nitrofurantoin, Amikacin, Colistin, Polymyxin B, Doxycycline, and Minocycline Revisited

Burke A. Cunha, MD[a,b,*]

[a]State University of New York School of Medicine, Stony Brook, NY, USA
[b]Infectious Disease Division, Winthrop-University Hospital, Mineola, NY 11501, USA

Antibiotics have been an important part of the therapeutic armamentarium against infectious diseases for decades. Although most practitioners have a penchant for using newer antimicrobials, some older antibiotics remain highly effective and underused. The side effects and drug interactions of older antibiotics are well known. Importantly, older antibiotics are invariably less expensive than most newer preparations with comparable activity.

Methicillin-sensitive *Staphylococcus aureus* (MSSA) is still the most commonly isolated colonizer or pathogen of hospitalized patients. Antibiotics effective against MSSA have retained their potency and remain the backbone of the anti-MSSA therapy (eg, antistaphylococcal penicillins [oxacillin, nafcillin], first-, second-, and third-generation cephalosporins [excluding ceftazidime], clindamycin). Because there has been increasing macrolide resistance with MSSA, macrolides should be avoided in penicillin-allergic patients who have MSSA infections. Methicillin-resistant *S aureus* (MRSA) strains have become more prevalent, but an increase has not been seen in methicillin resistance per se. The increased prevalence of MRSA is the result of extensive antibiotic use with a predominantly aerobic gram-negative bacillary spectrum and limited gram-positive coccal (*S aureus*) activity. Extensive use of such agents predisposes to MRSA colonization and infection, particularly in hospitalized patients in the ICU setting, where antibiotics with gram-negative activity are used intensively. Much

* Infectious Disease Division, Winthrop-University Hospital, 222 Station Plaza North, Suite 432, Mineola, NY 11501.

of the increase in the reported prevalence of MRSA represents colonization of respiratory secretions in intubated patients and colonization of urine in catheterized patients.

Although many antibiotics appear to be sensitive against MRSA in vitro, few antibiotics have had demonstrated effectiveness against MRSA in vivo. Antibiotics with proved clinical effectiveness against MRSA include vancomycin, quinupristin/dalfopristin, minocycline, tigecycline, linezolid, and daptomycin. Trimethoprim-sulfamethoxazole (TMP-SMX) is not reliably effective against systemic MRSA infections. Rifampin has anti–*S aureus* activity and has been used in combination with other antistaphylococcal agents. Adding rifampin to other MSSA/MRSA antibiotics yields no proved benefit. The same is true of aminoglycosides added to anti-MSSA antibiotics for enhanced *S aureus* activity. When a potent anti–*S aureus* antibiotic with demonstrated in vivo effectiveness is selected, the addition of rifampin or an aminoglycoside does not enhance effectiveness of the antistaphylococcal combination [1–3].

Older antibiotics revisited

The recent interest in "rediscovering" new applications for older antibiotics has developed because of changes in pathogen distribution and resistance. The use of some older antibiotics has increased because of an increase in infections for which the antibiotic was used, which leads to an increase in usage for some established indications [4,5]. Antibiotic resistance is one of the factors responsible for the resurgence of some older antimicrobials. Among gram-positive organisms, there has been an increase in MRSA colonization and infection. Although pneumococcal infections are not more prevalent, there has been some increase in minimal inhibitory concentrations and decrease in sensitivities. More importantly, a dramatic and serious increase in macrolide-resistant *Streptococcus pneumoniae* (MRSP) has occurred. Overuse of macrolides and TMP-SMX has resulted in an increase in penicillin-resistant *S pneumoniae* (PRSP) and MRSP, resulting in multi-drug-resistant pneumococci [3,6].

Among enterococci, there has been an increase in prevalence of vancomycin-resistant enterococci (VRE). Enterococci are part of the normal flora of the distal gastrointestinal tract. More than 95% of enterococci in feces are of the *Enterococcus faecalis* variety. For practical purposes, most *E faecalis* stains are vancomycin-sensitive enterococci (VSE) because of their sensitivity to vancomycin traditional antienterococcal drugs (ie, ampicillin). Most VRE strains are *E faecium*; for practical purposes they may be considered synonymous with VRE, because virtually all strains are vancomycin resistant. In general, VSE have not become more resistant over time, but there has been increased use of intravenous vancomycin over the past decades. The overuse of vancomycin has resulted in a decrease in normal colonic VSE flora, which has been accompanied by a commensurate increase in the VRE component of enterococci in the fecal flora. It is important to understand that the increase in VRE did not occur because *E faecium* strains have become more resistant per se, but because the prevalence of naturally or intrinsically resistant VRE has increased [2,7]. As with MRSA, the majority of enterococci isolated in hospitalized patients are colonizers rather than pathogens. As an infectious disease principle, colonization should not be treated but should be contained by infection control methods. In general, only infections that are due to MSSA/MRSA or VSE/VRE should be treated with antibiotics.

A increase in resistance in certain aerobic gram-negative pathogens has occurred worldwide, particularly *Enterobacter* species, *Klebsiella pneumoniae*, and *Pseudomonas aeruginosa*. There has also been an increase, for a variety of reasons, in the prevalence of colonization and infection due to certain naturally highly resistant aerobic gram-negative bacilli (ie, *Acinetobacter baumannii, Burkholderia [Pseudomonas] cepacia, Stenotrophomonas [Xanthomonas] maltophilia*). Because of the limited number of agents available with inherent activity against these organisms, therapeutic choices are limited. Few drugs have potent activity against resistant aerobic gram-negative bacillary pathogens (eg, meropenem, cefepime, respiratory quinolones). Of necessity, there has been a resurgence of interest in and use of older antibiotics with antiaerobic gram-negative activity and a "low resistance potential" (eg, amikacin, colistin, and polymyxin B) [3–5].

New uses for older antibiotics

The combination of increasing resistance among selected gram-positive and gram-negative pathogens has prompted a re-evaluation of the antibiotic armamentarium, because few antimicrobials are effective against previously or newly highly resistant micro-organisms. Among the tetracyclines, doxycycline and minocycline maintain their effectiveness in their traditional areas of use (eg, rickettsial infections, ehrlichiosis, Lyme and other spirochetal infections) and against bacterial zoonoses [1,3]. In addition, doxycycline has been useful in treating community-acquired pneumonia, including PRSP strains; as prophylaxis or therapy for chloroquine-resistant *P falciparum* malaria; and for treating natural or bioterrorist anthrax or plague. Minocycline has been an effective antistaphylococcal antibiotic. Minocycline has potent anti–*S aureus* activity and is clinically effective against both MSSA and MRSA. Aside from linezolid, minocycline is the only oral antibiotic preparation that has been shown to be clinically effective against MRSA [2,8].

Among the aminoglycosides, amikacin has a structure that renders it resistant to inactivation by aminoglycoside-inactivating enzymes. In the past, amikacin has been used to treat gram-negative bacillary infections, and it remains the aminoglycoside with the greatest degree of anti–*P aeruginosa* activity. At the present time, amikacin is being used more than ever as part of combination therapy for additive or synergistic effect against highly resistant strains of *P aeruginosa* and *Acinetobacter baumannii* [1,9,10].

Nitrofurantoin has long been used primarily to treat asymptomatic bacteriuria in pregnancy and to treat nosocomial urinary tract infections (ie, catheter-associated bacteriuria). Nitrofurantoin is active against all enterococcal isolates and gram-negative pathogens except *Proteus* species and *P aeruginosa*. It is not commonly appreciated that nitrofurantoin is highly active against both VSE and VRE strains. In hospitalized patients who have catheter-associated bacteriuria, which is most commonly due to either *Escherichia coli* or enterococci (VSE or VRE), the use of nitrofurantoin over the years has not diminished its effectiveness against VSE and VRE lower urinary tract infections. Nitrofurantoin has re-emerged as the preferred oral agent to treat cystitis or catheter-associated bacteriuria due to VSE/VRE [2,11,12].

Colistin and polymyxin B are antibiotics that were introduced in the 1950s and were highly effective against strains of *P aeruginosa*. From a pharmacokinetic perspective, polymyxin B and colistin were not studied extensively after their introduction, and they were believed to be highly nephrotoxic. Because of their unique detergent action on the cell membrane, there is virtually no acquired resistance to either colistin or polymyxin B in *P aeruginosa* or *A baumannii*. *Proteus* species are naturally resistant to colistin and polymyxin B. Because of the increase in multidrug-resistant (MDR) *A baumannii* and *P aeruginosa* strains, these antibiotics are often the only agents effective against those highly resistant pathogens [13,14]. It is now recognized that colistin and polymyxin B have minimal nephrotoxic potential when administered properly. As the pharmacokinetic and pharmacodynamic properties of these antibiotics are further delineated, dosing will be optimized in the treatment of *P aeruginosa* or *A baumannii* bloodstream infections, central nervous system infections, and nosocomial pneumonia [15,16].

Nitrofurantoin

Nitrofurantoin is an oral antibiotic used to treat lower urinary tract infections. Nitrofurantoin does not concentrate in the upper urinary tract and is only available for oral administration. It has been used to treat asymptomatic bacteria in pregnancy because it does not cross the placenta. Nitrofurantoin concentrates in the lower urinary tract. It is active against the most common uropathogens causing nosocomial catheter-associated bacteria (ie, *E coli* and enterococci). Nitrofurantoin is active against all gram-negative aerobic bacilli causing urinary tract infections, excluding *Proteus* species and *P aeruginosa*. The adverse effects of nitrofurantoin are both acute and chronic and are uncommon and overemphasized [12,17].

Nitrofurantoin is being used increasingly at present to treat VRE nosocomial urinary tract infections (ie, catheter-associated bacteria). It is one of the few non–ampicillin derivatives that is active against enterococci. Nitrofurantoin is active against both VSE and VRE. It is the preferred oral antibiotic for nosocomial VSE or VRE catheter-associated bacteriuria.

Prolonged and extensive use of nitrofurantoin over the past 50 years has not resulted in any resistance. Interestingly, its re-emergence as an important antibiotic in the therapeutic armamentarium is secondary to the increasing prevalence of VRE resulting from overuse of "high-resistance-potential" antibiotics (eg, intravenous vancomycin) (Box 1) [7,15,18–20].

Box 1. Nitrofurantoin

Drug class
Urinary antiseptic

Usual dose
100 mg (PO) every 12 h*

Pharmacokinetic parameters
- Peak serum level: 1 µg/mL
- Bioavailability: 80%
- Excreted unchanged: 25%
- Serum half-life (normal/end-stage renal disease): 0.5/1 h
- Plasma protein binding: 40%
- Volume of distribution (V_d): 0.8 L/kg

Primary mode of elimination
Renal

Comments
For urinary tract infections only, not systemic infection. Gastrointestinal upset minimal with microcrystalline preparations. No transplacental transfer. Chronic toxicities associated with prolonged use and renal insufficiency; avoid in renal insufficiency if CrCl ≤30 mL/min.

Traditional uses
- Gram-negative cystitis/catheter-associated bacteriuria (CAB) (not due to *Proteus* spp or *P aeruginosa*)
- Asymptomatic bacteriuria (in pregnancy)
- Enterococcal cystitis/CAB (penicillin-allergic patients)

Increased new uses
- VSE cystitis/CAB
- VRE cystitis/CAB

---

* In adults with normal hepatic/renal function, not intolerant/allergic to the drug.

Adapted from Cunha BA, editor. Antibiotic essentials. 5th edition. Royal Oak (MI): Physicians' Press; 2006.

Amikacin

Amikacin was the last aminoglycoside introduced and has been used primarily to treat systemic infections due to aerobic gram-negative bacilli. Amikacin's structure and kinetics distinguish it from the other commonly used aminoglycosides (ie, gentamicin, tobramycin). Because aminoglycosides display concentration-dependent killing kinetics, amikacin, like gentamicin or tobramycin, should optimally be given as a single daily dose. Of the aminoglycosides, amikacin has the highest degree of intrinsic anti–*P aeruginosa* activity and is also the aminoglycoside least likely to cause or develop *P aeruginosa* resistance. The use of gentamicin in particular, and to a lesser extent of tobramycin, has been associated with increased *P aeruginosa* resistance; this has not been the case with amikacin. The use of amikacin can prevent or eradicate *P aeruginosa* resistance. The structure of amikacin has only one location susceptible to enzymatic inactivation by aminoglycoside acetylating/adenylating enzymes, whereas gentamicin and tobramycin have six loci. In the past, because amikacin was more expensive than gentamicin or tobramycin, it was used less often. In the 1980s, when there was a nationwide increase in gentamicin-induced *P aeruginosa* resistance, amikacin was the aminoglycoside that could control or reverse *P aeruginosa* resistance [1–3,10,21–27].

The increased use of amikacin at the present time is due to an increased incidence of aminoglycoside-resistant *P aeruginosa* and *A baumannii*. Amikacin is rarely used as monotherapy and is used as a second agent in combination therapy. For gram-negative bacillary meningitis due to nonfermentative organisms, amikacin may be administered systemically and intrathecally to achieve therapeutic cerebrospinal fluid concentrations (Box 2) [15,28,29].

Colistin and polymyxin B

Polymyxins are a group of antibiotics that act on bacterial cell wall membranes, disrupting membrane function and causing cell death. The two polymyxin preparations used clinically are polymyxin E, simply termed colistin, and polymyxin B. Before aminoglycosides were used extensively, parenteral colistin and polymyxin B were used to treat serious gram-negative bacillary infections. Colistin and polymyxin B are active against all aerobic gram-negative bacilli except for *Proteus* species. Because colistin and polymyxin B work as a cell membrane detergent, antibiotic resistance does not develop to these antibiotics. Both colistin and polymyxin B were inadequately studied from a pharmacokinetic standpoint when they were introduced in the late 1950s. As a result of insufficient pharmacokinetic information, these antibiotics were administered using various dosing regimens. Hence nephrotoxicity was reported as a side effect of these drugs, and their use diminished as other, less potentially toxic antibiotics became available to treat aerobic gram-negative infections [1,14,30–45].

Box 2. Amikacin

Drug class
Aminoglycoside

Usual dose
15 mg/kg or 1 g (IV) every 24 h*

Pharmacokinetic parameters
- Peak serum level: 65–75 μg/mL (q 24 h dosing); 20–30 μg/mL (q 12 h dosing)
- Bioavailability: Not applicable
- Excreted unchanged: 95%
- Serum half-life (normal/end-stage renal disease): 2/50 h
- Plasma protein binding: <5%
- Volume of distribution (V_d): 0.25 L/kg

Primary mode of elimination
Renal

Comments
Dose for synergy is 7.5 mg/kg (IV) q 24 h or 500 mg (IV) q 24 h. Single daily dosing virtually eliminates nephrotoxic/ototoxic potential.

Therapeutic serum concentrations
- Peak (q 24 h dosing): 65–75 μg/mL
- Trough (q 24 h dosing): 0 μg/mL
- Intrathecal (IT) dose: 10–20 mg (IT) q 24 h

Cerebrospinal fluid penetration
- Noninflamed meninges: 15%
- Inflamed meninges: 20%

Traditional uses
Combination therapy for
- *P aeruginosa*
- Aerobic gram-negative bacilli

Increased/New uses
Combination therapy for
- MDR *P aeruginosa*
- MDR *Klebsiella pneumoniae*
- MDR *Acinetobacter baumannii*
- MDR *M tuberculosis*

---

* In adults with normal hepatic/renal function, not intolerant/allergic to the drug.
Adapted from Cunha BA, editor. Antibiotic essentials. 5th edition. Royal Oak (MI): Physicians' Press; 2006.

Because of the increase over the past decade in MDR *P aeruginosa*, *K pneumoniae*, and *A baumannii* strains, there has been renewed interest in and use of colistin and polymyxin B to treat infections due to these highly resistant aerobic gram-negative bacilli (GNB). Based on our current understanding of pharmacokinetics and pharmacodynamics, colistin and polymyxin B have been re-evaluated and dosing regimens optimized. Recent studies indicate that colistin and polymyxin B, dosed properly, have minimal nephrotoxic potential. Both colistin and polymyxin B display concentration-dependent killing kinetics (ie, the higher the dose, the more effective the microbial killing at nontoxic concentrations). Colistin and polymyxin B are increasingly relied on because there are so few antibiotics that have or maintain activity against these MDR GNB. Colistin and polymyxin B are antibiotics with a "low resistance potential" and argue against the common myth that resistance is inevitable with high volume and prolonged use of all antibiotics [1,3,15,30,32].

Pharmacokinetic principles have guided the determination of optimal dosing regimens for systemic infections in various body compartments. Intrathecal (IT) administration of colistin/polymyxin B is given with these antibiotics in full systemic doses. Administration of colistin/polymyxin B by the IT route does not lower the seizure threshold and is not epileptogenic [1,29,46–51]. To treat peritonitis in patients who have renal failure and chronic ambulatory peritoneal dialysis, intraperitoneal polymyxin B is supplemented with full systemic doses to maintain therapeutic concentrations in intraperitoneal fluid [52]. The uses and applications of colistin and polymyxin B for MDR GNB infections will grow in number (eg, ventilator-associated pneumonia, cystic fibrosis, orthopedic infections) [52–57]. The place of colistin and polymyxin B in the therapeutic armamentarium is assured, given that virtually no new anti-GNB antibiotics are in development. Few antibiotics are currently available against MDR GNB (eg, tigecycline against extended spectrum β-lactamase-producing *K pneumonia*, meropenem against MDR *P aeruginosa*, *A baumannii*) [15].

When colistin/polymyxin B is used for MDR GNB and synergy may be demonstrated, amikacin is the preferred aminoglycoside in combination therapy. Monotherapy with colistin and polymyxin B is usually used because of their high degree of anti-GNB activity and their "low resistance potential." If a nonaminoglycoside is added to colistin or polymyxin B for enhanced activity, rifampin may be synergistic against aerobic MDR GNB [1,2,58–60]. Polymyxin B also inhibits cytokines/endotoxin release from aerobic GNB (Box 3) [15,61].

Doxycycline and minocycline

Doxycycline

Doxycycline is effective against a wide variety of microbial pathogens, ranging from rickettsia to parasites [62–80]. Doxycycline is a second-generation extended spectrum tetracycline. It differs from conventional tetracyclines

Box 3. Colistin and polymyxin B

Colistin
Drug class: Cell membrane–altering antibiotic
Usual dose: 1.7 mg/kg (IV) every 8 h (1 mg = 12,500 U)*
Pharmacokinetic parameters
- Peak serum level: 5 µg/mL
- Bioavailability: Not applicable
- Excreted unchanged (urine): 90%
- Serum half-life (normal/end-stage renal disease): 3.5/48–72 h
- Plasma protein binding: <10%
- Volume of distribution (V_d): 15.8 L/kg
Primary mode of elimination: Renal
Comments
Colistin has less nephrotoxic potential than was previously
  thought. Particularly useful for multidrug-resistant *P*
  aeruginosa and *Acinetobacter* spp. For *P aeruginosa* or
  Acinetobacter meningitis, also give amikacin 10–40 mg (IT) q
  24 h, or colistin 10 mg (IT) q 24 h. IT colistin dose: 10 mg (IT) q
  24 h.
Cerebrospinal fluid penetration: 25%

Polymyxin B
Drug class: Cell membrane–altering antibiotic
Usual dose: 1–1.25 mg/kg (IV) q 12 h (1 mg = 10,000 U)*
Pharmacokinetic parameters
- Peak serum level: 8 µg/mL
- Bioavailability: Not applicable
- Excreted unchanged (urine): 60%
- Serum half-life (normal/end-stage renal disease): 6/48 h
- Plasma protein binding: <10%
- Volume of distribution (V_d): No data
Primary mode of elimination: Renal
Comments
Inhibits cytokine/endotoxin release from gram-negative bacilli. IT
  polymyxin B dose = 5 mg (50,000 U) q 24 h × 3 d, then q 48 h ×
  2 wk. Dissolve 50 mg (500,000 U) into 10 mL for IT
  administration.
Cerebrospinal fluid penetration: <10%

Colistin and polymyxin B
Traditional uses
- Gram-negative bacillary infections
Increased/New uses

(*continued on next page*)

- MDR *P aeruginosa*
- MDR *Klebsiella pneumoniae*
- MDR *Acinetobacter baumannii*
- Gram-negative bacillary meningitis

---

   * In adults with normal hepatic/renal function, not intolerant/allergic to the drug.
   Adapted from Cunha BA, editor. Antibiotic essentials. 5th edition. Royal Oak (MI): Physicians' Press; 2006.

in several important respects [1,81]. In contrast to tetracycline, doxycycline is highly active against *S pneumoniae*, including PRSP, *Hemophilus influenzae*, *Moraxella catarrhalis*, and *Legionella*. Doxycycline is effective monotherapy for community-acquired pneumonia [15,82–87]. It has good antistaphylococcal activity against MSSA but little activity against hospital-acquired MRSA (HA-MRSA). Recently, strains of community-acquired (CA) MRSA have been reported worldwide. Strains of CA-MRSA are sensitive to several commonly used antibiotics (eg, TMP-SMX, clindamycin, doxycycline) ineffective against HA-MRSA strains. Therefore, doxycycline may be used for CA-MRSA but not HA-MRSA [15].

Tetracyclines have little antienterococcal activity against most strains of *E faecalis* (ie, VSE strains) and most strains of *E faecium* (ie, VRE). Doxycycline has little or no anti-VSE activity but has shown effectiveness in systemic VRE infections [7,15].

Although doxycycline has been available for decades, its pharmacokinetic and pharmacodynamic attributes have not been fully exploited. Doxycycline displays concentration-dependent killing kinetics, that is, the higher the serum/tissue concentrations, the more effective the microbial killing. From a pharmacokinetic standpoint, doxycycline should optimally be dosed as a single daily dose rather than on a 12-hourly basis, as is conventionally done. Doxycycline has a long serum half-life of 18 to 22 hours and is highly lipid soluble. For practical purposes, this means that therapeutic steady state is not achieved until doxycycline has been administered for five half-lives, that is, approximately 4 to 5 days. Clinically, when doxycycline is given on a 100-mg (intravenous/per os), 12-hour basis, therapeutic concentrations and effect are not achieved until the fourth or fifth day of therapy. Clinicians sometimes report that after 72 hours of doxycycline therapy, patients have not improved, but doxycycline was not given in accordance with its pharmacokinetic and pharmacodynamic properties. For serious systemic infections, when a rapid therapeutic response is desired, doxycycline therapy should be initiated with a loading *regimen* (not loading dose). The doxycycline loading regimen should be administered as 200 mg (intravenous/per os [IV/PO]) every 12 hours for 3 days, then may be decreased to the usual

Box 4. Doxycycline and minocycline

Doxycycline
Drug class: Second-generation IV/PO tetracycline
Usual dose: 100–200 mg (IV/PO) q 12 h or 200 mg (IV/PO) q 24h*
Pharmacokinetic parameters
- Peak serum level: 100/200 mg = 4/8 μg/L
- Bioavailability: 93%
- Excreted unchanged: 40%
- Serum half-life (normal/end-stage renal disease): 18–22/18–22 h
- Plasma protein binding: 93%
- Volume of distribution (V_d): 0.75 L/kg
Primary mode of elimination: Hepatic
Comments
For serious systemic infection, begin therapy with a loading
   regimen of 200 mg (IV/PO) q 12 h × 3 d, then continue at same
   dose or decrease to 100 mg (IV/PO) q 12 h to complete therapy.
   May be useful for CA-MRSA, but not HA-MRSA. Meningeal
   dose = 200 mg (IV/PO) q 12h.
Cerebrospinal fluid penetration
Noninflamed meninges = 25%; inflamed meninges = 25%

Minocycline
Drug class: Second-generation tetracycline
Usual dose: 100 mg (IV/PO) q 12 h*
Pharmacokinetic parameters
- Peak serum level: 4 μg/L
- Bioavailability: 95%
- Excreted unchanged: 10%
- Serum half-life (normal/end-stage renal disease): 15/18–69 h
- Plasma protein binding: 75%
- Volume of distribution (V_d): 1.5 L/kg
Primary mode of elimination: Hepatic
Comments
MSSA and useful for HA-MRSA
Infuse slowly over 1 h. Dizziness due to high vestibular fluid
   levels. Meningeal dose = usual dose.
Cerebrospinal fluid penetration
Noninflamed meninges = 50%; inflamed meninges = 50%

Traditional uses of tetracyclines
Typical community-acquired pneumonia (CAP) pathogens
   Streptococcus pneumoniae
   Hemophilus influenzae
   Moraxella catarrhalis

(*continued on next page*)

Nonzoonotic atypical CAP pathogens
  Legionella
  Mycoplasma
  Chlamydia pneumoniae
Zoonotic atypical CAP pathogens
  Coxiella burnetii
  Chlamydia psittaci
  Francisella tularensis
Other pathogens
  Vibrio cholerae
  Bartonella
  Nocardia
Clinical syndromes
  Whipple's disease
  Melioidosis
  Lyme disease

Increased/New uses
Doxycycline
- Penicillin-resistant *S pneumoniae (PRSP)*
- *V vulnificus*
- *P falciparum* malaria
- Lymphatic filariasis
- Onchocerciasis
- Lyme disease
- Anthrax
- Plague
- VRE
- Community-acquired MRSA
Minocycline
- Community-acquired/hospital-associated MRSA
  Staphylococcal infections
  Osteomyelitis
  Acute bacterial endocarditis
  Central nervous system shunt infections
- *Stenotrophomonas (Xanthomonas) maltophilia*
- *Burkholderia (Pseudomonas) cepacia*
- MDR *Acinetobacter baumannii*
- Neuroborreliosis

---

* In adults with normal hepatic/renal function, not intolerant/allergic to the drug.
Adapted from Cunha BA, editor. Antibiotic essentials. 5th edition. Royal Oak (MI): Physicians' Press; 2006.

100 mg (IV/PO) every 12 hours. Alternatively, in keeping with its pharmacokinetic and pharmacodynamic characteristics, doxycycline may be administered as a single daily 400-mg IV/PO dose for 3 days, then decreased to the usual 100 mg (IV/PO) dose to complete the course of therapy [15,88–90].

Doxycycline is approximately five times more lipid soluble than conventional tetracycline, permitting good central nervous system penetration. Doxycycline is as effective as ceftriaxone in neuroborreliosis [91].

Minocycline

Minocycline has essentially the same spectrum of activity against microorganisms as doxycycline, with a few important exceptions. In contrast to doxycycline, minocycline has both excellent anti-MSSA and MRSA activity [1,81,92]. Aside from linezolid, minocycline is the only orally available antibiotic with a high degree of activity against MRSA [93–98]. Minocycline is also active against nonaeruginosa pseudomonads (ie, *S [Pseudomonas] maltophilia, Burkholderia [Pseudomonas/Xanthomonas] cepacia*). *S maltophilia* and *B cepacia* are low virulent organisms that commonly colonize secretions (eg, respiratory secretions in intubated patients), draining wounds, pleural fluid, and urine. These organisms rarely cause infections; when they do occur, it is usually in the setting of impaired host defenses or chronic lung diseases such as cystic fibrosis and bronchiectasis. These organisms rarely, if ever, cause ventilator-associated pneumonia in normal or compromised hosts. When treatment against *S maltophilia/B cepacia* is required, therapeutic options are limited to TMP-SMX, meropenem, cefepime, and minocycline. TMP-SMX and minocycline are the only orally administered antibiotics with activity against these organisms [99–102].

Although minocycline's spectrum of in vitro activity closely resembles that of doxycycline, because of its vestibular side effects, it has not been used extensively in all the infections where doxycycline has been used. Compared with doxycycline, minocycline has better central nervous system penetration [1,15,103]. On the basis of pharmacokinetic considerations, minocycline is the preferred tetracycline to use for central nervous system infections, namely shunt infections due to susceptible organisms (MSSA/MRSA or coagulase-negative staphylococci, central nervous system infections, or neuroborreliosis). Minocycline has also been used for the oral treatment of MSSA/MRSA acute bacterial endocarditis in intravenous drug abusers. It has been employed in IV-to-PO switch programs in the treatment of staphylococcal infections, when a potent, inexpensive oral anti–MSSA/MRSA agent is required (Box 4) [15,93,98,104].

Summary

Nitrofurantoin, amikacin, colistin, polymyxin B, doxycycline, and minocycline are antibiotics with proved effectiveness against selected pathogens. These antibiotics are associated with few adverse effects when used properly, and, importantly, they have not developed resistance over time. As "low-resistance-potential antibiotics" that are effective against an increasing number of infections due to resistant gram-positive or gram-negative pathogens, these antimicrobials remain an important part of the antibiotic armamentarium. They will be used increasingly in the future, as highly resistant organisms continue to be important clinically and therapeutic options remain limited.

References

[1] Kucers A, Crowe SM, Grayson ML, et al, editors. The use of antibiotics. A clinical review of antibacterial, antifungal and antiviral drugs. 5th edition. Oxford (UK): Butterworth Heinemann; 1997. p. 676–708.

[2] O'Grady F, Lambert HP, Finch RG, et al, editors. Antibiotics and chemotherapy. 2nd edition. New York: Churchill Livingstone; 1997.

[3] Bryskier A, editor. Antimicrobial agents. Washington, DC: ASM Press; 2005.

[4] Cunha BA. New uses for older antibiotics. Postgrad Med 1997;101:68–80.

[5] Klein NC, Cunha BA. New uses for older antibiotics. Med Clin North Am 2001;85:125–32.

[6] Cunha BA. Clinical relevance of penicillin-resistant Streptococcus pneumoniae. Semin Respir Infect 2002;17:204–14.

[7] Linden PK. Treatment options for vancomycin-resistant enterococcal infections. Drugs 2002;62:425–41.

[8] Cunha BA. Intravenous to oral antibiotic switch therapy. Drugs for Today 2001;37:311–9.

[9] Edson RS, Terrel CL. The aminoglycosides. Mayo Clin Proc 1999;74:519–28.

[10] Cunha BA. Aminoglycosides: current role in antimicrobial therapy. Pharmacotherapy 1988;8:334–50.

[11] Nicolle LE. Urinary tract infection: traditional pharmacologic therapies. Am J Med 2002;(Suppl 1A):35S–44S.

[12] Kucers A, Crowe SM, Grayson ML, et al, editors. The use of antibiotics. A clinical review of antibacterial, antifungal and antiviral drugs. 5th edition. Oxford (UK): Butterworth-Heinemann; 1997. p. 922–31.

[13] Jain R, Danziger LH. Multidrug-resistant Acinetobacter infections: an emerging challenge to clinicians. Ann Pharmacother 2004;38:1449–59.

[14] Evans ME, Feola DJ, Rapp RP. Polymyxin B sulfate and colistin: old antibiotics for emerging multiresistant gram-negative bacteria. Ann Pharmacother 1999;33:960–7.

[15] Cunha BA, editor. Antibiotic essentials. 5th edition. Royal Oak (MI): Physicians' Press; 2006.

[16] Ambrose P, Nightingale CH, editors. Principles of pharmacodynamics. New York: Marcel Dekker; 2001.

[17] Cunha BA. Nitrofurantoin: a review. Adv Ther 1989;6:213–36.

[18] Gordon KA, Jones RN. Susceptibility patterns of orally administered antimicrobials among urinary tract infection pathogens from hospitalized patients in North America: comparison report to Europe and Latin America. Results from the SENTRY Antimicrobial Surveillance Program (2000). Diagn Microbiol Infect Dis 2003;45:295–301.

[19] Zhanel GG, Laing NM, Nichol KA, et al. Antibiotic activity against urinary tract infection (UTI) isolates of vancomycin-resistant enterococci (VRE): results from the 2002 North American Vancomycin Resistant Enterococci Susceptibility Study (NAVRESS). J Antimicrob Chemother 2003;52:382–8.

[20] Lai KK. Treatment of vancomycin-resistant *Enterococcus faecium* infections. Arch Intern Med 1996;156:2579–84.

[21] Astal Z. Susceptibility patterns in *Pseudomonas aeruginosa* causing nosocomial infections. J Chemother 2004;16:264–8.

[22] Cunha BA. *Pseudomonas aeruginosa*: resistance and therapy. Semin Respir Infect 2002;17: 231–9.

[23] Friedland I, Gallagher G, King T, et al. Antimicrobial susceptibility patterns in *Pseudomonas aeruginosa*: data from a multicenter Intensive Care Surveillance Study (ISS) in the United States. J Chemother 2004;16:437–41.

[24] Karlowsky JA, Draghi DC, Jones ME, et al. Surveillance for antimicrobial susceptibility among clinical isolates of *Pseudomonas aeruginosa* and *Acinetobacter baumannii* from hospitalized patients in the United States, 1998 to 2001. Antimicrob Agents Chemother 2003; 47:1681–8.

[25] Karakoc B, Gerceker AA. In-vitro activities of various antibiotics, alone and in combination with amikacin against *Pseudomonas aeruginosa*. Int J Antimicrob Agents 2001;18: 567–70.

[26] Giamarellou-Bourboulis EJ, Kentepozidis N, Antonopoulos A, et al. Postantibiotic effect of antimicrobial combinations on multidrug-resistant *Pseudomonas aeruginosa*. Diagn Microbiol Infect Dis 2005;51:113–7.

[27] Savov E, Chankova D, Vatcheva R, et al. In vitro investigation of the susceptibility of *Acinetobacter baumannii* strains isolated from clinical specimens to ampicillin/sulbactam alone and in combination with amikacin. Int J Antimicrob Agents 2002;20: 390–2.

[28] Corpus KA, Weber KB, Zimmerman CR. Intrathecal amikacin for the treatment of pseudomonal meningitis. Ann Pharmacother 2004;38:992–5.

[29] Fulnecky EJ, Wright D, Scheld M, et al. Amikacin and colistin for treatment of *Acinetobacter baumannii* meningitis. J Infect 2005;51:e249–51.

[30] Stein A, Raoult D. Colistin: an antimicrobial for the 21st century? Clin Infect Dis 2002;35: 901–2.

[31] Berlana D, Llop JM, Fort E, et al. Use of colistin is the treatment of multidrug resistant gram-negative infections. Am J Health Syst Pharm 2005;62:39–47.

[32] Falagas ME, Kasiakou SK. Colistin: the revival of polymyxins for the management of multidrug-resistant gram-negative bacterial infections. Clin Infect Dis 2005;40: 1333–41.

[33] Levin AS, Barone AA, Penco J, et al. Intravenous colistin as therapy for nosocomial infections caused by multidrug-resistant *Pseudomonas aeruginosa* and *Acinetobacter baumannii*. Clin Infect Dis 1999;28:1008–11.

[34] Linden PK, Kusne S, Coley K, et al. Use of parenteral colistin for the treatment of serious infection due to antimicrobial-resistant *Pseudomonas aeruginosa*. Clin Infect Dis 2003;37: 154–60.

[35] Markou N, Apostolakos H, Koumoudiou C, et al. Intravenous colistin in the treatment of sepsis from multidrug-resistant gram-negative bacilli in critically ill patients. Crit Care 2003;7:78–83.

[36] Michalopoulos AS, Tsiodras S, Relios K, et al. Colistin treatment in patients with ICU-acquired infections caused by multiresistant gram-negative bacteria: the renaissance of an old antibiotic. Clin Microbiol Infect 2005;11:115–9.

[37] Michalopoulos AS, Kasiakou SK, Evangelos S, et al. Cure of multidrug-resistant *Acinetobacter baumannii* bacteraemia with continuous intravenous infusion of colistin. Clin Microbiol Infect 2005;11:119–21.

[38] Obritsch MD, Fish DN, MacLaren R, et al. Nosocomial infections due to multidrug-resistant *Pseudomonas aeruginosa*: epidemiology and treatment options. Pharmacotherapy 2005;25:1353–64.

[39] Murray CK, Hospenthal DR. Treatment of multidrug resistant *Acinetobacter*. Curr Opin in Infectious Disease 2005;18:502–6.

[40] Reina R, Estenssoro E, Saenz G, et al. Safety and efficacy of colistin in *Acinetobacter* and *Pseudomonas* infections: a prospective cohort study. Intensive Care Med 2005;31: 1058–65.

[41] Horton J, Pankey GA. Polymyxin B, colistin, and sodium colistimethate. Med Clin North Am 1982;66:135–42.

[42] Lee SY, Kuti JL, Nicolau DP. Polymyxins: older antibiotics for a new threat. Conn Med 2006;70:25–8.

[43] Menzies D, Minnaganti VR, Cunha BA. Polymyxin B. Antibiotics for Clinicians 2000;4: 33–40.

[44] Hermsen ED, Sullivan CJ, Rotschafer JC. Polymyxins: pharmacology, pharmacokinetics, pharmacodynamics, and clinical applications. Infect Dis Clin North Am 2003;17: 545–62.

[45] Tam VH, Schilling AN, Vo G, et al. Pharmacodynamics of polymyxin B against *Pseudomonas aeruginosa*. Antimicrob Agents Chemother 2005;49:3624–30.

[46] Sueke H, March H, Dhital A. Using intrathecal colistin for multidrug resistant shunt infection. Br J Neurosurg 2005;19:51–2.

[47] Gump WC, Walsh JW. Intrathecal colistin for treatment of highly resistant *Pseudomonas* ventriculitis. Case report and review of the literature. J Neurosurg 2005;102:915–7.

[48] Segal-Maurer S, Mariano N, Qavi A, et al. Successful treatment of ceftazidime-resistant *Klebsiella pneumoniae* ventriculitis with intravenous meropenem and intraventricular polymyxin B. Case report and review. Clin Infect Dis 1999;28:1134–8.

[49] Katragkou A, Roilides E. Successful treatment of multidrug-resistant *Acinetobacter baumannii* central nervous system infections with colistin. J Clin Microbiol 2005;43: 4916–7.

[50] Quinn AL, Parada JP, Belmares J, et al. Intrathecal colistin and sterilization of resistant *Pseudomonas aeruginosa* shunt infection. Ann Pharmacother 2005;39:949–52.

[51] Jimenez-Mejias ME, Pichardo-Guerrero C, Marque-Rivas FJ, et al. Cerebrospinal fluid penetration and pharmacokinetic/pharmacodynamic parameters of intravenously administered colistin in a case of multidrug-resistant *Acinetobacter baumannii* meningitis. Eur J Clin Microbiol Infect Dis 2002;21:212–4.

[52] Parchuri S, Mohan S, Young S, et al. Chronic ambulatory peritoneal dialysis associated peritonitis ESBL-producing *Klebsiella pneumoniae* successfully treated with polymyxin B. Heart Lung 2005;34:360–3.

[53] Kucers A, Crowe SM, Grayson ML, et al, editors. The use of antibiotics. A clinical review of antibacterial, antifungal and antiviral drugs. 5th edition. Oxford (UK): Butterworth-Heinemann; 1997. p. 667–75.

[54] Li H, Turnidge J, Milne R, et al. In vitro pharmacodynamic properties of colistin and colistin methanesulfonate against *Pseudomonas aeruginosa* isolates from patients with cystic fibrosis. Antimicrob Agents Chemother 2001;45:781–5.

[55] Kasiakou SK, Michalopoulos A, Soteriades ES, et al. Combination therapy with intravenous colistin for management of infections due to multidrug-resistant gram-negative bacteria in patients without cystic fibrosis. Antimicrob Agents Chemother 2005;49: 3136–46.

[56] Kasiakou SK, Fragoulis K, Tzagarakis G, et al. Cure of multidrug-resistant *Acinetobacter baumannii* fixation device–related orthopedic infections in two patients with intravenous colistin. Microb Drug Resist 2005;11:287–9.

[57] Garnacho-Montero J, Ortiz-Leyba C, Jimenez-Jimenez FJ, et al. Treatment of multidrug-resistant *Acinetobacter baumannii* ventilator-associated pneumonia (VAP) with intravenous colistin: a comparison with imipenem-susceptible VAP. Clin Infect Dis 2003;36: 1111–8.

[58] Petrosillo N, Chinello P, Proietti MF, et al. Combined colistin and rifampin therapy for carbapenem-resistant *Acinetobacter baumannii* infections: clinical outcome and adverse events. Clin Microbiol Infect 2005;11:682–3.

[59] Rynn C, Wooton M, Bowker KE, et al. In vitro assessment of colistin's antipseudomonal antimicrobial interactions with other antibiotics. Clin Microbiol Infect 1999;5:32–6.

[60] Morrison DC, Jacobs DM. Inhibition of lipopolysaccharide-initiated activation of serum complement by polymyxin B. Infect Immun 1976;13:298–301.

[61] Giamarellos-Bourboulis EJ, Xirouchaki E, Giamarellou H. Interactions of colistin and rifampin on multidrug-resistant *Acinetobacter-baumannii*. Diagn Microbiol Infect Dis 2001; 40:117–20.

[62] Solera J, Geijo P, Largo J, et al. A randomized, double-blind study to assess the optimal duration of doxycycline treatment for human brucellosis. Clin Infect Dis 2004;39: 1776–82.

[63] Pappas G, Akritidis N, Bosilkovski M, et al. Brucellosis. N Engl J Med 2005;352:2325–36.

[64] Bhattacharya SK. An evaluation of current cholera treatment. Expert Opin Pharmacother 2003;4:141–6.

[65] Chaowagul W, Chierakul W, Simpson AJ, et al. Open label randomized trial of oral trimethoprim-sulfamethoxazole, doxycycline, and chloramphenicol compared with trimethoprim-sulfamethoxazole and doxycycline for maintenance therapy of melioidosis. Antimicrob Agents Chemother 2005;49:4020–5.

[66] Rolain JM, Maurin M, Mallet MN, et al. Culture and antibiotic susceptibility of *Bartonella quintana* in human erythrocytes. Antimicrob Agents Chemother 2003;47:614–9.

[67] Perez-Castrillon JL, Bachiller-Luque P, Martin-Luquero M, et al. Tularemia epidemic in northwestern Spain: clinical description and therapeutic response. Clin Infect Dis 2001; 33:573–6.

[68] Rolain JM, Boulos A, Mallet MN, et al. Correlation between ratio of serum doxycycline concentration to MIC and rapid decline of antibody levels during treatment of Q fever endocarditis. Antimicrob Agents Chemother 2005;49:2673–6.

[69] Rolain JM, Mallet MN, Raoult D. Correlation between serum doxycycline concentrations and serologic evolution in patients with *Coxiella burnetii* endocarditis. J Infect Dis 2003; 188:1322–5.

[70] Calza L, Attard L, Manfredi R, et al. Doxycycline and chloroquine as treatment for chronic Q fever endocarditis. J Infect 2002;45:127–9.

[71] Bryskier A. *Bacillus anthracis* and antibacterial agents. Clin Microbiol Infect 2002;8: 467–78.

[72] Hernandez E, Girardet M, Ramisse F, et al. Antibiotic susceptibilities of 94 isolates of *Yersinia pestis* to 24 antimicrobial agents. J Antimicrob Chemother 2003;52:1029–31.

[73] Boulos A, Rolain JM, Raoult D. Antibiotic susceptibility of *Tropheryma whippleii* in MRC5 cells. Antimicrob Agents Chemother 2004;48:747–52.

[74] Newton PN, Chaulet JF, Brockman A, et al. Pharmacokinetics of oral doxycycline during combination treatment of severe falciparum malaria. Antimicrob Agents Chemother 2005; 49:1622–5.

[75] Taylor WR, Widjaja H, Richie TL, et al. Chloroquine/doxycycline combination versus chloroquine alone, and doxycycline alone for the treatment of *Plasmodium falciparum* and *Plasmodium vivax* malaria in northeastern Irian Jaya, Indonesia. Am J Trop Med Hyg 2001;64:223–8.

[76] Hoerauf A, Mand S, Adjei O, et al. Depletion of wolbachia endobacteria in *Onchocerca volvulus* by doxycycline and microfilaridermia after ivermectin treatment. Lancet 2001; 357:1415–6.

[77] Hoerauf A, Mand S, Volkmann L, et al. Doxycycline in the treatment of human onchocerciasis: kinetics of *Wolbachia endobacteria* reduction and of inhibition of embryogenesis in female *Onchocerca* worms. Microbes Infect 2003;5:261–73.

[78] Hoerauf A, Adjei O, Buttner DW. Antibiotics for the treatment of onchocerciasis and other filarial infections. Curr Opin Investig Drugs 2002;3:533–7.

[79] Stolk WA, de Vlas SJ, Habbema JD. Anti-Wolbachia treatment for lymphatic filariasis. Lancet 2005;365:2067–8.

[80] Taylor MJ, Makunde WH, McGarry HF, et al. Macrofilaricidal activity after doxycycline treatment of *Wuchereria bancrofti*: a double-blind, randomized placebo-controlled trial. Lancet 2005;365:2116–21.

[81] Klein NC, Cunha BA. Tetracyclines. Med Clin North Am 1995;79:789–801.

[82] Shea KW, Ueno Y, Abumustafa F, et al. Doxycycline activity against *Streptococcus pneumoniae*. Chest 1995;107:1775–6.

[83] Lederman ER, Gleeson TD, Driscoll T, et al. Doxycycline sensitivity of *S. pneumoniae* isolates. Clin Infect Dis 2003;36:1091.

[84] Johnson JR. Doxycycline for treatment of community-acquired pneumonia. Clin Infect Dis 2002;35:632–3.

[85] Jones RN, Sader HS, Fritsche TR. Doxycycline use for community-acquired pneumonia: contemporary in vitro spectrum of activity against *Streptococcus pneumoniae* (1999–2002). Diagn Microbiol Infect Dis 2004;49:147–9.

[86] Cunha BA. Doxycycline for community-acquired pneumonia. Clin Infect Dis 2003;37:870.

[87] Cunha BA. Empiric therapy of community-acquired pneumonia: guidelines for the perplexed? Chest 2004;125:1913–9.

[88] Cunha BA. Doxycycline. Antibiotics for Clinicians 1999;3:21–33.

[89] Cunha BA. Doxycycline re-visited. Arch Intern Med 1999;159:1006–7.

[90] Cunha BA, Domenico PD, Cunha CB. Pharmacodynamics of doxycycline. Clin Microbiol Infect Dis 2000;6:270–3.

[91] Borg R, Dotevall L, Hagberg L, et al. Intravenous ceftriaxone compared with oral doxycycline for the treatment of Lyme neuroborreliosis. Scand J Infect Dis 2005;37:449–54.

[92] Jonas M, Cunha BA. Minocycline. Ther Drug Monit 1982;4:137–45.

[93] Yuk JH, Dignani MC, Harris RL, et al. Minocycline as an alternative antistaphylococcal agent. Rev Infect Dis 1991;13:1023.

[94] Clumeck N, Marcelis L, Amiri-Lamraski MH, et al. Treatment of severe staphylococcal infections with rifampin-minocycline association. J Antimicrob Chemother 1984;13:71–2.

[95] Lewis S, Lewis B. Minocycline therapy of resistant *Staphylococcus aureus* infections. Infect Control Hosp Epidemiol 1993;14:423.

[96] Minuth JN, Holmes TM, Mushen DM. Activity of tetracycline, doxycycline and minocycline against methicillin-susceptible and resistant staphylococci. Antimicrob Agents Chemother 1974;6:411–4.

[97] Qadri SM, Halim M, Ueno Y, et al. Susceptibility of methicillin-resistant *Staphylococcus aureus* to minocycline and other antimicrobials. Chemotherapy 1994;40:26.

[98] Cunha BA. Methicillin-resistant *Staphylococcus aureus*: clinical manifestations and antimicrobial therapy. Clin Microbiol Infect 2005;11(Suppl 4):33–42.

[99] Yu W-L, Wang D-Y, Lin C-W, et al. Endemic *Burkholderia cepacia* bacteraemia: clinical features and antimicrobial susceptibilities of isolates. Scand J Infect Dis 1999;31:293–8.

[100] Thibault FM, Hernandez E, Vidal DR, et al. Antibiotic susceptibilities of 65 isolates of *Burkholderia pseudomallei* and *Burkholderia mallei* to 35 antimicrobial agents. J Antimicrob Chemother 2004;54:1134–8.

[101] Valdezate S, Vindel A, Loza E, et al. Antimicrobial susceptibilities of unique *Stenotrophomonas maltophilia* clinical strains. Antimicrob Agents Chemother 2001;45:1581–4.

[102] Wood GC, Hanes SD, Boucher BA, et al. Tetracyclines for treating multidrug-resistant *Acinetobacter baumannii* ventilator-associated pneumonia. Intensive Care Med 2003;29: 2072–6.

[103] Cunha BA. Minocycline vs. doxycycline for the antimicrobial therapy of Lyme neuroborreliosis. Clin Infect Dis 2000;30:237–8.

[104] Lawler MT, Sullivan MC, Levitz RE, et al. Treatment of prosthetic valve endocarditis due to methicillin-resistant *Staphylococcus aureus* with minocycline. J Infect Dis 1990;161: 812–4.

ELSEVIER
SAUNDERS

THE MEDICAL
CLINICS
OF NORTH AMERICA

Med Clin N Am 90 (2006) 1109–1124

Macrolide and Ketolide Resistance with *Streptococcus pneumoniae*

Gary V. Doern, PhD[a,b,*]

[a]*Clinical Microbiology Laboratories, University of Iowa Hospital and Clinics,
200 Hawkins Drive, Iowa City, IA 52242, USA*
[b]*University of Iowa College of Medicine, Iowa City, IA 52242, USA*

Antimicrobial agents in the macrolide family have long been considered drugs of potential utility in the management of infections caused by *Streptococcus pneumoniae*. However, with the emergence of macrolide resistance, the clinical value of macrolides in pneumococcal infections is threatened. In part, as a consequence of the development of macrolide resistance, recently the first agent in the ketolide antimicrobial class, telithromycin, was developed and introduced into clinical practice. The ketolides are macrolide antimicrobials whose chemistry has been modified in such a way as to avoid the effects of the most common mechanisms of macrolide resistance with *S pneumoniae*. The intent of this discussion is to review the current state of resistance to macrolides and ketolides with *S pneumoniae* in North America.

What's a macrolide or a ketolide?

Three macrolide antibiotics have been used extensively in North America, erythromycin, clarithromycin, and azithromycin. Their molecular structures are depicted in Fig. 1. Erythromycin and clarithromycin both have a 14-membered ring structure; the only difference between these two agents is a methoxy group substitution in clarithromycin for a hydroxyl group in erythromycin at the C-6 position. This substitution improves the oral bioavailability of clarithromycin and diminishes its upper gastrointestinal (GI) tract toxicity profile [1]. Azithromycin, an azalide derivative of

---

* Clinical Microbiology Laboratories (C606-GH), University of Iowa Hospital and Clinics, 200 Hawkins Drive Iowa City, Iowa 52242.
E-mail address: gary-doern@uiowa.edu

0025-7125/06/$ - see front matter © 2006 Elsevier Inc. All rights reserved.
doi:10.1016/j.mcna.2006.07.010

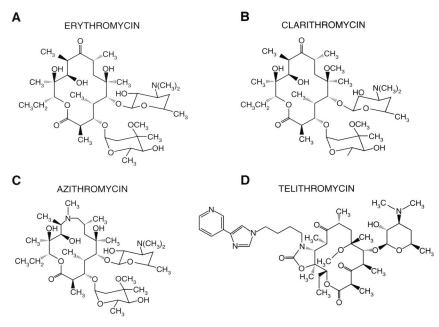

Fig. 1. Molecular structures of the 14-membered macrolides, erythromycin (*A*) and clarithromycin (*B*); the 15-membered azilide, azithromycin (*C*); and the ketolide antimicrobial, telithromycin (*D*).

erythromycin, has a 15-membered ring structure as a result of the insertion of a methyl-substituted nitrogen atom between the C-9 and C-10 positions of erythromycin; in addition, the ketone group at the C-9 position of erythromycin has been removed. The principal consequences of these changes are increased acid stability and a longer elimination half-life for azithromycin [1].

The ketolide antibiotic, telithromycin, is also depicted in Fig. 1. It has a 14-membered ring structure similar to erythromycin and clarithromycin. The cladinose moiety common to all three macrolides at C-3 has been replaced with a ketone functional group, thus the classification as a "ketolide" agent. In addition, with telithromycin, there is a methoxy substitution at C6 and importantly, the addition of a large, bulky side chain referred to as a carbamate extension at C11-C12. These alterations yield a molecule that at least partially escapes the effects of the two most common mechanisms of macrolide resistance in *S pneumoniae* [2].

Macrolide activity and resistance with *Streptococcus pneumoniae*

Macrolide antimicrobials bind primarily to a very specific site in domain V of the 50S subunit of the bacterial ribosome. This site is adjacent to an adenine residue at the 2058 position of 23S rRNA. By virtue of this binding, protein biosynthesis is diminished and growth of the bacterium ceases. The macrolides express a bacteriostatic effect.

The modal minimum inhibitory concentration (MIC) values for macrolide-susceptible strains of S pneumoniae are 0.03-0.06 µg/mL for clarithromycin, 0.06 µg/mL for erythromycin, and 0.12 µg/mL for azithromycin [3]. In other words, on a weight basis, clarithromycin is slightly more active than erythromycin, which in turn is twice as active as azithromycin. The Clinical and Laboratory Standards Institute (CLSI, formerly the NCCLS) has established the following MIC interpretive criteria for macrolides versus S pneumoniae: $\leq$ 0.25 (S), 0.5 (I), and $\geq$ 1 µg/mL (R) for erythromycin and clarithromycin and $\leq$ 0.5 (S), 1.0 (I), and $\geq$ 2 µg/mL (R) for azithromycin [4]. It is curious that the breakpoints for clarithromycin and erythromycin are lower (ie, more conservative) than those for azithromycin notwithstanding the fact that the first two agents are substantially more active than azithromycin. That said, use of the current CLSI macrolide breakpoints largely ensures that isolates of S pneumoniae categorized as being resistant to one agent in this family will also be classified as resistant to the other two. This is referred to as the class concept of testing. With the macrolides and S pneumoniae, erythromycin is most commonly used as the class testing agent.

We recently examined 1640 isolates of S pneumoniae obtained from patients with a variety of community-acquired respiratory tract infections from across the United States. Patients had been seen in 44 different US medical centers during the winter season of 2004-05. This represents the most recent survey in the multicenter GRASP (Global Resistance to Antimicrobials with Streptococcus Pneumoniae) surveillance project begun in 1994. Among the 1640 isolates, 2 (0.1%) had erythromycin MICs of 0.5 µg/mL and were classified as intermediate; 483 isolates (29.5%) had erythromycin MICs of $\geq$ 1 µg/mL and were classified as being macrolide resistant (Gary V. Doern, unpublished observations, 2005, data on file). In other words, 29.6% of this recent national collection of clinically significant isolates of S pneumoniae were found to be nonsusceptible to the macrolides.

Seen in Fig. 2 are MIC frequency distributions for erythromycin, clarithromycin, and azithromycin for the 485 macrolide nonsusceptible pneumococcal isolates from this survey. Note that approximately two thirds of these nonsusceptible isolates had intermediate MIC elevations (1-32 µg/mL); the remaining one third of strains had high-level resistance with MICs of $\geq$ 64 µg/mL. In other words, there exists a distinct bimodal macrolide MIC frequency distribution among macrolide nonsusceptible strains of S pneumoniae. This implies two different resistance mechanisms, which is indeed the case.

There are two dominant mechanisms of macrolide resistance with S pneumoniae: efflux mediated by the mefA gene product and mLS$_B$ resistance as a result of the ermB gene product [5,6]. The mefA protein is a surface determinant that actively extrudes macrolide antibiotics from the cytoplasm of S

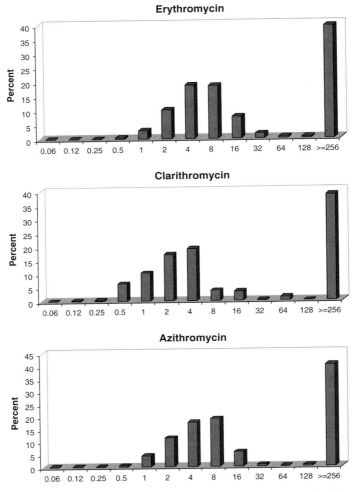

Fig. 2. MIC frequency distributions for 485 isolates of *Streptococcus pneumoniae* that were non-susceptible to erythromycin (*Data from* Gary V. Doern, PhD, unpublished observations.).

pneumoniae in an energy-dependent manner. Efflux-positive *S pneumoniae* typically have erythromycin MICs of 1 to 32 μg/mL but remain susceptible to clindamycin with MICs of ≤ 0.25 μg/mL. They are referred to as expressing the M phenotype.

The second major macrolide resistance determinant with *S pneumoniae* results from alteration of the principal ribosomal binding site of macrolides and is mediated by the *erm*B gene product. Specifically, the *erm*B gene product catalyzes methylation of the adenine residue at the 2058 position of 23S rRNA in domain V of the 50S ribosomal subunit. As noted above, it is at this site that macrolide antibiotics bind primarily to the pneumococcal ribosome thus inhibiting protein biosynthesis. Methylation of the A2058 site abrogates binding and results in high-level resistance not only to macrolides (MICs $\geq$ 64 µg/mL) but also to lincosamides such as clindamycin (MICs $\geq$ 8 µg/mL) and streptogramin B antimicrobials (MICs $\geq$ 8 µg/mL). This is referred to as the macrolide-lincosamide-streptogrammin B or mLS$_B$ phenotype. In the pneumococcus, *erm*B-mediated mLS$_B$ resistance may be inducible but usually exists in the constitutive state.

Rarely, other *erm* genes such as *erm*A have been recognized as accounting for macrolide resistance in *S pneumoniae* [5,6]. In addition, spontaneous point mutations in 23S rRNA have been described at the A2058 and A2059 loci and in various other positions that result in macrolide MIC increases [7–12]. Finally, mutations in ribosomal proteins, in particular L4 and L22, resulting in elevated MICs, have been recognized [7,8,11–15]. None of these determinants of macrolide resistance occur frequently, however, and there is no evidence of clonal expansion of isolates harboring these resistance mechanisms.

In the laboratory, the mechanism of macrolide resistance with an isolate of *S pneumoniae* can be readily deduced by use of either a full-range MIC test or by use of a nonquantitative category susceptibility test method such as a disk diffusion procedure. One of the three macrolides and clindamycin should be tested. High-level macrolide-resistant strains due to *erm*B are resistant to clindamycin as well as the macrolides. Efflux-positive isolates with low-level macrolide resistance will test as being resistant to the macrolides but susceptible to clindamycin [16,17].

Ketolide activity and resistance with *Streptococcus pneumoniae*

Because of its molecular structure, telithromycin binds to two distinct sites on the 50S subunit of the pneumococcal ribosome. One of these is the same site used by macrolides adjacent to the A2058 residue of 23S rRNA in domain V. In addition, telithromycin binds to a second site in domain II of the 50S ribosomal subunit adjacent to an adenine residue at the 752 position of 23S rRNA. Binding at either of these sites leads to inhibition of protein biosynthesis and antibacterial effect. In distinction to the macrolides, telithromycin is bactericidal for *S pneumoniae*.

Fig. 3 depicts an MIC frequency distribution for telithromycin versus the entire collection of 1640 pneumococci from 2004 to 2005. The CLSI MIC breakpoints for telithromycin versus *S pneumoniae* are $\leq$ 1 (S), 2 (I), and $\geq$ 4 (R) [4]. As can be seen in Fig. 3, all but 2 of the 1640 isolates from 2004 to 2005 had telithromycin MICs of $\leq$ 1 and would have been classified as being susceptible. The remaining two isolates had MICs of 2 µg/mL and would have been considered intermediate. To wit, no telithromycin resistant strains were recognized.

Note, however, that the telithromycin distribution is characterized by one population of organisms with extremely low MICs (modal MIC

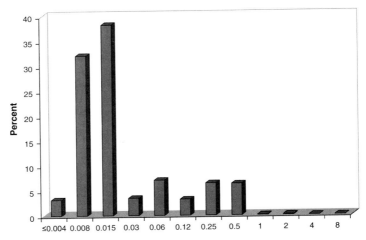

Fig. 3. Telithromycin MIC frequency distribution for 1640 isolates of *Streptococcus pneumoniae* (*Data from* Gary V. Doern, PhD, unpublished observations.).

0.008-0.015) and then a second distinct population of organisms with conspicuously higher telithromycin MICs. This second population of organisms represents approximately 30% of the total and consists primarily of strains that are macrolide resistant. Clearly, macrolide resistance determinants do diminish the activity of the ketolides such as telithromycin but simply not to the extent that the organisms would be classified as being telithromycin resistant based on an MIC breakpoint of $\geq$ 4 µg/mL. Interestingly, macrolide-resistant *S pneumoniae* with the mLS$_B$ phenotype, ie, those with erythromycin MICs of $\geq$ 64 µg/mL, typically have lower telithromycin MICs than do pneumococci with the M phenotype [18]. Evidently, *mef*A-mediated efflux has a greater impact on telithromycin activity than does *erm*B-mediated altered ribosomes.

Rare ketolide-resistant strains of *S pneumoniae* have, however, been described [19–22]. Such strains are often *erm*B positive and may also harbor 23S rRNA mutations and or have altered L4 and L22 ribosomal proteins. The question arises, as ketolides are used more extensively in the management of community-acquired respiratory tract infections, will resistance emerge and if so, what will be the dominant resistance determinants? This issue is discussed further below.

The prevalence and epidemiology of macrolide resistance

Before 1990 in North America, macrolide resistance was very uncommon with *S pneumoniae* [23,24]. During the decade of the 1990s, however, overall macrolide resistance rates rose to levels of approximately 27% in the United States (Table 1). During the past 5 to 6 years, macrolide resistance rates

Table 1
Overall macrolide resistance rates with *Streptococcus pneumoniae* in the United States during the decade of the 1990s and into the new millenium

Year	Number of centers	Number of isolates	Percentage macrolide resistant*	Study [ref]
1987–88	15	487	0.2	Jorgensen et al [24]
1992–93	19	799	5.0	Barry et al [25]
1994–95	30	1527	10.0	GRASP I [26]
1997–98	34	1601	19.3	GRASP II [27]
1997–98	96	2950	20.9	TRUST I [28]
1998–99	96	4296	23.5	TRUST II [28]
1999–00	33	1531	26.2	GRASP III [29]
1999–00	239	9499	26.5	TRUST III [30]
2000–01	240	6362	28.0	TRUST IV [31]
2001–02	45	1925	27.9	GRASP IV [32]
2001–02	239	7671	27.7	TRUST V [31]
2002–03	44	1817	29.5	GRASP V [32]
2004–05	41	1640	29.6	GRASP VI[†]

* Percentage intermediate + resistant.
[†] *Data from* Gary V. Doern, PhD, unpublished observations.

seem to have stabilized and currently exist at an overall rate of approximately 30%. More than 85% of the time, macrolide resistance with *S pneumoniae* occurs in strains that are coresistant to β-lactams, tetracycline, or TMP-SMX [29–32]. As noted above, 60% to 70% of macrolide-resistant strains in the United States have *mef*A-mediated efflux as their resistance mechanism; the remaining 30% to 40% are of the mLS$_B$ phenotype as a result of harboring the *erm*B gene. This proportion has remained remarkably constant over the 15-year period that macrolide resistance has emerged with *S pneumoniae* in the United States [32]. In Canada, although absolute rates of macrolide resistance with *S pneumoniae* are 10% to 12% lower than in the United States, the relative proportion of efflux versus mLS$_B$ is essentially the same [33–40]. Interestingly, in other parts of the world, mLS$_B$ is encountered far more frequently than efflux. This is especially true in certain Western European countries such as Spain, France, and Italy as well as in Hong Kong, Singapore, and South Africa [41–43]. These differences may be the result of different profiles of antibiotic usage in different countries.

In the past, *erm*B-positive isolates of *S pneumoniae* that were also *mef*A-positive were recognized only infrequently. As recently as the mid-1990s, such strains were very uncommon in North America [18]. Today, however, in the United States, nearly half of *erm*B-positive isolates of *S pneumoniae* also harbor the *mef*A gene (G.V. Doern, unpublished observations, data on file). It is highly likely that these organisms emerged as a result of *mef*A-positive strains acquiring the *erm*B gene, rather than vice versa. Interestingly, pneumococci harboring both *mef*A and *erm*B are far less prevalent in other parts of the world than they are in North America [44].

Macrolide resistance, like β-lactam and multidrug resistance with *S pneumoniae*, occurs most frequently among isolates from pediatric patients and in certain geographic areas [29–32]. For instance, in the United States, highest rates of resistance are typically encountered in the southeastern region of the country [30,32]. Certain pneumococcal serotypes including 6B, 9V, 14, 19F, and 23F are most often found to be resistant [45–47]. Further, as with resistance to other antimicrobial classes among *S pneumoniae*, the expansion of macrolide resistance has been largely the result of spread of a limited number of clonal groups that have the selective advantage of being macrolide resistant [45].

Importantly, it is now evident that use of recently introduced pediatric pneumococcal vaccines, while generally being effective [48], does not reduce the prevalence of pediatric infections caused by the 19F serotypes (included in the vaccine) and may unwittingly promote the emergence of serotype 19A strains (not included in the vaccines) [49]. Both 19F and 19A strains of *S pneumoniae* are typically macrolide resistant [45,49].

Independent risk factors for infection due to macrolide-resistant strains of *S pneumoniae* include age younger than 5 years or older than 65 years, recent hospitalization, residence in a long-term care facility, day care attendance, and previous receipt of antimicrobial therapy [50]. Regarding the last issue, antibiotic exposures, previous macrolide use is clearly associated with a higher likelihood of subsequent infection in an individual patient being caused by a macrolide-resistant strain of *S pneumoniae* [51–53]. It is also clear, however, that agents in different antibiotic classes can drive resistance not only to themselves but also to other, unrelated agents [51,52,54]. This is not surprising in view of the frequency with which *S pneumoniae* is found to be stably multiply drug resistant, including coresistance to β-lactams, macrolides, TMP-SMX, and other antimicrobial agents.

Perhaps a more important question pertains to drivers of resistance in a broader epidemiologic context, ie, what is happening at the level of populations? First of all, among all *S pneumoniae* across the United States, both as causes of infection and as respiratory tract commensals, nearly 30% are now macrolide resistant. To wit, the pool of pneumococci is presently nearly two-thirds full of strains that are macrolide resistant. Further, the two principal resistance determinants are encoded for by genes that are not endogenous to *S pneumoniae*, ie, the *mef*A or *erm*B genes. These genes were acquired in the first place from other organisms as a result of exogenous genetic events but today they exist stably inserted into the pneumococcus genome. Under these circumstances, it seems prudent to consider drivers of resistance from a broader population-based perspective rather than only in the context of factors associated with resistance in individual patient infections.

Substantial evidence points to the importance of overall antibiotic usage profiles as the main driver of the general problem of resistance when viewed from a population perspective [51,55–60]. Accepting this, it may also be that different antibiotics within a given family behave differently in promoting the emergence of resistance, perhaps owing to their different antibacterial and pharmacokinetic properties, properties such as potency and elimination half-life. Macrolides and *S pneumoniae* represent a case in point.

As noted above, azithromycin is the least active macrolide versus *S pneumoniae*. In addition, levels of azithromycin achievable both in plasma and in sites such as epithelial lining fluid following administration of standard dosage amounts are substantially lower than those achieved with erythromycin and clarithromycin [61–64]. Potency, or effect, is clearly a product of both activity and levels of drug to which a pathogen is exposed. In this regard, azithromycin is clearly the least potent of the macrolides versus *S pneumoniae*. Add to this the fact that azithromycin has an elimination half-life of nearly 3 days and use of this agent results in a situation where the pneumococcus either at the site of infection in the respiratory tract or residing as a commensal on the epithelial surfaces of airways, is exposed to low levels of a relatively inactive drug for a prolonged period of time. What better way to select for resistance?

Numerous peer-reviewed publications [52,53,65–68] and several commentaries [69–71] have made the point that different macrolides are distinguishable from one another in terms of their likelihood of promoting the emergence of macrolide resistance with *S pneumoniae* and further, among the macrolides, azithromycin usage has been most responsible for the emergence of macrolide resistance. Unfortunately, irrespective of how an isolate of *S pneumoniae* got to be macrolide resistant in the first place, if that organism harbors the *erm*B gene and as a result, expresses the mLS$_B$ phenotype, it is resistant from a clinical perspective to all the macrolides. This is referred to as the class killer concept. If we continue to use specific agents in a given antimicrobial family with a propensity for driving resistance, we run the risk of losing that entire family of agents.

The clinical significance of macrolide resistance

From an epidemiologic perspective, *S pneumoniae* has clearly changed with respect to macrolide resistance. The question arises, what does macrolide resistance mean clinically? At least some patients infected with macrolide-resistant *S pneumoniae* appear to fail therapy when treated with a macrolide. A recent case control study from four different centers described 86 patients with pneumococcal bacteremia as a result of macrolide-resistant strains and in 19 cases, patients had received a macrolide before developing bacteremia [72]. Conversely, none of 136 carefully matched control patients infected with macrolide-susceptible strains of *S pneumoniae* were receiving a macrolide at the time they developed bacteremia. In other words, macrolide resistance appeared to be associated with failure in some patients. These observations are consistent with the findings of two other published studies [73,74] and were recently summarized in an editorial commentary [75].

Of note, failure occurs far more often when the infecting strain has high-level *erm*B-mediated macrolide resistance with MICs of ≥ 64 μg/mL than with strains that have mid-level resistance due to efflux (MICs 1-16 μg/mL). In addition, failures have been recognized most often in patients receiving azithromycin therapy.

This latter observation may to related to the fact that, as noted above, azithromcyin is substantially less potent than clarithromycin versus *S pneumoniae*. Specifically, when considered in the context of bronchopulmonary infections, clarithromycin is 20 to 30 times more potent than azithromycin. This is the result of the enhanced in vitro activity of clarithromycin, being 2 to 4 times more active than azithromycin in the test tube, combined with this agent's more favorable pharmacokinetic profile in the lung, ie, 5 to 10 times higher drug concentrations present in epithelial lining fluid. It might be that clarithromycin's potency advantage explains why macrolide failures when they do occur in patients with pneumococcal bronchopulmonary infections occur far more often with azithromycin than clarithromycin. Further, this would be consistent with the observations from three animal model studies that indicated that only organisms with clarithromycin MICs of ≥ 16 μg/mL are likely to fail therapy with this agent [76–78]. As seen in Fig. 2 and as noted above, only approximately 10% of pneumococcal isolates in the United States have MICs of ≥ 16 μg/mL to clarithromycin and nearly all of these express high-level macrolide resistance as a result of *erm*B.

This apparent disconnect in at least some patients between macrolide resistance as it is defined in the laboratory and failure, especially when clarithromycin is used, has been referred to as the "in vitro-in vivo paradox" [79]. This is not, however, to imply that macrolide resistance with *S pneumoniae* is unimportant. It is very important. It clearly accounts for failure in certain patients and mitigates against use of macrolides in the management of patients with infections likely to be caused by macrolide-resistant *S pneumoniae*. Rather the point is simply that resistance does not always result in failure particularly when the most potent agent in the family, clarithromycin, is used.

Will ketolide resistance emerge with *S pneumoniae*?

As stated above, ketolide resistance with *S pneumoniae* is distinctly uncommon in North America. This may be because the one ketolide thus far introduced into clinical practice in North America, telithromycin, has only been available for about 2 years. It remains, however, that more than 4,000,000 perscriptions for telithromycin have already been written in North America. Further, this antimicrobial has been available in some countries in Europe for as long as 5 years. Total ex-US usage of telithromycin is estimated to have approached 22,000,000 perscriptions. Despite this extensive usage profile both in North America and worldwide, telithromycin resistance remains distinctly uncommon with *S pneumoniae*. In this regard, the following statement seems to be true. While ketolide resistance may ultimately become a problem with *S pneumoniae*, it has not happened yet and it is unlikely to emerge as quickly as has occurred with certain other agents in the past.

From a purely teleological perspective, to completely escape the effect of telithromycin, an isolate of *S pneumoniae* would have to substantially change both of the ribosomal binding sites used by this agent in expressing its antibacterial effect, the A2058 site in domain V and the A752 site in domain II. Obviously both of these sites are important to the pneumococcus in manufacturing protein, otherwise telithromycin would not retain activity in the face of changes to the A2058 residue in *erm*B-positive isolates, or for that matter, in the face of other 23S rRNA mutations. One wonders whether the pneumococcus could survive changes at both of the telithromycin ribosomal binding sites so as to escape the effect of the drug and become resistant while still remaining viable. This speaks to the issue of the fitness costs of resistance.

Numerous different antimicrobial agents are characterized as having multiple different targets within bacteria, all of which are important simultaneously. Two obvious examples are β-lactams and fluoroquinolones. The ketolides are unique, however, in having two different binding sites both present on the same target. This property, taken in the context of the foregoing discussion, may be an important means for this antimicrobial class to avoid the problems of developing resistance with *S pneumoniae* in the future.

Summary

Macrolide resistance has emerged as a major problem with *S pneumoniae* in North America, particularly in the United States, with overall resistance rates approaching 30%. Most of this change occurred during the 1990s. Interestingly, during the past 5 to 6 years in North America, the rate of increase in the overall prevalence of macrolide resistance with *S pneumoniae* seems to have plateaued. Two mechanisms of macrolide resistance dominate: midrange resistance due to *mef*A-mediated efflux (MICs 1-32 μg/mL) and high-level *erm*B-mediated mLS$_B$ resistance (MICs $\geq$ 64 μg/mL). Approximately two thirds of resistant strains have efflux as their resistance mechanism; the remainder express high-level mLS$_B$ resistance. The epidemiology of macrolide resistance is well understood, resistance being seen most often in select pneumococcal serotypes, in a defined number of clonal groups, and very often in the background of strains of *S pneumoniae* that are stably resistant to multiple different antibiotic classes.

The macrolides vary in terms of their potency for *S pneumoniae*, with clarithromycin being the most potent, azithromycin being the least potent. These differences are not apparent when conventional in vitro susceptibility tests are performed because current CLSI interpretive criteria used to define susceptibility categories with *S pneumoniae* fail to delineate the potency distinctions. These differences, however, may be important in terms of the likelihood of use of a specific agent promoting the emergence of resistance in the first place, and in terms of the likelihood of a given macrolide being effective in the management of a respiratory tract infection caused by an isolate of *S pneumoniae* defined as being nonsusceptible in the laboratory.

The ketolide antimicrobial, telithromycin, was introduced into clinical practice in North America, 2 years ago. Because of its molecular structure, telithromycin retains sufficient activity against macrolide-resistant strains of *S pneumoniae* to be effective clinically even in the face of high-level *erm*B-mediated resistance. While rare, telithromycin-resistant strains have been recognized worldwide; currently in North America, telithromycin resistance with *S pneumoniae* remains vanishingly uncommon.

Dedication

This review is dedicated with love and admiration to my mother, Shirley Mae Doern, who passed away during its preparation. I have been the life-long beneficiary of her counsel, her encouragement, her love, and her example. I will miss her deeply. Gareth V. Doern.

References

[1] Nightingale CH. Macrolides: new questions, new insights. Infect Med 1998;15(Suppl A):8–9.
[2] Balfour JAB, Figgitt DP. Telithromycin. Drugs 2001;61(6):815–29.
[3] Doern GV, Heilmann KP, Huynh HK, et al. Antimicrobial resistance among clinical isolates of *Streptococcus pneumoniae* in the United States during 1999–2000, including a comparison of resistance rates since 1994–1995. Antimicrob Agents Chemother 2001;45(6):1721–9.
[4] Clinical and Laboratory Standards Institute (CLSI). Performance standards for antimicrobial susceptibility testing; fifteenth informational supplement: approved standard M100–S15. Wayne, PA: CLSI; 2005.
[5] Leclercq R, Courvalin P. Resistance to macrolides and related antibiotics in *Streptococcus pneumoniae*. Antimicrob Agents Chemother 2002;46(9):2727–34.
[6] Roberts MC, Sutcliffe J, Courvalin P, et al. Nomenclature for macrolide and macrolide-lincosamide-streptogramin B resistance determinants. Antimicrob Agents Chemother 1999;43(12):2823–30.
[7] Farrell DJ, Morrissey I, Bakker S, et al. In vitro activities of telithromycin, linezolid, and quinupristin-dalfopristin against *Streptococcus pneumoniae* with macrolide resistance due to ribosomal mutations. Antimicrob Agents Chemother 2004;48(8):3169–71.
[8] Farrell DJ, Douthwaite S, Morrissey I, et al. Macrolide resistance by ribosomal mutation in clinical isolates of *Streptococcus pneumoniae* from the PROTEKT 1999–2000 study. Antimicrob Agents Chemother 2003;47(6):1777–83.
[9] Canu A, Malbruny B, Coquemont M, et al. Diversity of ribosomal mutations conferring resistance to macrolides, clindamycin, streptogramin, and telithromycin in *Streptococcus pneumoniae*. Antimicrob Agents Chemother 2002;46(1):125–31.
[10] Tait-Kamradt A, Davies T, Appelbaum PC, et al. Two new mechanisms of macrolide resistance in clinical strains of *Streptococcus pneumoniae* from Eastern Europe and North America. Antimicrob Agents Chemother 2000;44(12):3395–401.

[11] Davies TA, Bush K, Sahm D, et al. Predominance of 23S rRNA mutants among non-erm, non-mef macrolide-resistant clinical isolates of *Streptococcus pneumoniae* collected in the United States in 1999–2000. Antimicrob Agents Chemother 2005;49(7):3031–3.

[12] Reinert RR, Wild A, Appelbaum P, et al. Ribosomal mutations conferring resistance to macrolides in *Streptococcus pneumoniae* clinical strains isolated in Germany. Antimicrob Agents Chemother 2003;47(7):2319–22.

[13] Pihlajamäki M, Kataja J, Seppälä H, et al. Ribosomal mutations in *Streptococcus pneumoniae* clinical isolates. Antimicrob Agents Chemother 2002;46(3):654–8.

[14] Wolter N, Smith AM, Farrell DJ, et al. Novel mechanism of resistance to oxazolidinones, macrolides, and chloramphenicol in ribosomal protein L4 of the *Pneumococcus*. Antimicrob Agents Chemother 2005;49(8):3554–7.

[15] Jones RN, Farrell DJ, Morrissey I. Quinupristin-dalfopristin resistance in *Streptococcus pneumoniae*: novel L22 ribosomal protein mutation in two clinical isolates from the SENTRY Antimicrobial Surveillance Program. Antimicrob Agents Chemother 2003;47(8):2696–8.

[16] Waites K, Johnson C, Gray B, et al. Use of clindamycin disks to detect macrolide resistance mediated by *erm*B and *mef*E in *Streptococcus pneumoniae* isolates from adults and children. J Clin Microbiol 2000;38(5):1731–4.

[17] Shortridge V, Doern GV, Brueggemann AB, et al. Prevalence of macrolide resistance mechanisms in *Streptococcus pneumoniae* isolates from a multicenter antibiotic resistance surveillance study conducted in the United States in 1994–1995. Clin Infect Dis 1999;29:1186–8.

[18] Farrell DJ, Jenkins SG. Distribution across the USA of macrolide resistance and macrolide resistance mechanisms among *Streptococcus pneumoniae* isolates collected from patients with respiratory tract infections: PROTEKT US 2001–2002. J Antimicrob Chemother 2004;54(Suppl. S1):i17–22.

[19] Reinert RR, van der Linder M, Al-Lahham A. Molecular characterization of the first telithromycin-resistant *Streptococcus pneumoniae* isolate in Germany. Antimicrob Agents Chemother 2005;49(8):3520–2.

[20] Rantala M, Haanperä-Heikkinen M, Lindgren M, et al. *Streptococcus pneumoniae* isolates resistant to telithromycin. Antimicrob Agents Chemother 2006;50(5):1855–8.

[21] Faccone D, Andres P, Galas M, et al. Emergence of a *Streptococcus pneumoniae* clinical isolate highly resistant to telithromycin and fluoroquinolones. J Clin Microbiol 2005;43(11): 5800–3.

[22] Farrell DJ, Felmingham D. Activities of telithromycin against 13,874 *Streptococcus pneumoniae* isolates collected between 1999 and 2003. Antimicrob Agents Chemother 2004;48(5): 1882–4.

[23] Spika JS, Facklam RR, Plikaytis BD, et al, and the Pneumococcal Surveillance Working Group. Antimicrobial resistance of *Streptococcus pneumoniae* in the United States, 1979–1987. J Infect Dis 1991;163:1273–8.

[24] Jorgensen JH, Doern GV, Maher LA, et al. Antimicrobial resistance among respiratory isolates of *Haemophilus influenzae*, *Moraxella catarrhalis*, and *Streptococcus pneumoniae* in the United States. Antimicrob Agents Chemother 1990;34(11):2075–80.

[25] Barry AL, Pfaller MA, Fuchs PC, et al. In vitro activities of 12 orally administered antimicrobial agents against four species of bacterial respiratory pathogens from US medical centers in 1992 and 1993. Antimicrob Agents Chemother 1994;38(10):2419–25.

[26] Doern GV, Brueggemann A, Holley HP Jr, et al. Antimicrobial resistance of *Streptococcus pneumoniae* recovered from outpatients in the United States during the winter months of 1994 to 1995: results of a 30-center national surveillance study. Antimicrob Agents Chemother 1996;40(5):1208–13.

[27] Doern GV, Brueggemann AB, Huynh H, et al. Antimicrobial resistance with *S pneumoniae* in the United States, 1997–98. Emerg Infect Dis 1999;5(6):757–65.

[28] Sahm DF, Karlowsky JA, Kelly LJ, et al. Need for annual surveillance of antimicrobial resistance in *Streptococcus pneumoniae* in the United States: 2-year longitudinal analysis. Antimicrob Agents Chemother 2001;45(4):1037–42.

[29] Doern GV, Heilmann KP, Huynh HK, et al. Antimicrobial resistance among clinical isolates of *Streptococcus pneumoniae* in the United States during 1999–2000, including a comparison of resistance rates since 1994–1995. Antimicrob Agents Chemother 2001; 45(6):1721–9.

[30] Thornsberry C, Sahm DF, Kelly LJ, et al. Regional trends in antimicrobial resistance among clinical isolates of *Streptococcus pneumoniae*, *Haemophilus influenzae*, and *Moraxella catarrhalis* in the United States: results from the TRUST Surveillance Program, 1999–2000. Clin Infect Dis 2002;34(Suppl 1):S4–16.

[31] Karlowsky JA, Thornsberry C, Jones ME, et al. Factors associated with relative rates of antimicrobial resistance among *Streptococcus pneumoniae* in the United States: results from the TRUST Surveillance Program. Clin Infect Dis 2003;36:963–70.

[32] Doern GV, Richter SS, Miller A, et al. Antimicrobial resistance among *Streptococcus pneumoniae* in the United States: have we begun to turn the corner on resistance to certain antibiotic classes? Clin Infect Dis 2005;41:139–48.

[33] Simor AE, Louie M, Low DE. Canadian national survey of prevalence of antimicrobial resistance among clinical isolates of *Streptococcus pneumoniae*. The Canadian Bacterial Surveillance Network. Antimicrob Agents Chemother 1996;40(9):2190–3.

[34] Davidson RJ. Canadian Bacterial Surveillance Network, Low DE. A cross-Canada surveillance of antimicrobial resistance in respiratory tract pathogens. Can J Infect Dis 1999;10(2): 128–33.

[35] Zhanel GG, Karlowsky JA, Palatnick L, et al. The Canadian Respiratory Infection Study Group. Prevalence of antimicrobial resistance in respiratory tract isolates of *Streptococcus pneumoniae*: results of a Canadian National Surveillance Study. Antimicrob Agents Chemother 1999;43(10):2504–9.

[36] Low DE, de Azavedo J, Weiss K, et al. Antimicrobial resistance among clinical isolates of *Streptococcus pneumoniae* in Canada during 2000. Antimicrob Agents Chemother 2002; 46(5):1295–301.

[37] Zhanel GG, Palatnick L, Nichol KA, et al. Antimicrobial resistance in respiratory tract *Streptococcus pneumoniae* isolates: results of the Canadian Respiratory Organism Susceptibility Study, 1997 to 2002. Antimicrob Agents Chemother 2003;47(6):1867–74.

[38] Powis J, McGeer A, Green K, et al. In vitro antimicrobial susceptibilities of *Streptococcus pneumoniae* clinical isolates obtained in Canada in 2002. Antimicrob Agents Chemother 2004;48(9):3305–11.

[39] Wierzbowski AK, Swedlo D, Boyd D, et al. Molecular epidemiology and prevalence of macrolide efflux genes *mef*(A) and *mef*(E) in *Streptococcus pneumoniae* obtained in Canada from 1997 to 2002. Antimicrob Agents Chemother 2005;49(3):1257–61.

[40] Hoban DJ, Wierzbowski AK, Nichol K, et al. Macrolide-resistant *Streptococcus pneumoniae* in Canada during 1998–1999: Prevalence of *mef*(A) and *erm*(B) and susceptibilities to ketolides. Antimicrob Agents Chemother 2001;45(7):2147–50.

[41] Farrel DJ, Morrissey I, Bakker S, et al. Molecular characterization of macrolide resistance mechanisms among *Streptococcus pneumoniae* and *Streptococcus pyogenes* isolated from the PROTEKT 1999–2000 study. J Antimicrob Chemother 2002;50(Suppl S1): 39–47.

[42] Felmingham D, Reinert RR, Hirakata Y, et al. Increasing prevalence of antimicrobial resistance among isolates of *Streptococcus pneumoniae* from the PROTEKT surveillance study, and comparative in vitro activity of the ketolide, telithromycin. J Antimicrob Chemother 2002;50(Suppl S1):25–37.

[43] Reinert RR, Ringelstein A, van der Linden M, et al. Molecular epidemiology of macrolide-resistant *Streptococcus pneumoniae* isolates from Europe. J Clin Microbiol 2005;43(3): 1294–300.

[44] Farrell DJ, Morrissey I, Bakker S, et al. Molecular epidemiology of multiresistant *Streptococcus pneumoniae* with both *erm*(B)- and *mef*(A)-mediated macrolide resistance. J Clin Microbiol 2004;42(2):764–8.

[45] Richter SS, Heilmann KP, Coffman SL, et al. The molecular epidemiology of penicillin-resistant *Streptococcus pneumoniae* in the United States, 1994–2000. Clin Infect Dis 2002;34: 330–9.

[46] Munford RS, Murphy TV. Antimicrobial resistance in *Streptococcus pneumoniae*: can immunization prevent its spread. J Investig Med 1994;42:613–21.

[47] Joloba ML, Windau A, Bajaksouzian S, et al. Pneumococcal conjugate vaccine serotypes of *Streptococcus pneumoniae* isolates and the antimicrobial susceptibility of such isolates in children with otitis media. Clin Infect Dis 2001;333:1498–2004.

[48] Pelton SI, Daga R, Gaines BM, et al. Pneumococcal conjugate vaccines: proceedings from an interactive symposium at the 41st Interscience Conference on antimicrobial agents and chemotherapy. Vaccine 2003;21:1562–71.

[49] McEllistrem MC, Adams JM, Patel K, et al. Acute otitis media due to penicillin-nonsusceptible *Streptococcus pneumoniae* before and after the introduction of the pneumococcal conjugate vaccine. Clin Infect Dis 2005;40:1738–44.

[50] Lynch JP, Martinez FJ. Clinical relevance of macrolide-resistant *Streptococcus pneumoniae* for community-acquired pneumonia. Clin Infect Dis 2002;34(Suppl 1):S27–46.

[51] Doern GV. Antimicrobial use and the emergence of antimicrobial resistance with *Streptococcus pneumoniae* in the United States. Clin Infect Dis 2001;33(Suppl 3):S187–92.

[52] Vanderkooi OG, Low DE, Green K, et al. for the Toronto Invasive Bacterial Disease Network. Predicting antimicrobial resistance in invasive pneumococcal infections. Clin Infect Dis 2005;40:1288–97.

[53] Beekmann SE, Diekema DJ, Heilmann KP, et al. Macrolide use identified as risk factor for macrolide-resistant *Streptococcus pneumoniae* in a 17-center case-control study. Eur J Clin Microbiol Infect Dis 2006. Available at: http://www.springerlink.com/openurl.asp?genre=article&id=. Accessed April 13, 2006.

[54] Ghaffar F, Muniz LS, Katz K, et al. Effects of large dosages of amoxicillin/clavulanate or azithromycin on nasopharyngeal carriage of *Streptococcus pneumoniae*, *Haemophilus influenzae*, nonpneumococcal α-hemolytic streptococci, and *Staphylococcus aureus* in children with acute otitis media. Clin Infect Dis 2002;34:1301–9.

[55] Diekema DJ, Brueggemann AB, Doern GV. Antimicrobial-drug use and changes in resistance to *Streptococcus pneumoniae*. Emerg Infect Dis 2000;6(5):552–6.

[56] Bronzwaer SL, Cars O, Buchholz U, et al. A European study on the relationship between antimicrobial use and antimicrobial resistance. Emerg Infect Dis 2002;8(3):278–82.

[57] García-Rey C, Aguilar L, Baquero F, et al. Importance of local variations in antibiotic consumption and geographical differences of erythromycin and penicillin resistance in *Streptococcus pneumoniae*. J Clin Microbiol 2002;40(1):159–64.

[58] Kristinsson KG. Effect of antimicrobial use and other risk factors on antimicrobial resistance in pneumococci. Microb Drug Resist 1997;3(2):117–23.

[59] Hyde TB, Gay K, Stephens DS, et al. Macrolide resistance among invasive *S pneumoniae* isolates. JAMA 2001;286(15):1857–62.

[60] Hennessy TW, Petersen KM, Bruden D, et al. Changes in antibiotic-prescribing practices and carriage of penicillin-resistant *Streptococcus pneumoniae*: a controlled intervention trial in rural Alaska. Clin Infect Dis 2002;34:1543–50.

[61] Conte JE Jr, Golden JA, Duncan S, et al. Intrapulmonary pharmacokinetics of clarithromycin and of erythromycin. Antimicrob Agents Chemother 1995;39(2):334–8.

[62] Conte JE Jr, Golden J, Duncan S, et al. Single-dose intrapulmonary pharmacokinetics of azithromycin, clarithromycin, ciprofloxacin, and cefuroxime in volunteer subjects. Antimicrob Agents Chemother 1996;40(7):1617–22.

[63] Patel KB, Xuan D, Tessier PR, et al. Comparison of bronchopulmonary pharmacokinetics of clarithromycin and azithromycin. Antimicrob Agents Chemother 1996;40(10):2375–9.

[64] Rodvold KA, Gotfried MH, Danziger LH, et al. Intrapulmonary steady-state concentrations of clarithromycin and azithromycin in healthy adult volunteers. Antimicrob Agents Chemother 1997;41(6):1399–402.

[65] Guggenbichler JP, Kastner H. The influence of macrolide antibiotics on the fecal and oral flora. Infect Med 1998;15:17–25.

[66] Gray GC, Witucki PJ, Gould MT, et al. Randomized, placebo-controlled clinical trial of oral azithromycin prophylaxis against respiratory infections in a high-risk, young adult population. Clin Infect Dis 2001;33:983–9.

[67] Leach AJ, Shelby-James TM, Mayo M, et al. A prospective study of the impact of community-acquired azithromycin treatment of trachoma on carriage and resistance of *Streptococcus pneumoniae*. Clin Infect Dis 1997;24:356–62.

[68] Ghaffar F, Muniz LS, Katz K, et al. Effects of amoxicillin/clavulanate or azithromycin on nasopharyngeal carriage of *Streptococcus pneumoniae* and *Haemophilus influenzae* in children with acute otitis media. Clin Infect Dis 2000;31:875–80.

[69] Blondeau JM. Differential impact of macrolide compounds in the selection of macrolide nonsusceptible *Streptococcus pneumoniae*. Therapy 2005;2(6):813–8.

[70] Doern GV. Correspondence – reply to: Predicting the emergence of antimicrobial resistance. Clin Infect Dis 2002;34:1418–20.

[71] Ambrose PG. Antimicrobial susceptibility breakpoints; PK-PD and susceptibility breakpoints. Treat Respir Med 2005;4(Suppl 1):5–11.

[72] Lonks JR, Garau J, Gomez L, et al. Failure of macrolide antibiotic treatment in patients with bacteremia due to erythromycin-resistant *Streptococcus pneumoniae*. Clin Infect Dis 2002; 35:556–64.

[73] Van Kerkhoven D, Peetermans WE, Verbist L, et al. Breakthrough pneumococcal bacteraemia in patients treated with clarithromycin or oral β-lactams. J Antimicrob Chemother 2003; 51:691–6.

[74] Kelley MA, Weber DJ, Gilligan P, et al. Breakthrough pneumococcal bacteremia treated with azithromycin and clarithromycin. Clin Infect Dis 2000;31:1008–11.

[75] Jacobs MR. In vivo veritas: in vitro macrolide resistance in systemic *Streptococcus pneumoniae* infections does result in clinical failure. Clin Infect Dis 2002;35:565–9.

[76] Hoffman HL, Klepser ME, Ernst EJ, et al. Influence of macrolide susceptibility on efficacies of clarithromycin and azithromycin against *Streptococcus pneumoniae* in a murine lung infection model. Antimicrob Agents Chemother 2003;47(2):739–46.

[77] Maglio D, Capitano B, Banevicius MA, et al. Efficacy of clarithromycin against *Streptococcus pneumoniae* expressing *mef*(A)-mediated resistance. Int J Antimicrob Agents 2004;23: 498–501.

[78] Noreddin AM, Roberts D, Nichol K, et al. Pharmacodynamic modeling of clarithromycin against macrolide-resistant [PCR-positive *mef*(A) or *erm*(B)] *Streptococcus pneumoniae* simulating clinically achievable serum and epithelial lining fluid free-drug concentrations. Antimicrob Agents Chemother 2002;46(12):4029–34.

[79] Nuermberger E, Bishai WR. The clinical significance of macrolide-resistant *Streptococcus pneumoniae*: it's all relative. Clin Infect Dis 2004;38:99–103.

ELSEVIER
SAUNDERS

THE MEDICAL
CLINICS
OF NORTH AMERICA

Med Clin N Am 90 (2006) 1125–1140

Antibiotic Therapy
for *Helicobacter pylori*

Jason Collins, MD, Amira Ali-Ibrahim, MD,
Duane T. Smoot, MD, FACP, FACG*

*Gastroenterology Section, Department of Medicine, Howard University College of Medicine,
Washington, DC 20059, USA*

Helicobacter pylori has been one of the most studied pathogens in recent times. Literature searches will yield nearly 22,000 results for studies and papers published on the subject. The excitement began in 1983, the year Drs. J.R. Warren and B. Marshall published their findings concerning an "unidentified curved bacilli on gastric epithelium" [1]. Their description was quite thorough and made a case for the association of this bacterium with gastric inflammation. Salient features were pointed out, such as their near ubiquity in active chronic gastritis yet absence when there was no inflammation and their distribution in relation to the mucous layer and adjacent to the gastric epithelial cells. Twenty-three years later, what is most compelling about the initial publication is the last sentence, which reads, "They may have a part to play in other poorly understood, gastritis associated diseases" (i.e., peptic ulcer and gastric cancer). Warren and Marshall were awarded the 2005 Nobel Prize in Medicine for their discovery of the bacterium *H pylori* and its role in gastritis and peptic ulcer disease.

H pylori are spiral, flagellated, gram-negative rods [2]. Characteristics important to their survival include motility, urease production, and the ability to bind to gastric epithelial cells. Urease is produced in great abundance by *H pylori* because this enzyme breaks down urea, producing ammonia, and creates a buffered pH zone around the pathogen. Recent research has also identified bacterial virulence factors that play a critical role in clinical disease [3]. Virulence factors implicated in disease include the cag pathogenicity island (PAI), vacuolizing cytotoxin A (vacA), and outer membrane protein-encoding genes [4]. Cag PAI–containing *H pylori* strains are associated with

---

* Corresponding author. Department of Medicine, Howard University Hospital, 2041 Georgia Avenue, NW, Washington, DC 20060.
E-mail address: dsmoot@howard.edu (D.T. Smoot).

doi:10.1016/j.mcna.2006.07.002

a higher inflammatory response and an increased risk for peptic ulcer disease and gastric cancer. VacA induces cell vacuolization, membrane channel formation, disruption of endosomal/lysosomal function, apoptosis, and immunomodulation [5]. It is likely to be involved in the pathogenesis of peptic ulcer formation and gastric cancer. Several outer membrane proteins—BabA, SabA, and AlpAB—are well-known adherence factors [4]. Bacterial adherence is important in preventing clearance of the bacteria from the stomach.

Epidemiology

Approximately 50% of the world's population is infected with *H pylori* [6]. Various risk factors identified include lower socioeconomic group, younger age, ethnicity, and geographic location [6,7]. The frequency of infection has begun to decrease in developed countries, but infection is still quite prevalent there [8]. The United States has a 30% to 40% prevalence of *H pylori* [9]. However, certain racial and ethnic groups (Hispanics and African Americans) have a higher prevalence than the general population [10]. A higher prevalence of *H pylori*–specific IgG antibody has also been found among Alaska native residents, with a 75% seropositivity rate [11]. The exact mode of transmission from person to person is unknown. The most likely modes of transmission include the oral–oral and fecal–oral routes. Evidence for fecal–oral transmission is based on the presence of *H pylori* in feces detected by culture and polymerase chain reaction (PCR) [12]. Evidence supporting the oral–oral spread of the bacterium is based on studies identifying *H pylori* DNA in saliva of adults and in gastric contents of children who vomit in day care centers [13,14].

Clinical manifestations

H pylori has a complex relationship with nonmalignant diseases of the stomach. These include peptic ulcer disease (PUD), nonsteroidal anti-inflammatory drug (NSAID)–induced gastropathy, gastroesophageal reflux disease (GERD), and nonulcer dyspepsia (NUD). Whether *H pylori* infection results in clinically significant manifestations of disease depends on variables such as bacterial virulence, host genetics, and environmental factors [3].

H pylori continues to be the most common cause of PUD [15]. Thus, the most effective therapy for peptic ulcers is eradication of *H pylori*. The association between *H pylori* and NSAID-induced gastropathy has not been fully elucidated. Animal studies have shown that eradication of *H pylori* before NSAID use results in reduced gastric damage [16]. In a study evaluating the risks of NSAIDS in the elderly, when adjusted for *H pylori* infection, use of proton pump inhibitors was the only factor associated with a decreased risk for ulcer disease [17]. Although *H pylori* eradication prior to NSAID use may be advisable, the association has not been substantiated by human trials. Concomitant use of proton pump inhibitors has been shown to decrease the risk and recurrence of ulcer disease [18].

The literature offers conflicting data regarding the need to eradicate *H pylori* in patients who have NUD and no history of PUD. In a Cochrane Review combining 14 trials, *H pylori* eradication therapy was associated with a small but statistically significant reduction in symptoms in *H pylori*–positive patients with NUD [19]. Given this modest clinical benefit, an economic model suggests that treating *H pylori* in patients who have NUD may be cost-effective [19]. Thus, for patients presenting with NUD and no alarm symptoms, the "test and treat" strategy is appropriate [20].

The interactions between *H pylori* and GERD have been recently studied, thus far with no firm conclusion. A meta-analysis, which included 14 case-control studies and 10 clinical trials, concluded that there was a positive association between successful treatment of *H pylori* infection and the occurrence of both de novo and rebound/exacerbated GERD [21]. However, other reviews of this topic have not concluded that there is a definite indirect relationship between *H pylori* infection and GERD [22–24]. The data suggest that people who develop GERD after being treated for *H pylori* infection may have had significant corpus gastritis with reduced acid secretion and hence have been at higher risk for gastric cancer. The risk of gastric cancer associated with *H pylori* is well documented. People who are infected with *H pylori* are three to six times more likely to develop gastric cancer [25,26]. A population-based intervention study performed in China with an average follow-up of 7.5 years showed a nonstatistical reduction in incidence of gastric cancer by 37% in people who were treated for *H pylori* infection [27]. *H pylori* is also clearly culpable in gastric mucosa-associated lymphoid tissue (MALT) lymphomas. *H pylori* eradication is the initial treatment for Stage I MALT, with an approximate remission rate of 70% [25,26]. Long-term follow-up shows a favorable outcome after successful treatment of *H pylori* [28,29].

Diagnosis of *Helicobacter pylori*

The decision to test is often prompted by patients' presenting with dyspeptic symptoms. Population screening has not yet been recommended. When patients present with upper abdominal pain or dyspepsia, it is important to evaluate the patient for alarm symptoms when deciding between invasive and noninvasive testing. Alarm symptoms include gastrointestinal bleeding, anemia, weight loss, difficulty swallowing, palpable mass, evidence of malabsorption, long duration of symptoms, and so on. If no alarm symptoms are present and the patient's symptoms are consistent with dyspepsia, then noninvasive testing followed by treatment is recommended [30,31]. Noninvasive tests include serologic assays, urea breath tests, and stool antigen tests.

Serologic tests identify the presence of anti–*H pylori* antibody (IgG) in the serum. They have a sensitivity and specificity of approximately 85%

and 80%, respectively [32]. These tests indicate prior exposure to *H pylori* and do not indicate that the person is currently infected with *H pylori*. The advantages of serology are the relatively low cost and the noninvasive aspect. If a patient has not been treated previously for *H pylori* infection or has not received antibiotics (for other reasons) that may treat *H pylori* infection, then blood antibody tests are reliable. The major disadvantage of the antibody-based assays is the likelihood of false-positive results in patients previously treated with antibiotics, because *H pylori* antibodies circulate for some time after an infection has been cleared [32].

Alternatives to serologic assays include urea breath tests and the stool antigen test. Both of these tests detect current *H pylori* infection and may be used for both the initial diagnosis and for evaluating treatment success, when performed 4 to 6 weeks after the completion of antibiotic therapy [33–35]. Two carbon-labeled urea breath tests (^{13}C and ^{14}C) have been developed that make use of *H pylori*'s urease enzyme, which is produced in great abundance [33,34]. The urea breath test is one of the more accurate tests available, with a sensitivity of 95% and specificity of 96% [33,34,36]. False negatives may occur in patients who are being treated with antibiotics or proton pump inhibitors. Stool antigen testing detects the presence of *H pylori* antigen in the stool by means of a polyclonal anti–*H pylori* antibody [35]. Its sensitivity ranges from 89% to 92%, and its specificity ranges from 87% to 93% [35].

Invasive tests include histologic identification of *H pylori*, the rapid urease tests (RUT), bacterial culture, and PCR. Histologic identification of *H pylori* is widely used and provides the benefit of assessing for the presence of *H pylori*, as well as for the pattern of gastritis or dysplastic changes. A plethora of staining methods are available to identify *H pylori*, including Giemsa, Warthin-Starry, Genta, immunohistochemical *H pylori* antibody staining, and traditional hematoxylin and eosin staining [37–39]. The RUTs are dependent on *H pylori*'s ability to split urea. This chemical reaction is detected and indicates presence of the pathogen. The sensitivity of RUTs ranges from 80% to 95%, and their specificity varies from 95% to 100% [36,40]. The advantages of urease assays are their low cost, rapid results (usually within hours), and high reliability. False positives are uncommon but may occur with excessive salivation, reflux of alkaline bile into the stomach, and use of proton pump inhibitors [40]. False negatives may occur when patients have taken bismuth or certain antibiotics within 24 hours of testing [40]. Culture, though not considered the gold standard, is 100% specific [41,42]. Unfortunately, culturing the pathogen is technically demanding and infrequently successful. Hence sensitivity varies widely, depending on the technique and the laboratory [41,42]. PCR is primarily used for research and is not practical in the clinical setting.

Treatment of *Helicobacter pylori*

Treating peptic ulcers with antibiotics was an idea that was ridiculed 20 years ago, yet it has become the standard of care for most patients who have peptic ulcers [43,44]. Because rates of *H pylori* re-infection are low, the goal of *H pylori* treatment has always been complete eradication of the organism. Ideal antibiotic regimens should have cure rates of 80% or greater (intent-to-treat analysis) or 90% or greater (per-protocol analysis), without major side effects and with minimal induction of bacterial resistance [43]. The recommended *H pylori* treatment regimens include the combination of two or more antimicrobial agents. Using multiple antibiotics increases the eradication rates and reduces the risk for resistance. Overall, the antibiotic dosages are higher than the dosages used for other non–life-threatening infections; this is necessary to achieve a higher concentration of the medication in the mucous layer where the organism lives [44]. A proton pump inhibitor (PPI) or histamine receptor inhibitor (H_2 blocker) is combined with antibiotics to prevent their degradation at acidic pHs. Because PPIs and H_2 blockers are not able to raise the gastric pH to 7 in most people, antibiotics used to treat *H pylori* must be able to work in a minimally acidic environment.

The National Institutes of Health Consensus Panel was the first to propose generalized guidelines for the management of *H pylori* infection in February 1994 [45]. The Consensus Panel recommended that diagnostic testing for *H pylori* infection only be performed when treatment is intended. The panel also recommended that all *H pylori*–infected patients who had duodenal or gastric ulcer be treated with an eradication regimen, whether it was a new ulcer or a relapse. It advised that patients who have *H pylori* and who are receiving maintenance antisecretory treatment be given anti–*H pylori* treatment. The panel concluded that there was insufficient evidence to support treatment of patients who have NUD, if *H pylori* infection is documented.

These guidelines were updated in 1998 by an Ad Hoc Committee on Practice Parameters of the American College of Gastroenterology [46]. Its guidelines recommend testing for *H pylori* only when there is an intention to treat. Indications for testing in these guidelines include active PUD, history of documented PUD, and history of documented gastric MALT lymphoma. Testing is not indicated in long-term PPI therapy for GERD and in asymptomatic patients with a past history of PUD. No recommendations were issued regarding patients who are taking NSAIDs. Patients who have NUD may be tested on a case-by-case basis and treatment offered to those with a positive result [46]. More recently, a European panel, the European Maastricht 2-2000 panel, organized guidelines for testing and treating *H pylori* infection into two levels [47]. Its recommendations are listed in Box 1.

First-line therapy

The two types of first-line therapy are PPI-based triple therapies and bismuth-based triple therapies.

> **Box 1. Recommendations for the treatment of *Helicobacter pylori* infection, according to the Maastricht 2000 Consensus report**
>
> *Treatment is strongly recommended for*
> - Duodenal or gastric ulcer (active or not, including complicated PUD)
> - MALT lymphoma
> - Atrophic gastritis
> - Recent resection of gastric cancer
> - First-degree relative of patient with gastric cancer
> - Desire of the patient (after full consultation with the physician)
>
> *Treatment is advised for*
> - Functional dyspepsia
> - GERD (in patients requiring long-term profound acid suppression)
> - Use of NSAIDs (*H pylori* infection and the use of NSAIDs or aspirin are independent risk factors for PUD)
>
> ---
>
> *Data from* Bazzoli F. Key points from the revised Maastricht Consensus Report: the impact on general practice. Eur J Gastroenterol Hepatol 2001;13:S3–7.

Proton-pump-inhibitor–based triple therapies

These regimens include 500 mg of clarithromycin twice a day, 1 g of amoxicillin twice a day, and a PPI once or twice a day. The duration of treatment ranges from 10 days to 2 weeks, depending on which combination is used. The PPIs most frequently used include omeprazole, 20 mg twice daily or 40 mg once daily, lansoprazole, 30 mg twice or three times daily, and esomeprazole, 40 mg once daily (Box 2) [48–56]. To date, no studies have shown that larger doses of PPIs are more effective [57]. Metronidazole, 500 mg twice a day, may be substituted for either clarithromycin or amoxicillin. Clarithromycin, 500 mg, is frequently used with metronidazole, 500 mg, in patients who have an allergy to penicillin. Although the use of this combination is effective, there is a high likelihood that the *H pylori* strain will become resistant to both clarithromycin and metronidazole if the patient is not treated successfully [58]. *H pylori* resistance to amoxicillin is rare; therefore, this antibiotic is frequently chosen in first-line and second-line therapies. Table 1 shows the eradication rates for these different combinations in the United States. Similar rates of bacterial eradication have been seen with shorter durations of therapy in European trials. A recent meta-analysis that included mostly European studies showed that, in terms of eradication rates, the 10-day course does not offer a significant advantage

> ## Box 2. Recommended initial treatment options for *Helicobacter pylori*
>
> - PPI plus clarithromycin, 500 mg twice daily, or metronidazole, 500 mg twice daily, plus amoxicillin, 1 g twice daily for 10 days
> - PPI plus metronidazole, 500 mg twice daily, plus clarithromycin, 500 mg twice daily for 10 days
> - Bismuth subsalicylate, 525 mg four times daily, metronidazole, 250 mg four times daily, plus tetracycline, 500 mg four times daily for 2 weeks, plus H_2-receptor antagonist therapy as directed for 4 weeks
> - Bismuth subsalicylate, 525 mg four times daily, metronidazole, 250 mg four times daily, plus tetracycline, 500 mg four times daily, plus a PPI for 2 weeks
>
> PPI = esomeprazole, 40 mg daily, or omeprazole, 20 mg twice daily, or lansoprazole, 30 mg twice daily.

over the 7-day course. However, this has not been the case in most of the United States studies [59]. The recommended duration of treatment of *H pylori*–infected patients is 7 days in Europe, whereas it is 10 to 14 days in the United States [59,60].

Bismuth-based triple therapies

This combination most frequently includes bismuth subsalicylate, 525 mg, metronidazole, 250 mg, and tetracycline, 500 mg, all four times a day,

Table 1
Eradication rate in studies in the United States

Study	Regimen	Duration of therapy (d)	Intent to treat Eradication rate %
Laine et al., [56]	EAC	10	78
Laine et al., [48]	OAC	10	88
	OBMT	10	83
Laine et al., [64]	OAC	10	75
Fennerty et al., [53]	LAC	10	81
	LAC	14	82
Bochenek et al., [54]	PAC	7	65
	PCM	7	77
Vakil et al., [55]	RAC	7	77
	RAC	10	78
	OAC	10	73

Abbreviations: A, amoxicillin; B, bismuth; C, clarithromycin; E, esomeprazole; L, lansoprazole; M, metronidazole; O, omeprazole; P, pantoprazole; R, rabeprazole; T, tetracycline.

plus an H_2 blocker twice a day for 14 days. When low-cost therapy is important, this treatment is recommended, because metronidazole, bismuth, and tetracycline are inexpensive, and using an H_2 blocker further reduces the cost when compared with that of PPI-based triple therapies. Metronidazole resistance is common in some parts of the United States and may negatively affect the efficacy of this regimen. Tetracyline resistance is rare and does not alter the regimen's efficacy. Eradication rates in the United States with this regimen are approximately 82%, whereas in Europe eradication rates are approximately 95% [60]. In 1999, the Latin American Consensus Conference recommended furazolidone, a nitrofuran derivative, to be used as an alternative [61]. Furazolidone was given for 2 weeks at a dose of 100 mg four times daily, combined with amoxicillin, omeprazole, and bismuth with intention-to-treat (ITT) rates of 92%. However, substantial side effects were associated with this combination, including headache, nausea, vomiting, hypotension, and skin rash [61]. To avoid side effects, lower doses of furazolidone 100 mg twice daily were used, but they yielded an eradication rate of 54% [61]. Currently, this combination is more frequently used as a "rescue" therapy when one is considering third-line treatment options in patients resistant to clarithromycin and metronidazole.

Second-line therapy

An optimal strategy for retreatment after failure of the initial treatment regimen has not yet been established [43,44]. The major causes of failure of initial therapy are antibiotic resistance and poor patient compliance. Controlled trials, however, have suggested that antimicrobial sensitivity testing is not essential for clinical management of initial eradication failure [49]. Quadruple therapy has been used with good success as an optimal second-line therapy. These therapies combine a PPI with bismuth-based triple therapy. The eradication rate for this regimen is approximately 80% [62–64]. A regimen of 7 days of bismuth, tetracycline, metronidazole, and a PPI has been suggested as useful in improving eradication rates when used as first-line therapy. However, a meta-analysis of five well-designed "head-to-head" comparison studies failed to find a significant difference in eradication rates between this regimen and the standard PPI triple therapy (80% versus 79%) [62]. This pooled analysis supports the use of a repeat triple therapy with avoidance of one of the previously used antimicrobial agents [62]. For example, people who were initially treated with omeprazole, amoxicillin, and clarithromycin would be retreated with omeprazole, amoxicillin, and metronidazole. Metronidazole resistance may be overcome by increasing the dose of metronidazole given when retreating [65]. Clarithromycin resistance is the major reason for lack of success in second-line therapy. Clarithromycin resistance is relatively common (see further discussion), and it cannot be overcome by increasing the dose of clarithromycin. However, bismuth-based quadruple therapy as a second-line therapy may be more effective when the dose of metronidazole is increased from 1 g/d to 1.5 g/d in three divided doses, or 2 g in four divided doses [65]. One example of a stepwise approach to treating *H pylori* infection is given in Fig. 1.

Third-line rescue therapy

Patients who fail two treatment trials are a challenge. European guidelines recommend bacterial culture in these patients to select a third-line treatment according to microbial sensitivity to antibiotics [66,67]. Because cultures are often performed only in research centers, the routine use of this procedure in patients who failed several treatments is not feasible. In 2001, Perri and colleagues [66] published a randomized trial of two "rescue" therapies for use after failure of standard triple therapy. Patients were given rifabutin, 300 mg daily, in combination with amoxicillin, 1 g twice daily, and pantoprazole, 40 mg twice daily for 10 days. The success rate was 86%. Several other studies combined rifabutin at 150 mg twice daily with omeprazole, 20 mg twice daily, or lansoprazole, 30 mg twice daily. Their eradication rates varied between 60% and 79% [67–69]. Another study by Perri and colleagues [70] in 2001 showed that an 80% eradication rate was also achieved by using azithromycin, 1000 mg daily for three days, tinidazole for 1 week,

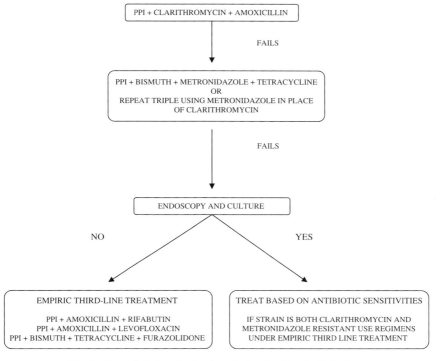

Fig. 1. Suggested stepwise treatment plan for *H pylori* infection.

and omeprazole for 1 month. A 14-day quadruple therapy has achieved still better results. It includes omeprazole, 20 mg, tetracycline, 500 mg, metronidazole, 500 mg, and bismuth subcitrate caplets, 240 mg, all twice daily [70]. Graham and colleagues [65] performed a pilot study in the United States using the aforementioned regimen as a first-line therapy with metronidazole-resistant strains, which yielded an eradication rate of 88.9%. This study was followed by that of Dore and colleagues [71] of 74 Italian patients from Sardinia, a region with a 14% to 26% resistance rate to tetracycline and amoxicillin. They documented a 93% eradication rate with twice-daily quadruple therapy containing esomeprazole, tetracycline, metronidazole, and bismuth subcitrate [71].

In some parts of the United States and around the world, "rescue"therapy with a quadruple combination of PPI, bismuth, tetracycline, and metronidazole has a failure rate of approximately 20% to 30%. This situation has caused a therapeutic dilemma, because patients who are not cured with these two consecutive treatments including clarithromycin and metronidazole will have at least single, and usually double, resistance [72]. In a study conducted in Hong Kong with 109 patients who failed previous therapies and who had resistance to both clarithromycin and metronidazole, the authors used a combination of a PPI twice daily, rifabutin, 300 mg once daily, and levofloxacin, 500 mg once daily for 7 days [73]. They documented an eradication rate of 91% [73]. One of the more recent studies, conducted by Javier and colleagues [74], used an eradication regimen with levofloxacin, 500 mg, amoxicillin, 1 g, and omeprazole, 20 mg, all twice daily prescribed for 10 days, with a documented eradication rate of 60% to 66%. Before this study, Gatta and colleagues [75] had used the same combination but with levofloxacin 250 mg twice daily and found an eradication rate of 76%. In areas where levofloxacin is widely used for respiratory infections, high prevalences of resistance strains have been reported [75]. The use of high-dose amoxicillin, 750 mg daily, with high-dose omeprazole, 40 mg daily for 14 days, in patients with strains resistant to both metronidazole and clarithromycin yielded an eradication rate of 76% [76]. Finally, the use of furazolidone-based rescue regimens has been suggested in the literature. This regimen consists of furazolidone combined with tetracycline, bismuth, and a PPI in a quadruple therapy with an eradication rate of 90%. Furazolidone has also been used in a triple-therapy format with no PPI and an eradication rate of 86% [77,78].

Penicillin allergy

Usually when penicillin allergy is documented, metronidazole and clarithromycin are used instead of amoxicillin. When a patient fails such a therapy, it presents a therapeutic challenge. In a recent study by Gisbert and colleagues [79], *H pylori*–infected patients who were allergic to penicillin were treated initially with a PPI, clarithromycin, and metronidazole, resulting in an eradication rate of 58%. This low rate was attributed to metronidazole resistance. In case of failure, rescue treatment options include a third-line therapy with levofloxacin, clarithromycin, and omeprazole [79]. Additionally, rifabutin, clarithromycin, and omeprazole for 10 days may be used [79]. However, this therapy may not be well tolerated; in one study, 89% of patients had adverse effects, including gastrointestinal symptoms, abnormal liver function tests, leucopenia, and thrombocytopenia [79].

Antimicrobial resistance

After patients have tested positive for *H pylori* and the decision to treat has been made, the approach to treatment must take into consideration patient compliance, potential side effects, and prior antibiotic therapies for other infections. The patients' countries of origin must be considered, because patterns of resistance to different antibiotics vary among the United States, Europe, and other countries around the world. Resistance is primarily a result of point mutations that occur in *H pylori* [80]. The *H pylori* Antimicrobial Resistance Monitoring Program (HARP) is a prospective, multicenter United States network that tracks national prevalence rates of *H pylori* antimicrobial resistance [72]. HARP collected 347 isolates from December 1998 through 2002. Prevalence of metronidazole resistance was approximately 25.1% (although in some parts of the United States it is greater than 35%), clarithromycin resistance was 12.9%, and amoxicillin resistance was 0.9% [72]. In Europe, resistance to clarithromycin is about 10% [80]. Higher resistance to metronidazole exists in developing countries (20% to 30%), which is attributed to the frequent use of metronidazole to treat other conditions [72]. Poor patient compliance is due to the number of pills required per day and to side effects [81]. These side effects may include nausea, taste disturbance, diarrhea, cramps, and headache. Retesting to confirm eradication is not practiced as often in the United States as in Europe, where it is common practice. It is only recommended in patients who have a history of ulcer complications, gastric MALT lymphoma, or early gastric cancer. Patients who have recurrent symptoms after treatment of *H pylori* infection also need further evaluation.

Summary

H pylori is a genetically diverse organism that can quickly develop resistance to antibiotics. This factor, together with its location in the stomach mucus, makes *H pylori* a difficult organism to treat. Initial treatment of this bacterium is successful more than 80% of the time, but with growing resistance, initial treatment success rates are falling below 80% in many parts of the United States. It is recommended that, after two unsuccessful attempts to treat *H pylori*, upper gastrointestinal endoscopy with gastric biopsy for bacterial culture and antimicrobial resistance testing be sought to guide further treatment. In addition to the new antibiotic treatments that are being developed for people with multiresistant strains, several companies are looking at the prospects of a therapeutic *H pylori* vaccine that would easily treat everyone infected with this bacterium. Therapeutic vaccines are currently being studied in animal models with some success [82,83].

References

[1] Marshall BJ, Warren JR, et al. Unidentified curved bacilli in the stomach of patients with gastritis and peptic ulceration. Lancet 1984;16:1311–5.
[2] Dunn BE, Cohen H. *Helicobacter pylori*. Clin Microbiol Rev 1997;10:720–41.
[3] Arents NL, van Zwet AA, Thijs JC, et al. The importance of vacA, cagA, and iceA genotypes of Helicobacter pylori infection in peptic ulcer disease and gastroesophageal reflux disease. Am J Gastroenterol 2001;96:2603–8.
[4] Figueiredo C, Machado JC, Yamaoka Y. Pathogenesis of *Helicobacter pylori* infection. Helicobacter 2005;10:14–20.
[5] Cover TL, Blanke SR, et al. *Helicobacter pylori* VacA, a paradigm for toxin multifunctionality. Nat Rev Microbiol 2005;3:320–32.
[6] Go MF. Review article: natural history and epidemiology of *Helicobacter pylori* infection. Aliment Pharmacol Ther 2002;16:3–15.
[7] Klein PD, Graham DY, et al. Water source as risk factor for *Helicobacter pylori* infection in Peruvian children. Lancet 1991;337:1503–7.
[8] Gold BD. *Helicobacter pylori* infection in children. Curr Probl Pediatr Adolesc Health Care 2001;31:247–66.
[9] Dooley CP, Cohen H, Fitzgibbons PL, et al. Prevalence of *Helicobacter pylori* infection and histologic gastritis in asymptomatic persons. N Engl J Med 1989;321: 1562–6.
[10] Everhart JE, Kruszon-Moran D, Perez-Perez GI, et al. Seroprevalence and ethnic differences in *Helicobacter pylori* infection among adults in the United States. J Infect Dis 2000;18: 1359–63.
[11] Parkinson AJ, Gold BD, Bulkow L, et al. High prevalence of *Helicobacter pylori* in the Alaska Native population and association with low serum ferritin levels in young adults. Clin Diagn Lab Immunol 2000;7:885–8.
[12] Thomas JE, Gibson GR, Darboe MK, et al. Isolation of *Helicobacter pylori* from human faeces. Lancet 1992;340:1194–5.
[13] Young KA, Aryon Y, Rampton DS, et al. Quantitative culture of *Helicobacter pylori* from gastric juice: the potential for transmission. J Med Microbiol 2000;49:343–7.
[14] Parsonnet J, Shmuely H, Haggerty T, et al. Fecal and oral shedding of *Helicobacter pylori* from healthy infected adults. JAMA 1999;282:2240–5.
[15] Rosenstock S, Jorgensen T, Bonnevie O, et al. Risk factors for peptic ulcer disease: a population based prospective cohort study comprising 2416 Danish adults. Gut 2003;52: 186–93.
[16] Chang CC, Chen SH, Lien GS, et al. Eradication of *Helicobacter pylori* significantly reduced gastric damage in nonsteroidal anti-inflammatory drug–treated Mongolian gerbils. World J Gastroenterol 2005;11:104–8.
[17] Pilotto A, Pranceschi M, Leandro G, et al. Proton-pump inhibitors reduce the risk of uncomplicated peptic ulcer in elderly either acute or chronic users of aspirin/non-steroidal anti-inflammatory drugs. Aliment Pharmacol Ther 2004;20:1091–7.
[18] Ford A, Delaney B, Forman D, et al. Eradication therapy for peptic ulcer disease in *Helicobacter pylori* positive patients. Cochrane Database Syst Rev 2006;2CD003840.
[19] Moayyedi P, Soo S, Deeks J, et al. Eradication of *Helicobacter pylori* for non-ulcer dyspepsia. Cochrane Database Syst Rev 2006;2CD002096.

[20] Malfertheiner P, Megraud F, O'Moran C, et al. Current concepts in the management of *Helicobacter pylori* infection—the Maastricht 2-2000 Consensus Report. Aliment Pharmacol Ther 2002;16:167–80.

[21] Cremonini F, Di Caro S, Delgado-Aros S, et al. Meta-analysis: the relationship between *Helicobacter pylori* infection and gastro-oesophageal reflux disease. Aliment Pharmacol Ther 2003;18(3):279–89.

[22] Raghunath A, Pali A, Hungin S, et al. Prevalence of *Helicobacter pylori* in patients with gastro-oesophageal reflux disease: systemic review. BMJ 2003;326:737.

[23] Sharma P, Vakil N. Review article: *Helicobacter pylori* and reflux disease. Aliment Pharmacol Ther 2003;17(3):297–305.

[24] Raghunath AS, Hungin AP, Wooff D, et al. Systematic review: the effect of *Helicobacter pylori* and its eradication on gastro-oesophageal reflux disease in patients with duodenal ulcers or reflux oesophagitis. Aliment Pharmacol Ther 2004;20(7):733–44.

[25] Nomura AM, Kolonel LN, Miki K, et al. *Helicobacter pylori*, pepsinogen, and gastric adenocarcinoma in Hawaii. J Infect Dis 2005;191:2075–81.

[26] Parsonnet J, Friedman GD, Vandersteen DP, et al. *Helicobacter pylori* infection and the risk of gastric carcinoma. N Engl J Med 1991;325:1127–31.

[27] Wong BC, Lam SK, Wong WM, et al. *Helicobacter pylori* eradication to prevent gastric cancer in a high-risk region of China: a randomized controlled trial. JAMA 2004;291:187–94.

[28] O'Rourke JL, Dixon MF, Jack A, et al. Gastric B-cell mucosa-associated lymphoid tissue (MALT) lymphoma in an animal model of *Helicobacter heilmannii* infection. J Pathol 2004;203:896–903.

[29] Fischbach W, Goebeler-Kolve ME, Dragosics B, et al. Long-term outcome of patients with gastric marginal zone B-cell lymphoma of mucosa-associated lymphoid tissue (MALT) following exclusive *Helicobacter pylori* eradication therapy: experience from a large prospective series. Gut 2004;53:34–7.

[30] You JHS, Wong P, Wu JCY, et al. Cost-effectiveness of *Helicobacter pylori* "test and treat" for patients with typical reflux symptoms in a population with a high prevalence of *H. pylori* infection: a Markov model analysis. Scand J Gastroenterol 2006;41:21–9.

[31] Allison JE, Hurley LB, Hiatt RA, et al. A randomized controlled trial of test-and-treat strategy for *Helicobacter pylori*: clinical outcomes and health care costs in a managed care population receiving long-term acid suppression therapy for physician-diagnosed peptic ulcer disease. Arch Intern Med 2003;163:1165–71.

[32] Loy CT, Irwig LM, Katelaris PH, et al. Do commercial serological kits for *Helicobacter pylori* infection differ in accuracy? A meta-analysis. Am J Gastroenterol 1996;91: 1138–44.

[33] Peura DA, Pambianco DJ, Dye KR, et al. Microdose ^{14}C-urea breath test offers diagnosis of *Helicobacter pylori* in 10 minutes. Am J Gastroenterol 1996;91:233–8.

[34] Slomianski A, Schubert T, Cutler AF. [^{13}C] urea breath test to confirm eradication of *Helicobacter pylori*. Am J Gastroenterol 1995;90:224–6.

[35] Vaira D, Malfertheiner P, Megraud F, et al and the HpSA European study group. Diagnosis of *Helicobacter pylori* infection with a new non-invasive antigen-based assay. Lancet 1999;354:30–3.

[36] Cutler AF, Havstad S, Ma CK, et al. Accuracy of invasive and noninvasive tests to diagnose *Helicobacter pylori* infection. Gastroenterology 1995;109:136–41.

[37] Aston-Key M, Diss TC, Isaacson PG, et al. Detection of *Helicobacter pylori* in gastric biopsy and resection specimens. J Clin Pathol 1996;49:107–11.

[38] Laine L, Levin DN, Naritoku W, et al. Prospective comparison of H&E, Giemsa and Genta stains for the diagnosis of *Helicobacter pylori*. Gastrointest Endosc 1997;45:463–7.

[39] Rotimi O, Cairns A, Gray S, et al. Histological identification of *Helicobacter pylori*: comparison of staining methods. J Clin Pathol 2000;53:756–9.

[40] Midolo P, Marshall B. Accurate diagnosis of Helicobacter pylori. Urease test. Gastroenterol Clin North Am 2000;29:871–8.

[41] van der Wouden EJ, Thijs JC, van Zwet AA, et al. Reliability of biopsy-based diagnostic tests for *Helicobacter pylori* after treatment aimed at its eradication. Eur J Gastroenterol Hepatol 1999;11(11):1255–8.

[42] Cutler AF. Diagnostic tests for *Helicobacter pylori* infection. Gastroenterologist 1997;5:202–12.

[43] Suerbaum S, Michetti P. *Helicobacter pylori* infection. N Engl J Med 2002;347(15):1175–86.

[44] Vakil N. Treatment of *Helicobacter pylori*. Am J Ther 1998;5:197–202.

[45] National Institutes of Health Consensus Development Panel on Helicobacter pylori in Peptic Ulcer Disease. Helicobacter pylori in peptic ulcer disease. JAMA 1994;272:65–9.

[46] Howden CW, Hunt RH. Guidelines for the management of *Helicobacter pylori* infection. Am J Gastroenterol 1998;93:2330–8.

[47] Bazzoli F. Key points from the revised Maastricht Consensus Report: the impact on general practice. Eur J Gastroenterol Hepatol 2001;13:S3–7.

[48] Laine L, Suchower L, Frantz J, et al. Twice daily 10 day triple therapy with esomeprazole, amoxicillin and clarithromycin for *Helicobacter pylori* eradication in duodenal ulcer disease: results of three multicenter, double blind, United States trials. Am J Gastroenterol 1998;93: 2106–12.

[49] Lind T, Veldhuyzen van Zanten S, Unge P, et al. Eradication of *Helicobacter pylori* using one-week triple therapies combining omeprazole with two antimicrobials: the MACH I Study. Helicobacter 1996;1:138–44.

[50] Lind T, Megraud F, Unge P, et al. The MACH2 study: role of omeprazole in eradication of *Helicobacter pylori* with 1-week triple therapies. Gastroenterology 1999;116:248–53.

[51] Malfertheiner P, Bayerdorffer E, Diete U, et al. The GU-MACH study: the effect of 1-week omeprazole triple therapy on *Helicobacter pylori* infection in patients with gastric ulcer. Aliment Pharmacol Ther 1999;13:703–12.

[52] Zanten SJ, Bradette M, Farley A, et al. The DU-MACH study: eradication of *Helicobacter pylori* and ulcer healing in patients with acute duodenal ulcer using omeprazole based triple therapy. Aliment Pharmacol Ther 1999;13:289–95.

[53] Fennerty MB, Kovacs TO, Krause R, et al. A comparison therapy of 10 and 14 days of lansoprazole triple therapy for eradication of *Helicobacter pylori*. Arch Intern Med 1998;158: 1651–6.

[54] Bochenek WJ, Peters S, Fraga PD, et al. *Helicobacter pylori* Pantaprazole Eradication (HELPPE) Study group. Eradication of *H. pylori* by 7-day triple therapy regimens combining pantoprazole with clarithromycin, metronidazole, or amoxicillin in patients with peptic ulcer disease: results of two double-blinded, randomized studies. Helicobacter 2003;8:626–42.

[55] Vakil N, Lanza F, Schwartz H, et al. Seven-day therapy for *Helicobacter pylori* in the United States. Aliment Pharmacol Ther 2004;20:99–107.

[56] Laine L, Fennerty MB, Osato M, et al. Esomeprazole-based *Helicobacter pylori* eradication therapy and the effect of antibiotic resistance: results of three US multicenter, double-blind trials. Am J Gastroenterol 2000;95:3393–8.

[57] Laheij RJ, Rossum LG, Jansen JB, et al. Evaluation of treatment regimens to cure *Helicobacter pylori* infection—a meta-analysis. Aliment Pharmacol Ther 1999;13:857–64.

[58] Peitz U, Hackelsberger A, Malfertheiner P, et al. A practical approach to patients with refractory *Helicobacter pylori* infection, or who are re-infected after standard therapy. Drugs 1999;57:905–20.

[59] Calvet X, Garcia N, Lopez T, et al. A meta-analysis of short versus long therapy with a proton pump inhibitor, clarithromycin and either metronidazole or amoxicillin for treating *Helicobacter pylori* infection. Aliment Pharmacol Ther 2000;14:603–9.

[60] Fennerty MB, Lieberman DA, Vakil N, et al. Effectiveness of *Helicobacter pylori* therapies in a clinical practice setting. Arch Intern Med 1999;159:1562–6.

[61] Coelho LG, Leon-Barua R, Quigley EM, et al. Latin-American Consensus Conference on *Helicobacter pylori* infection. Am J Gastroenterol 2000;95:2688–91.

[62] Gene E, Calvet X, Azagra R, et al. Triple vs. quadruple therapy for treating *Helicobacter pylori* infection: an updated meta analysis. Aliment Pharmacol Ther 2003;18:543–4.

[63] Graham DY, Hoffman J, el-Zimaity HM, et al. Twice a day quadruple therapy (bismuth sub-salicylate, tetracycline, metronidazole plus lansoprazole) for treatment of *Helicobacter pylori* infection. Aliment Pharmacol Ther 1997;11:935–8.

[64] Laine L, Hunt R, El-Zimaity H, et al. Bismuth-based quadruple therapy using a single cap-sule of bismuth subcitrate, metronidazole, and tetracycline given with omeprazole versus omeprazole, amoxicillin, and clarithromycin for eradication of *Helicobacter pylori*: a prospective, randomized, multicenter, North American trial. Am J Gastroenterol 2003; 98:562–7.

[65] Graham DY, Osato MS, Hoffman J, et al. Metronidazole containing quadruple therapy for infection with metronidazole resistance *Helicobacter pylori*: a prospective study. Aliment Pharmacol Ther 2000;14:745–50.

[66] Perri F, Festa V, Clemente R, et al. Randomized study of two "rescue" therapies for *Helico-bacter pylori*–infected patients after failure of standard triple therapies. Am J Gastroenterol 2001;96:58–62.

[67] Gisbert JP, Pajares JM. Review article: *Helicobacter pylori* "rescue" therapy after failure of two eradication treatments. Helicobacter 2005;10:363–72.

[68] Bock H, Koop H, Lehn N, et al. Rifabutin-based triple therapy after failure of *Helicobacter pylori* eradication treatment: preliminary experience. J Clin Gastroenterol 2000;31:222–5.

[69] Canducci F, Ojetti V, Pola P, et al. Rifabutin-based *Helicobacter pylori* eradication rescue therapy. Aliment Pharmacol Ther 2001;15:143.

[70] Perri F, Cillani MR, Quitadamo M, et al. Ranitidine bismuth citrate–based triple therapies after failure of the standard "Maastricht triple therapy": a promising alternative to the qua-druple therapy? Aliment Pharmacol Ther 2001;15:1017–22.

[71] Dore MP, Graham DY, Mele R, et al. Colloidal bismuth subcitrate–based twice-a-day quadruple therapy as primary or salvage therapy for *Helicobacter pylori* infection. Am J Gas-troenterol 2002;97:857–60.

[72] Meyer JM, Silliman NP, Wang W, et al. Risk factors for *Helicobacter pylori* resistance in the United States: the Surveillance of *H. pylori* Antimicrobial Resistance Partnership (SHARP) study, 1993–1999. Ann Intern Med 2002;136:13–24.

[73] Wong WM, Gu Q, Lam SK, et al. Randomized controlled study of rabeprazole, levofloxacin and rifabutin triple therapy vs. quadruple therapy as second line treatment for *Helicobacter pylori* infection. Aliment Pharmacol Ther 2003;17:553–60.

[74] Gisbert JP, Castro-Fernández M, Bermejo F, et al. The *H. pylori* Study Group of the Aso-ciación Española de Gastroenterología. Third-line rescue therapy with levofloxacin after two *H. pylori* treatment failures. Am J Gastroenterol 2006;101:243–7.

[75] Gatta L, Zullo A, Perna F, et al. A 10 day levofloxacin-based triple therapy in patients who failed two eradication courses. Aliment Pharmacol Ther 2005;22:45–9.

[76] Miehlke S, Kirsch C, Schneider-Brachert W, et al. A prospective, randomized study of quadruple therapy and high dose dual therapy for treatment of *Helicobacter pylori* resistant to both metronidazole and clarithromycin. Helicobacter 2003;8:310–9.

[77] Isakov V, Domareva I, Koudryavtseva L, et al. Furazolidone-based triple "rescue" therapy vs. quadruple "rescue therapy" for the eradication of *Helicobacter pylori* resistant to metro-nidazole. Aliment Pharmacol Ther 2002;16:1277–82.

[78] Treiber G, Ammon S, Malfertheiner P, et al. Impact of furazolidone-based quadruple therapy for eradication of *Helicobacter pylori* after previous treatment failure. Helicobacter 2002;7:225–31.

[79] Gisbert JP, Gisbert JL, Marcos S, et al. *Helicobacter pylori* first line and rescue options in patients allergic to penicillin. Aliment Pharmacol Ther 2005;22:1041–6.

[80] Mégraud F, Hazell S. Antibiotic susceptibility and resistance. In: Mobley HLT, Mendz GL, Hazell SL, editors. *Helicobacter pylori*: physiology and genetics. Washington, DC: ASM Press; 2001. p. 511–30.

[81] Cutler AF, Schubert TT. Patient factors affecting *H. pylori* eradication with triple therapy. Am J Gastroenterol 1993;88:505–9.

[82] Michetti P, Kreiss C, Kotloff KL, et al. Oral immunization with urease and *Escherichia coli* heat-labile enterotoxin is safe and immunogenic in *Helicobacter pylori*–infected adults. Gastroenterology 1999;116:804–12.

[83] Blanchard TG, Czinn SJ. Immunology of *Helicobacter pylori* and prospects for vaccine. Gastroenterol Clin North Am 2000;29:671–85.

ELSEVIER
SAUNDERS

THE MEDICAL
CLINICS
OF NORTH AMERICA

Med Clin N Am 90 (2006) 1141–1163

Antimicrobial Therapy of *Clostridium difficile*-Associated Diarrhea

Emilio Bouza, MD, PhD[a],*,
Almudena Burillo, MD, PhD[b],
Patricia Muñoz, MD, PhD[a]

[a]*Department of Clinical Microbiology and Infectious Diseases,
Hospital General Universitario Gregorio Marañón, Universidad Complutense,
Dr. Esquerdo 46, 28007 Madrid, Spain*
[b]*Servicio de Microbiología Clínica, Hospital de Madrid-Monteprincipe,
Avda. Monteprincipe, 25, 28660 Madrid, Spain*

Clostridium difficile-associated diarrhea (CDAD) is the most common etiologically defined cause of hospital-acquired diarrhea. Caused by the toxins of certain strains of *C difficile*, CDAD represents a growing concern, with epidemic outbreaks in some hospitals where very aggressive and difficult-to-treat strains have been found recently [1–9].

Incidence of CDAD varies ordinarily between 1 and 10 cases in every 1,000 admissions, raising rates of morbidity and significantly increasing costs [10,11]. Length of stay of in-patients with CDAD is prolonged from 18 to 30 days [12,13] and the disease has an estimated extra cost per episode for the hospital budget of £4,107, as calculated by a British group, and $3,340, as calculated by a group in the United States [14,15].

C difficile is a gram-positive sporulated rod that grows in strict anaerobic conditions, forming colonies that are circular to irregular [16] (Fig. 1), with a characteristic odor redolent of horse feces (a smell "like a horse stable") [17].

Strains with clinical interest are the toxin-producing ones. Two main toxins are responsible for virulence in most *C difficile* isolates. These are named toxin A and toxin B [18–20]. Although traditionally toxin A has been considered as enterotoxic and toxin B as cytotoxic, both are cytotoxic for a variety of cellular types, both induce an increase in vascular permeability, and both cause hemorrhage [21]. Besides, both toxins may act

* Corresponding author. Servicio de Microbiología Clínica y Enfermedades Infecciosas, Hospital General Universitario Gregorio Marañón, Dr. Esquerdo 46, 28007 Madrid, Spain.
E-mail address: ebouza@microb.net (E. Bouza).

0025-7125/06/$ - see front matter
doi:10.1016/j.mcna.2006.07.011

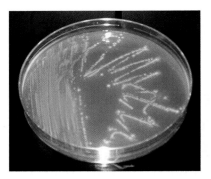

Fig. 1. Growth of *C difficile* on agar medium.

sinergically in the destruction of digestive-tract cells [22]. Researchers have identified toxin-A–negative and toxin-B–positive strains that still retain their ability to produce disease [23,24].

In approximately 5% of strains at some institutions, a third toxin or group of toxins, named binary toxins, is present. The pathogenic meaning of this toxin or toxins is still not well defined, though the toxin or toxins might be responsible for increasing disease severity [25–31].

Clinical manifestations of *C difficile*-associated disease

Clinical manifestations of infection by *C difficile* are numerous and range from asymptomatic carrier status to fulminant colitis, including the most common of all, CDAD, with or without pseudo-membranes in the wall of the colon [32–34]. The severity of the disease depends on two factors. These are the host characteristics, especially immune status, and the pathogen characteristics, especially virulence, inoculum, and ability to produce toxins.

CDAD may present as a mild disease, similar to antimicrobial-related diarrhea not due to *C difficile*, which usually comes to an end on the withdrawal of antibiotic administration, most frequently acquired in hospital but occasionally in the community [35–38].

The most common clinical presentation of CDAD is a moderate-to-severe nosocomial diarrhea. Patients with CDAD usually present with malaise, abdominal cramps or pain, nausea, vomiting, brown or clear watery diarrhea, fever, and leukocytosis. In these cases, endoscopic examination of the colon commonly reveals unspecific inflammatory lesions (unspecific colitis) [34].

In more severe cases (<20% of CDAD), pseudo-membranes are present in the wall of the colon and endoscopy shows white-yellowish plaques (2–10 mm) in any segment of the colon [34]. Small bowel or other segments of the digestive tract are very rarely involved [32].

One of the most severe clinical presentations of CDAD is as an impending fulminant colitis with a sudden rise in the peripheral white blood count to between 30,000 and 50,000 per cubic millimeter (leukemoid reaction) [39–41]. In a very elegant and clarifying work by Wanahita et al [41] involving 400 inpatients with leucocytosis $>15,000/mm^3$ in an institution, the investigators showed that *C difficile* was a very frequent underlying condition, often in the absence of diarrhea. Patients with a leukemoid reaction have a mortality rate of approximately 50%, significantly higher than that of other forms of CDAD [41].

The isolation of *C difficile* from nonfecal samples is very uncommon and its final clinical significance unclear [42–44].

Risk factors for CDAD

The main risk factor associated with symptomatic infection by *C difficile* is antimicrobial treatment within the previous 6 to 8 weeks, which occurs in over 90% of patients. The administration of antibiotics decreases the "resistance to colonization," diminishing microbial competence [45,46]. The antimicrobials most frequently associated with CDAD are summarized in Table 1 [47,48]. Anti-microbials least associated with CDAD are aminoglycosides, cotrimoxazole, benzyl penicillin, and ureido or piperacil penicillins.

There seems to be an obvious difference among quinolones with low antianaerobic activity, which do not alter the intestinal microflora, and those with antianaerobic activity, though not active against *C difficile*. The latter have been associated with epidemic outbreaks of CDAD as once happened in a hospital after substituting treatment with levofloxacin for treatment with gatifloxacin [49,50] (see Table 1). On the other hand, levofloxacin has been described as a potentially responsible factor in an epidemic outbreak described in 2005 [7].

Other therapeutic drugs, such as antineoplasic agents (5-fluoruracil), antifungal agents (amphotericin B or fluconazole) or antiviral agents, have also been described as predisposing to CDAD, though the exact pathogenic mechanism remains unknown. The authors have examined CDAD

Table 1
Antimicrobials predisposing to *Clostridium difficile* associated diarrhea

Very commonly related	Commonly related	Uncommonly related
Clindamycin	Other penicillins	Aminoglycosides
Ampicillin	Sulphonamides	Bacitracin
Amoxicillin	Trimethoprim	Metronidazole
Cephalosporins	Cotrimoxazole	Teicoplanin
	Quinolones	Rifampin
		Chloramphenicol
		Tetracyclines
		Carbapenems
		Daptomycin
		Tigecycline

patients who were only being administered antituberculous drugs containing rifampin.

Advanced age is another risk factor for the infection and a very high proportion of patients with CDAD are over 65 years old [51–54]. The increased susceptibility of the elderly to the infection may be related to the presence of underlying diseases, to the higher exposure to antimicrobials, or to the presence of lower antibody titers against *C difficile*.

Oncologic diseases, hemodialysis, immunosuppression, ulcerative colitis, malnutrition, solid-organ transplantation and HIV infection are among the predisposing conditions to CDAD [2,55–68].

Prolonged hospital stay also increases the risk of CDAD. Incidence is lower among patients with a higher titer of anti-*Clostridium* antibodies in serum and in these patients relapses are less frequent [69–73].

Confirmation of *C difficile*-associated disease

Five issues should be taken into consideration when CDAD is suspected:

- Diarrhea that occurs 48 hours or more after the beginning of the hospital stay may also be community-acquired.
- The diarrhea is related to previous use of antimicrobials, though not necessarily to a simultaneous use.
- Diagnosis should exclude other entities that present with diarrhea, such as parenteral nutrition and enteropathogens.
- Diagnosis requires *C difficile* toxin in feces, either directly in the sample, or in *C difficile* strains isolated from samples with a negative direct cell culture assay, retested for toxin production.
- Good therapeutic response to treatment with oral vancomycin or metronidazole is now being reconsidered because some healthcare centers report an increasing percentage of patients with a low response to metronidazole.

Laboratory methods

The choice sample for the diagnosis of CDAD is a fresh sample of diarrheic stools, readily sent to the laboratory [17,74–79]. The benefit of sending several stool samples for toxin detection per episode is very limited [80,81].

The gold standard for the diagnosis of the disease is the toxin-B cytotoxicity test in cell cultures [82,83]. An alternative technique for laboratories without cell cultures is the use of enzyme-linked immunosorbent assays (ELISAs) [76,84,85]. They have an excellent specificity, although their sensitivity allows for the detection of toxin quantities over 100 to 1000 pg (the cellular culture detects 10–20 pg of toxin A and 1 pg of toxin B when used with the appropriate antisera). Therefore, the false-negative rate amounts to 10% to 40%. There are ELISA assays that detect either toxin A or both toxins A and B [86].

Molecular techniques have also been successfully employed in the diagnosis of CDAD [87–90]. Their complexity and cost prevent them from being adopted in the laboratory on a routine basis, so they should be used for confirmation only, or be restricted to highly qualified reference laboratories.

The Infectious Diseases Society of America [91] and the Society for Health Care and Epidemiology of America [92] have published guidelines for the correct use of detection techniques of *C difficile* [45]. According to these guidelines:

- With few exceptions, only diarrheic stools should be examined.
- Microbiological tests, except those required for epidemiological studies, are not needed to confirm that the patient has been cured once the symptoms have subsided.
- Only samples from patients over the age of 1 year should be examined.
- ELISA techniques are an alternative to the standard method, although their sensitivity is quite lower.
- Diarrhea that develops after 3 days of hospitalization should be tested only for *C difficile* toxin (the "3-day rule"), with the exception of elderly patients, patients with HIV, or neutropenic patients.

Several culture media allow for the easy isolation of *C difficile* from feces [17,93,94], but culture is not frequently performed in CDAD cases and is considered unnecessary by many laboratories around the world. The authors recommend the complementary use of culture for the isolation of *C difficile* because it is highly sensitive and allows for the isolation of strains in patients with negative direct assay test. The use of culture permits a "second look" cytotoxicity assay, which, in the authors' institution, has improved the diagnosis of CDAD by 15% [95]. The isolation of *C difficile* also enables antimicrobial susceptibility testing and facilitates epidemiologic studies [95,96].

In most cases, endoscopy is not required to confirm the diagnosis of CDAD and is therefore an unnecessary risk for the patient.

Image techniques can be useful for the diagnosis of CDAD. The prevalence of an abnormal colon on CT in adult inpatients with *C difficile* colitis is close to 50%. Segmental colonic wall thickness (>4 mm) is the main finding. The areas most commonly involved are the rectum and sigmoid colon. Positive scans are associated with increased white blood cell count, abdominal pain, and diarrhea, but specific CT findings could not predict surgical treatment [97].

Antimicrobial activity of different drugs against *C difficile*

A high percentage of *C difficile* strains are resistant to antimicrobials, such as cephalosporins, clindamycin, macrolides, telithromycin, aminoglycosides, tetracyclines, cotrimoxazole, ertapenem, imipenem, and chloramphenicol [98–106]. Most fluoroquinolones now in use have a low activity against this pathogen, though some of the most recently synthesized, with a good antianaerobic coverage, show lower minimal inhibiting concentration, as compared with those already in use [99,107–115]. Meanwhile, the microorganism shows in vitro susceptibility to ampicillin, meropenem, metronidazole, penicillin, piperacillin, piperacillin–tazobactam, teicoplanin, and vancomycin [98,99,103,116,117].

Among new antimicrobials, ramoplanin is particularly interesting. It is a new peptide that inhibits the synthesis of the cell wall by sequestrating peptidoglycan biosynthesis lipid intermediates. It is poorly absorbed by the digestive tract and cannot be administered intravenously. Therefore, it is a good choice for endoluminal dispensing in CDAD. Ramoplanin demonstrates excellent in vitro activity against *C difficile*, including strains resistant to metronidazole and with intermediate resistance to vancomycin [118,119]. Daptomycin and telavancin also show good activity against *C difficile* [120–122] as also do linezolid and the newer oxazolidinones, which are at present in different research phases [123–125].

Nitazoxanide, a nitrothiazolic compound with antimicrobial activity against *C difficile* comparable to that of metronidazole and vancomycin, has shown very good results in experimental animal models infected with *C difficile* [126,127].

Until recently, the activity of vancomycin and metronidazole, both first-line drugs for the therapy of CDAD, was not questioned and susceptibility testing was not even recommended. However, resistance to metronidazole, present in some equine isolates, was reported in 1997 [128]. Reviewing antimicrobial susceptibility profiles of 415 clinical *C difficile* isolates obtained during an 8-year period, the authors found a resistance rate to metronidazole (minimal inhibiting concentration >16 micrograms/mL) of 6.3%. The authors did not find any strains with full resistance to vancomycin, although strains with intermediate resistance amounted to 3.1%. Resistance was more frequent in isolates from HIV patients and clonal dissemination could not be proved among the isolates with decreased susceptibilities to the antimicrobials tested in any of the cases [62]. The authors believe that resistance to metronidazole is heterogeneous and can be lost in strains after a prolonged period of storage (due to freezing and defrosting) [129]. The authors do not know the clinical interpretation of this resistance and its influence in the poor response to metronidazole or in recurrent disease.

Antimicrobial treatment of CDAD

The first step in the treatment of patients with CDAD is to withdraw antimicrobials whenever possible. Up to 25% of CDAD episodes may resolve with this simple measure [70,130,131]. The therapeutic response usually involves the resolution of fever on the first day and of diarrhea on the fourth or fifth day. It is not feasible to predict which subset of patients will respond to the withdrawal of antibiotics. On the other hand, for hospitalized patients who are especially ill, it is hardly possible to stop antimicrobial therapy altogether. Thus, this is not a common practice in the health care setting. Patients for whom antimicrobial therapy cannot be discontinued are less likely to overcome diarrhea when treated with metronidazole [132].

The second step is the administration of either metronidazole or vancomycin, first-line drugs for the treatment of CDAD. Oral metronidazole (500 mg thrice daily or 250 mg four times per day) and oral vancomycin (125 mg every 6 h) have similar efficacy, with response rates near 90% to 97%, according to commonly cited reports [131,133,134]. However, in the last few years, response rates have changed in some hospitals in certain geographic areas [135]. The normal duration of therapy is 10 to 14 days, although no well-performed studies have established the possible advantage of shortening or lengthening this course. Some investigators advocate longer therapy (14 days) to avoid recurrence. All antimicrobials should be administered orally because C difficile is in the lumen of the colon. If the intravenous route is required, only metronidazole is effective, as intravenous vancomycin achieves only low concentrations in the colon lumen [136]. The therapeutic response usually involves the resolution of fever and of diarrhea on the fourth or fifth day [136].

In patients who are not critically ill, metronidazole is preferred to vancomycin because of metronidazole's lower cost and because it minimizes the risk of selecting vancomycin-resistant enterococci. The indications for oral vancomycin are pregnancy, breast-feeding, metronidazole intolerance, or therapeutic failure of metronidazole after 3 to 5 days of treatment.

In a Cochrane analysis that included nine prospective and comparative studies in patients with CDAD, metronidazole, bacitracin, teicoplanin, fusidic acid, and rifaximin were each as effective as vancomycin for initial symptomatic resolution [137].

Most infections by C difficile respond to either treatment with vancomycin or metronidazole, and the lack of therapeutic response requires the confirmation of the diagnosis and the exclusion of ileitis or toxic megacolon, as these conditions may prevent the drugs from reaching sufficiently high levels in the colon lumen. Patients with ileitis may benefit from increasing the transport of the antibiotic to the colon lumen by using high doses of oral vancomycin (500 mg four times per day) or by the instillation of vancomycin or metronidazole in the colon lumen by means of enemas.

Other drugs to be used

Bacitracin was used in the treatment of CDAD in the 1980s. However, since then, vancomycin has been preferred because persistence of toxins in the stools is higher in patients on bacitracin than for those on vancomycin. Nevertheless, the rate of recurrence in patients treated with bacitracin is not higher than that in patients on vancomycin [138–140].

Teicoplanin is an alternative to vancomycin though with no clear benefit and with the disadvantage of not being available at present in the United States [133,141,142]. Fusidic acid is associated with more recurrences, is worse tolerated by patients when compared with vancomycin [133], and shows similar results when compared with metronidazole [143].

Nitazoxanide, an antihelminthic and antiprotozoal agent with activity against a broad range of parasites, also shows in vitro activity against *C difficile* [126,127,144,145]. After its oral administration, nitazoxanide reaches high concentrations in the lumen of the colon. It has achieved cure rates of 75% in patients who failed metronidazole treatment. However, relapse occurs in one out of three patients. In a recently published prospective, randomized, double-blind study, nitazoxanide (500 mg two times per day) was compared with metronidazole (250 mg four times per day) for 10 days in treating hospitalized patients with *C difficile* colitis. The study found that nitazoxanide was at least as effective as metronidazole in treating *C difficile* colitis [134,146,147].

Tiacumicins B and C are members of a novel group of 18 macrolide antibiotics with in vitro activity against *C difficile*. The in vivo activities of the tiacumicins were favorably compared with that of vancomycin in a hamster model of antibiotic-associated colitis [148,149].

Rifaximin is a synthetic antibiotic derived from rifamycin to achieve low gastrointestinal absorption while retaining good antibacterial activity. It has a broad spectrum of antibacterial action, including action against aerobic and anaerobic gram-positive and gram-negative microorganisms. Potential indications include *C difficile* infections [117,149–151].

Nonantimicrobial treatment

Antimotility agents (eg, loperamide) are not indicated, since they impair response and increase the risk of toxic megacolon [152,153].

Intravenous immunoglobulins have been used in patients with severe disease or multiple recurrences, but no prospective and comparative studies establish their role in the treatment of this disease [154–156]. In spite of this, the administration of 200 to 500 mg/kg, in one or more doses, has been used in patients with refractory disease as an adjuvant therapy to conventional treatment.

A hyperimmune bovine gammaglobuline that neutralizes the effects of *C difficile* toxins has been studied, but it only prevents the disease in rodents [157–159]. The feasibility of 40% immune whey protein concentrate (immune WPC-40) to aid in the prevention of relapse of *C difficile* diarrhea has also been evaluated. Immune WPC-40 was made from milk after immunization of Holstein-Frisian cows with *C difficile*-inactivated toxins and killed whole-cell *C difficile*. Immune WPC-40 contained a high concentration of specific sIgA antibodies and was effective in neutralizing the cytotoxic effect of *C difficile* toxins in cell assays in vitro [160–162]. WPC-40 was administered to 11 patients who failed treatment or had a history of relapsing *C difficile* after a 14-day treatment course. All patients were cured and none of them suffered another episode of diarrhea. The potential use of monoclonal antibodies has also been evaluated [163].

Colestipol, colestyramine and other exchange resins able to bind to *C difficile* toxin, may also bind to antimicrobials used to treat CDAD. Therefore, their clinical use is not recommended [164–167]. Nothing can be established from studies in which patients have received corticosteroids as part of the treatment for CDAD [168].

Data regarding the role of oligofructose in the prevention of CDAD relapses are still conflicting [169,170]. In a study performed by Lewis et al [169], consecutive inpatients with CDAD were randomly assigned to receive oligofructose or placebo for 30 days, in addition to specific antibiotic treatment. Relapses were more common in those taking placebo. The oligosaccharide is well tolerated and increases fecal bifidobacterial concentrations [170].

Another promising line of research explores the use of synthetic oligosaccharide sequences that are attached to an inert support and are able to bind to toxin A in the lumen of the colon. One of them is Synsorb 90, which can effectively neutralize toxin-A activity from stool samples [171]. Tolevamer (GT160-246), a polyanionic polymer chain with a high molecular weight, has been evaluated in vitro and in animal models. These evaluations show that tolevamer neutralizes the activity of *C difficile* toxin A [172,173].

Tolevamer has already been administered to humans [174,175] both for the treatment of a first episode as well as for the treatment of recurrent disease. In a recently published multicenter, double-blind, study, patients with CDAD were randomized to receive 3 g of tolevamer per day (n = 97), 6 g of tolevamer per day (n = 95), or 500 mg of vancomycin per day (n = 97). Tolevamer administered at a dosage of 6 g per day was found to be no less effective than vancomycin with regard to time-to-resolution of diarrhea and was associated with a trend toward a lower recurrence rate [176]. A second international study is taking place.

Surgery is a last resort for the treatment of unmanageable CDAD with toxic megacolon or colon perforations. Fulminant *C difficile* colitis can result in bowel perforation and peritonitis with a high mortality rate. The indications for surgery are systemic toxicity and peritonitis, radiological and clinical evidence of progressive toxic colonic dilatation, and progressive colonic dilatation with bowel perforation. The most frequent surgical techniques are either hemicolectomy or total colectomy. In both cases, the postoperative mortality may be > 30% [177,178]. Very occasionally, colonic surgery may complicate with *C difficile* enteritis [179–182].

Treatment of relapsing episodes

One of the main complications of CDAD is recurrence, which is described in 8% to 50% of cases [11,131,139,141,183–192]. Recurrences are multiple in a significant percentage of the patients. Risk factors for recurrence are (1) advanced age, (2) remaining on antimicrobial therapy after a first CDAD episode, (3) low albumin levels, (4) a long hospital stay, (5) admittance to an intensive care unit, and (6) a severe underlying disease [72,187,193–195]. It is essential to know whether the relapse is a result of a reactivation of the disease by a previous clon or if it is due to the acquisition of a new clon. Different typing techniques have shown that 10% to 50% of recurrences are caused by a new strain ("re-infections") [196–199]. In a series of HIV patients with CDAD, a third of the recurrences were reinfections [184].

One of the major explanations for recurrences is the patient's inability to produce a good immune response [70,72,73]. The risk of recurrence is similar for patients on metronidazole or on vancomycin [183,200]. Recurrence appears 3 to 21 days (mean: 6 days) after completion of therapy. Most patients with a relapse respond to another 10-day course of therapy with the same antimicrobial agent but 3% to 5% of patients may have up to five subsequent relapses [201].

In patients with a poor response or with a third relapse, both the patient and the patient's family require a therapeutic alternative [202]. An option is to keep on using the same agent, though on a different dosage or with a longer duration. Some protocols recommend a double dose of vancomycin for 10 days; others prolong the administration of vancomycin for 3 weeks; and still others follow a decreasing dosage scheme on vancomycin 500 mg daily during the first week, 250 mg daily during the second week, 125 mg daily during the third week, followed by 125 mg every 3 days for 21 days [202]. There are no reports on prolonged or intermittent use of metronidazole.

A different approach is the use of a different drug or the use of nonanti-microbial agents. Bacitracin, fusidic acid, teicoplanin, and rifampin have been used mostly for the treatment of first episodes of CDAD and their use has been mentioned.

A meta-analysis from six randomized trials showed that probiotics had significant efficacy for CDAD (relative risk = 0.59, 95% CI 0.41, 0.85, $P = .005$) [203]. Two randomized studies of patients with CDAD recurrences evaluated intestinal recolonization with *Saccharomyces boulardii* [200,204]. In one of them, *S. boulardii* was administered for 4 weeks after treatment with vancomycin (2 g daily) for 10 days. Recurrences decreased but only when van-comycin was administered at such a high dose [204]. The efficacy of *S boulardii* to decrease recurrences has been shown in several studies [64,200]. This probi-otic has been widely prescribed because it is inexpensive and many believe it has no risks. The authors' group has recently published a study on one of its complications, fungemia by *Saccharomyces*, that may present as small epi-demic outbreaks, particularly in intensive care unit patients with intravascular catheters [205].

Following studies of several small groups of patients, some investigators reported that the administration of *Lactobacillus rhamnosus* or *Lactobacillus plantarum* stopped recurrences [206,207]. However, in two prospective and comparative studies with this probiotic and placebo, recurrences did not decrease [208,209].

Local bacteriotherapy is the name for the lavage of the lumen of the colon or for the administration of enemas prepared with fresh feces from healthy volunteers [210–213]. Related reports almost always concern isolated cases or short series. No relevant study supports recommendations on this method, which has obvious drawbacks, including the additional risk of transmitting other infectious agents.

Characteristics of aggressive recent epidemic outbreaks

In 1998, Ya Nair et al [187] reported a series of 8 out of 36 patients (22%) on metronidazole who did not have a good response to the treatment, and 7 patients had a relapse within 2 months. In 2004, Noren et al [196] found a 25% recurrence rate in patients on metronidazole in Sweden.

The most severe recent event has been the emergence of a new epidemic *C difficile* strain in Canada and the United States. In 2004, Pépin et al reported a spectacular rise in especially virulent CDAD cases, with a high fatality rate in a hospital in Quebec [214]. They reviewed the progression of CDAD in the period from January 1991 through December 2003. Incidence increased from 35.6 per 100,000 population in 1991 to 156.3 per 100,000 population in 2003. In the subgroup of patients aged 65 years or more, the increase was from 102.0 to 866.5 per 100,000 inhabitants. The percentage of complicated cases rose from 7.1% (12:169) in 1991 and 1992 to 18.2% (71:390) in 2003 ($P < .001$), and the proportion of patients who died within 30 days after the CDAD episode rose from 4.7% (8:169) in 1991 and 1992 to 13.8% (54:390) in 2003 ($P < .001$). The investigators, after adjusting for age and other confounding factors, suggest that the evolution was worse in patients on metronidazole [214]. Pépin et al also published a second study [193] in which failure rates (poor response or relapse) dramatically increased in patients on metronidazole during the period from 2003 to 2004. Among the patients initially treated with metronidazole, the proportion of those who had to switch to vancomycin or for whom vancomycin was added because of a disappointing response was steady between 1991 and 2002 (9.6%), though it rose to 25.7% from 2003 to 2004 ($P < .001$). The rate of poor outcome (failure plus recurrence) increased from 20.8% to 47.2% ($P < .001$) and was particularly dramatic in patients over 65 years old (58.4%). This was also the case in other hospitals in the area and has raised a great concern, leading Canadian health authorities to include *C difficile* and its related illnesses in the group of compulsory communicable diseases [215–219].

In a later study, the same Canadian group [220] showed that metronidazole was as effective as vancomycin for the treatment of patients with a first recurrence of CDAD, yet the risk of complications with any treatment of CDAD may be higher than has previously been documented.

The same findings have been reported in the United States. In a prospective observational study of 207 patients who developed CDAD in a Houston, Texas, hospital and who were treated with metronidazole, only 103 (50%) were cured by the initial course of therapy, 46 (22%) presented with a therapeutic failure with persistence of symptoms despite treatment for more than 10 days, and 58 (28%) responded initially but had a recurrence within the ensuing 90 days. Mortality in patients with CDAD reached 27% and was higher among those with a poor response during the initial course of therapy (33% versus 21%; $P < .05$) [221].

The epidemic in Quebec was caused by a particular clone (toxinotype III, North American PFGE type 1/PCR, ribotype 27 (NAP1/027)) that is a hyperproducer of toxins A and B. This same strain was found in several states of the United States, in the United Kingdom, in the Netherlands, in Belgium, and in France [135,221,222].

Neither the Canadian nor the American research reported the systematic isolation of *C difficile* strains. Thus, susceptibility testing to metronidazole or genotyping of isolates on a large scale has not been possible.

The present epidemic strain is a toxin hyperproducer, shows an increased resistance to fluoroquinolones, and is responsible for the outbreaks at more than seven American hospitals in different states from 2001 to 2004 [6,7,135,223–225]. This same strain was the one that caused the Quebec outbreak [215,219] and an additional outbreak in England [226].

Preliminary results from a study of *C difficile* strains isolated during a 2-month period in 2005 from 38 hospitals of 14 European countries were presented in 2006 at the European Congress of Clinical Microbiology and Infectious Diseases meeting in Nice, France [227]. Barbut et al found that 25 out of 486 isolates collected in Europe were toxinotype III, and 20 of those belonged to ribotype 27. All of these were isolated in Belgium and the Netherlands, but for one that was recovered in Ireland. The polymerase chain reaction ribotype 027, toxinotype III strain has a characteristic antimicrobial susceptibility pattern, since it is resistant to the newer fluoroquinolones (moxifloxacin) and to erythromycin, but susceptible to clindamycin.

References

[1] Barbut F, Petit JC. Epidemiology of Clostridium difficile-associated infections. Clin Microbiol Infect 2001;7(8):405–10.
[2] Bouza E, Muñoz P, Alonso R. Clinical manifestations, treatment and control of infections caused by Clostridium difficile. Clin Microbiol Infect 2005;11(Suppl 4):57–64.
[3] Quirk M. Clostridium difficile epidemic strain far reaching. Lancet Infect Dis 2006;6(2):74.
[4] Musher DM, Logan N, Mehendiratta V. Epidemic Clostridium difficile. N Engl J Med 2006;354(11):1199–203 [author reply 203].
[5] Beaulieu M, Thirion DJ, Williamson D, et al. Clostridium difficile-associated diarrhea outbreaks: the name of the game is isolation and cleaning. Clin Infect Dis 2006;42(5):725 [author reply 7–9].

[6] McDonald LC. Clostridium difficile: responding to a new threat from an old enemy. Infect Control Hosp Epidemiol 2005;26(8):672–5.

[7] Muto CA, Pokrywka M, Shutt K, et al. A large outbreak of Clostridium difficile-associated disease with an unexpected proportion of deaths and colectomies at a teaching hospital following increased fluoroquinolone use. Infect Control Hosp Epidemiol 2005;26(3):273–80.

[8] Bartlett JG, Perl TM. The new Clostridium difficile—what does it mean? N Engl J Med 2005;353(23):2503–5 [Epub December 1, 2005].

[9] Loo VG, Poirier L, Miller MA, et al. A predominantly clonal multi-institutional outbreak of Clostridium difficile-associated diarrhea with high morbidity and mortality. N Engl J Med 2005;353(23):2442–9 [Epub December 1, 2005].

[10] Lai KK, Melvin ZS, Menard MJ, et al. Clostridium difficile-associated diarrhea: epidemiology, risk factors, and infection control. Infect Control Hosp Epidemiol 1997;18(9):628–32.

[11] Olson MM, Shanholtzer CJ, Lee JT Jr, et al. Ten years of prospective Clostridium difficile-associated disease surveillance and treatment at the Minneapolis VA Medical Center, 1982–1991. Infect Control Hosp Epidemiol 1994;15(6):371–81.

[12] Macgowan AP, Brown I, Feeney R, et al. Clostridium difficile-associated diarrhoea and length of hospital stay. J Hosp Infect 1995;31(3):241–4.

[13] Riley TV, Codde JP, Rouse IL. Increased length of hospital stay due to Clostridium difficile associated diarrhoea. Lancet 1995;345(8947):455–6.

[14] Wilcox MH, Cunniffe JG, Trundle C, et al. Financial burden of hospital-acquired Clostridium difficile infection. J Hosp Infect 1996;34(1):23–30.

[15] Kofsky P, Rosen L, Reed J, et al. Clostridium difficile—a common and costly colitis. Dis Colon Rectum 1991;34(3):244–8.

[16] Cato EP, George WL, Finegold SM. Genus Clostridium Prazmowski. In: Sneath PHA, Mair NS, Sharpe ES, et al, editors. Bergey's manual of systematic bacteriology, vol. 2. Baltimore: Williams and Wilkins; 1986. p. 1141–2000.

[17] Brazier JS. The diagnosis of Clostridium difficile-associated disease. J Antimicrob Chemother 1998;41(Suppl C):29–40.

[18] Barroso LA, Wang SZ, Phelps CJ, et al. Nucleotide sequence of Clostridium difficile toxin B gene. Nucleic Acids Res 1990;18(13):4004.

[19] Dove CH, Wang SZ, Price SB, et al. Molecular characterization of the Clostridium difficile toxin A gene. Infect Immun 1990;58(2):480–8.

[20] Hammond GA, Johnson JL. The toxigenic element of Clostridium difficile strain VPI 10463. Microb Pathog 1995;19(4):203–13.

[21] Borriello SP, Davies HA, Kamiya S, et al. Virulence factors of Clostridium difficile. Rev Infect Dis 1990;12(Suppl 2):S185–91.

[22] Lyerly DM, Saum KE, MacDonald DK, et al. Effects of Clostridium difficile toxins given intragastrically to animals. Infect Immun 1985;47(2):349–52.

[23] Lyerly DM, Barroso LA, Wilkins TD, et al. Characterization of a toxin A-negative, toxin B-positive strain of Clostridium difficile. Infect Immun 1992;60(11):4633–9.

[24] Martirosian G, Szczesny A, Cohen SH, et al. Analysis of Clostridium difficile-associated diarrhea among patients hospitalized in tertiary care academic hospital. Diagn Microbiol Infect Dis 2005;52(2):153–5.

[25] Barth H, Aktories K, Popoff MR, et al. Binary bacterial toxins: biochemistry, biology, and applications of common Clostridium and Bacillus proteins. Microbiol Mol Biol Rev 2004; 68(3):373–402 [table of contents].

[26] McEllistrem MC, Carman RJ, Gerding DN, et al. A hospital outbreak of Clostridium difficile disease associated with isolates carrying binary toxin genes. Clin Infect Dis 2005;40(2): 265–72 [Epub December 15, 2004].

[27] Barbut F, Decre D, Lalande V, et al. Clinical features of Clostridium difficile-associated diarrhoea due to binary toxin (actin-specific ADP-ribosyltransferase)-producing strains. J Med Microbiol 2005;54(Pt 2):181–5.

[28] Terhes G, Urban E, Soki J, et al. Community-acquired Clostridium difficile diarrhea caused by binary toxin, toxin A, and toxin B gene-positive isolates in Hungary. J Clin Microbiol 2004;42(9):4316–8.

[29] Goncalves C, Decre D, Barbut F, et al. Prevalence and characterization of a binary toxin (actin-specific ADP-ribosyltransferase) from Clostridium difficile. J Clin Microbiol 2004; 42(5):1933–9.

[30] Alonso R, Martin A, Pelaez T, et al. Toxigenic status of Clostridium difficile in a large Spanish teaching hospital. J Med Microbiol 2005;54(Pt 2):159–62.

[31] Geric B, Rupnik M, Gerding DN, et al. Distribution of Clostridium difficile variant toxino-types and strains with binary toxin genes among clinical isolates in an American hospital. J Med Microbiol 2004;53(Pt 9):887–94.

[32] Hurley BW, Nguyen CC. The spectrum of pseudomembranous enterocolitis and anti-biotic-associated diarrhea. Arch Intern Med 2002;162:2177–84.

[33] Ozaki E, Kato H, Kita H, et al. Clostridium difficile colonization in healthy adults: transient colonization and correlation with enterococcal colonization. J Med Microbiol 2004; 53(Pt 2):167–72.

[34] Kelly CP, LaMont JT. Clostridium difficile infection. Annu Rev Med 1998;49:375–90.

[35] Gopal Rao G, Mahankali Rao CS, Starke I. Clostridium difficile-associated diarrhoea in patients with community-acquired lower respiratory infection being treated with levoflox-acin compared with beta-lactam-based therapy. J Antimicrob Chemother 2003;51(3): 697–701.

[36] Hirschhorn LR, Trnka Y, Onderdonk A, et al. Epidemiology of community-acquired Clos-tridium difficile-associated diarrhea. J Infect Dis 1994;169(1):127–33.

[37] Kyne L, Merry C, O'Connell B, et al. Community-acquired Clostridium difficile infection. J Infect 1998;36(3):287–8.

[38] Riley TV, Cooper M, Bell B, et al. Community-acquired Clostridium difficile-associated diarrhea. Clin Infect Dis 1995;20(Suppl 2):S263–5.

[39] Bartlett JG. Leukocytosis and Clostridium difficile-associated diarrhea. Am J Gastroenterol 2000;95(11):3023–4.

[40] Bulusu M, Narayan S, Shetler K, et al. Leukocytosis as a harbinger and surrogate marker of Clostridium difficile infection in hospitalized patients with diarrhea. Am J Gastroenterol 2000;95(11):3137–41.

[41] Marinella MA, Burdette SD, Bedimo R, et al. Leukemoid reactions complicating colitis due to Clostridium difficile. South Med J 2004;97(10):959–63.

[42] Garcia-Lechuz JM, Hernangomez S, Juan RS, et al. Extra-intestinal infections caused by Clostridium difficile. Clin Microbiol Infect 2001;7(8):453–7.

[43] Simpson AJ, Das SS, Tabaqchali S. Nosocomial empyema caused by Clostridium difficile. J Clin Pathol 1996;49(2):172–3.

[44] Watt B. Extra-intestinal Clostridium difficile. Microbiol Sci 1987;4(11):337.

[45] Bartlett JG. Clinical practice. Antibiotic-associated diarrhea. N Engl J Med 2002;346(5): 334–9.

[46] Johnson S, Gerding DN. Clostridium difficile–associated diarrhea. Clin Infect Dis 1998; 26(5):1027–34 [quiz 35–6].

[47] Lusk RH, Fekety R, Silva J, et al. Clindamycin-induced enterocolitis in hamsters. J Infect Dis 1978;137(4):464–75.

[48] Johnson S, Samore MH, Farrow KA, et al. Epidemics of diarrhea caused by a clindamycin-resistant strain of Clostridium difficile in four hospitals. N Engl J Med 1999;341(22):1645–51.

[49] Gaynes R, Rimland D, Killum E, et al. Outbreak of Clostridium difficile infection in a long-term care facility: association with gatifloxacin use. Clin Infect Dis 2004;38(5):640–5 [Epub February 11, 2004].

[50] Gerding DN. Clindamycin, cephalosporins, fluoroquinolones, and Clostridium difficile-associated diarrhea: this is an antimicrobial resistance problem. Clin Infect Dis 2004; 38(5):646–8 [Epub February 11, 2004].

[51] Moshkowitz M, Ben Baruch E, Kline Z, et al. Clinical manifestations and outcome of Pseudomembranous colitis in an elderly population in Israel. Isr Med Assoc J 2004;6(4):201–4.

[52] Simor AE, Bradley SF, Strausbaugh LJ, et al. Clostridium difficile in long-term-care facilities for the elderly. Infect Control Hosp Epidemiol 2002;23(11):696–703.

[53] Brandt LJ, Kosche KA, Greenwald DA, et al. Clostridium difficile-associated diarrhea in the elderly. Am J Gastroenterol 1999;94(11):3263–6.

[54] Simor AE, Yake SL, Tsimidis K. Infection due to Clostridium difficile among elderly residents of a long-term-care facility. Clin Infect Dis 1993;17(4):672–8.

[55] Wongwanich S, Ramsiri S, Kusum M, et al. Clostridium difficile infections in HIV-positive patients. Southeast Asian J Trop Med Public Health 2000;31(3):537–9.

[56] Anastasi JK, Capili B. HIV and diarrhea in the era of HAART: 1998 New York State hospitalizations. Am J Infect Control 2000;28(3):262–6.

[57] Barbut F, Meynard JL, Guiguet M, et al. Clostridium difficile-associated diarrhea in HIV-infected patients: epidemiology and risk factors. J Acquir Immune Defic Syndr Hum Retrovirol 1997;16(3):176–81.

[58] Cozart JC, Kalangi SS, Clench MH, et al. Clostridium difficile diarrhea in patients with AIDS versus non-AIDS controls. Methods of treatment and clinical response to treatment. J Clin Gastroenterol 1993;16(3):192–4.

[59] Saddi VR, Glatt AE. Clostridium difficile-associated diarrhea in patients with HIV: a 4-year survey. J Acquir Immune Defic Syndr 2002;31(5):542–3.

[60] Pulvirenti JJ, Gerding DN, Nathan C, et al. Difference in the incidence of Clostridium difficile among patients infected with human immunodeficiency virus admitted to a public hospital and a private hospital. Infect Control Hosp Epidemiol 2002;23(11):641–7.

[61] Pulvirenti JJ, Mehra T, Hafiz I, et al. Epidemiology and outcome of Clostridium difficile infection and diarrhea in HIV infected inpatients. Diagn Microbiol Infect Dis 2002;44(4):325–30.

[62] Pelaez T, Alcala L, Alonso R, et al. Reassessment of Clostridium difficile susceptibility to metronidazole and vancomycin. Antimicrob Agents Chemother 2002;46(6):1647–50.

[63] Tacconelli E, Tumbarello M, de Gaetano Donati K, et al. Clostridium difficile-associated diarrhea in human immunodeficiency virus infection—a changing scenario. Clin Infect Dis 1999;28(4):936–7.

[64] Altiparmak MR, Trablus S, Pamuk ON, et al. Diarrhoea following renal transplantation. Clin Transplant 2002;16(3):212–6.

[65] Munoz P, Palomo J, Yanez J, et al. Clinical microbiological case: a heart transplant recipient with diarrhea and abdominal pain. Recurring C. difficile infection. Clin Microbiol Infect 2001;7(8):451–2, 8–9.

[66] Avery R, Pohlman B, Adal K, et al. High prevalence of diarrhea but infrequency of documented Clostridium difficile in autologous peripheral blood progenitor cell transplant recipients. Bone Marrow Transplant 2000;25(1):67–9.

[67] West M, Pirenne J, Chavers B, et al. Clostridium difficile colitis after kidney and kidney–pancreas transplantation. Clin Transplant 1999;13(4):318–23.

[68] Keven K, Basu A, Re L, et al. Clostridium difficile colitis in patients after kidney and pancreas–kidney transplantation. Transpl Infect Dis 2004;6(1):10–4.

[69] Mulligan ME, Miller SD, McFarland LV, et al. Elevated levels of serum immunoglobulins in asymptomatic carriers of Clostridium difficile. Clin Infect Dis 1993;16(Suppl 4):S239–44.

[70] Kyne L, Warny M, Qamar A, et al. Asymptomatic carriage of Clostridium difficile and serum levels of IgG antibody against toxin A. N Engl J Med 2000;342(6):390–7.

[71] Shim JK, Johnson S, Samore MH, et al. Primary symptomless colonisation by Clostridium difficile and decreased risk of subsequent diarrhoea. Lancet 1998;351(9103):633–6 [see comments].

[72] Kyne L, Warny M, Qamar A, et al. Association between antibody response to toxin A and protection against recurrent Clostridium difficile diarrhoea. Lancet 2001;357(9251):189–93.

[73] Warny M, Vaerman JP, Avesani V, et al. Human antibody response to Clostridium difficile toxin A in relation to clinical course of infection. Infect Immun 1994;62(2):384–9.

[74] Snell H, Ramos M, Longo S, et al. Performance of the TechLab C. DIFF CHEK-60 enzyme immunoassay (EIA) in combination with the C. difficile Tox A/B II EIA kit, the Triage C. difficile panel immunoassay, and a cytotoxin assay for diagnosis of Clostridium difficile-associated diarrhea. J Clin Microbiol 2004;42(10):4863–5.

[75] Alfa MJ, Swan B, VanDekerkhove B, et al. The diagnosis of Clostridium difficile-associated diarrhea: comparison of Triage C. difficile panel, EIA for Tox A/B and cytotoxin assays. Diagn Microbiol Infect Dis 2002;43(4):257–63.

[76] Lozniewski A, Rabaud C, Dotto E, et al. Laboratory diagnosis of Clostridium difficile-associated diarrhea and colitis: usefulness of Premier Cytoclone A + B enzyme immunoassay for combined detection of stool toxins and toxigenic C. difficile strains. J Clin Microbiol 2001;39(5):1996–8.

[77] Fekety R. Guidelines for the diagnosis and management of Clostridium difficile-associated diarrhea and colitis. American College of Gastroenterology, Practice Parameters Committee. Am J Gastroenterol 1997;92(5):739–50.

[78] Silletti RP, Lee G, Ailey E. Role of stool screening tests in diagnosis of inflammatory bacterial enteritis and in selection of specimens likely to yield invasive enteric pathogens. J Clin Microbiol 1996;34(5):1161–5.

[79] Peterson LR, Kelly PJ, Nordbrock HA. Role of culture and toxin detection in laboratory testing for diagnosis of Clostridium difficile-associated diarrhea. Eur J Clin Microbiol Infect Dis 1996;15(4):330–6.

[80] Mohan SS, McDermott BP, Parchuri S, et al. Lack of value of repeat stool testing for Clostridium difficile toxin. Am J Med 2006;119(4):356 [e7–8].

[81] Borek AP, Aird DZ, Carroll KC. Frequency of sample submission for optimal utilization of the cell culture cytotoxicity assay for detection of Clostridium difficile toxin. J Clin Microbiol 2005;43(6):2994–5.

[82] Thelestam M, Bronnegard M. Interaction of cytopathogenic toxin from Clostridium difficile with cells in tissue culture. Scand J Infect Dis Suppl 1980;(Suppl 22):16–29.

[83] Chang TW, Lauermann M, Barlett JG. Cytotoxicity assay in antibiotic-associated colitis. J Infect Dis 1979;140:765–70.

[84] Laughon BE, Viscidi RP, Gdovin SL, et al. Enzyme immunoassays for detection of Clostridium difficile toxins A and B in fecal specimens. J Infect Dis 1984;149(5):781–8.

[85] Jacobs J, Rudensky B, Dresner J, et al. Comparison of four laboratory tests for diagnosis of Clostridium difficile-associated diarrhea. Eur J Clin Microbiol Infect Dis 1996;15(7):561–6.

[86] Johnson S, Kent SA, O'Leary KJ, et al. Fatal pseudomembranous colitis associated with a variant clostridium difficile strain not detected by toxin A immunoassay. Ann Intern Med 2001;135(6):434–8.

[87] Wren B, Clayton C, Tabaqchali S. Rapid identification of toxigenic Clostridium difficile by polymerase chain reaction. Lancet 1990;335(8686):423.

[88] Kato H, Kato N, Watanabe K, et al. Identification of toxin A-negative, toxin B-positive Clostridium difficile by PCR. J Clin Microbiol 1998;36(8):2178–82.

[89] Alonso R, Munoz C, Pelaez T, et al. Rapid detection of toxigenic Clostridium difficile strains by a nested PCR of the toxin B gene. Clin Microbiol Infect 1997;3(1):145–7.

[90] Alonso R, Munoz C, Gros S, et al. Rapid detection of toxigenic Clostridium difficile from stool samples by a nested PCR of toxin B gene. J Hosp Infect 1999;41(2):145–9.

[91] Guerrant RL. Practise guidelines for the management of infectious diarrhea. Clin Infect Dis 2001;32:331–51.

[92] Gerding DN, Johnson S, Peterson LR, et al. Clostridium difficile-associated diarrhea and colitis. Infect Control Hosp Epidemiol 1995;16(8):459–77.

[93] Hafiz S, Oakley CL. Clostridium difficile: isolation and characteristics. J Med Microbiol 1976;9(2):129–36.

[94] George WL, Sutter VL, Citron D, et al. Selective and differential medium for isolation of Clostridium difficile. J Clin Microbiol 1979;9(2):214–9.

[95] Bouza E, Pelaez T, Alonso R, et al. "Second-look" cytotoxicity: an evaluation of culture plus cytotoxin assay of Clostridium difficile isolates in the laboratory diagnosis of CDAD. J Hosp Infect 2001;48(3):233–7.

[96] Delmee M, Van Broeck J, Simon A, et al. Laboratory diagnosis of Clostridium difficile-associated diarrhoea: a plea for culture. J Med Microbiol 2005;54(Pt 2):187–91.

[97] Ash L, Baker ME, O'Malley CM Jr, et al. Colonic abnormalities on CT in adult hospitalized patients with Clostridium difficile colitis: prevalence and significance of findings. AJR Am J Roentgenol 2006;186(5):1393–400.

[98] Baverud V, Gunnarsson A, Karlsson M, et al. Antimicrobial susceptibility of equine and environmental isolates of Clostridium difficile. Microb Drug Resist 2004;10(1):57–63.

[99] Jamal WY, Mokaddas EM, Verghese TL, et al. In vitro activity of 15 antimicrobial agents against clinical isolates of Clostridium difficile in Kuwait. Int J Antimicrob Agents 2002; 20(4):270.

[100] Goldstein EJ, Citron DM, Merriam CV, et al. Comparative in vitro activities of ertapenem (MK-0826) against 469 less frequently identified anaerobes isolated from human infections. Antimicrob Agents Chemother 2002;46(4):1136–40.

[101] Wexler HM, Molitoris E, Molitoris D, et al. In vitro activity of telithromycin (HMR 3647) against 502 strains of anaerobic bacteria. J Antimicrob Chemother 2001;47(4): 467–9.

[102] Livermore DM, Carter MW, Bagel S, et al. In vitro activities of ertapenem (MK-0826) against recent clinical bacteria collected in Europe and Australia. Antimicrob Agents Chemother 2001;45(6):1860–7.

[103] Barbut F, Decré D, Burghoffer B, et al. Antimicrobial susceptibilities and serogroups of clinical strains of Clostridium difficile isolated in France in 1991 and 1997. Antimicrob Agents Chemother 1999;43(11):2607–11.

[104] Wust J, Hardegger U. Studies on the resistance of Clostridium difficile to antimicrobial agents. Zentralbl Bakteriol Mikrobiol Hyg [A] 1988;267(3):383–94.

[105] Wexler H, Carter WT, Harris BH, et al. In vitro activity of cefbuperazone against anaerobic bacteria. Antimicrob Agents Chemother 1985;27(4):674–6.

[106] Jones RN. Review of the in vitro spectrum of activity of imipenem. Am J Med 1985;78(6A): 22–32.

[107] Liebetrau A, Rodloff AC, Behra-Miellet J, et al. In vitro activities of a new des-fluoro(6) quinolone, garenoxacin, against clinical anaerobic bacteria. Antimicrob Agents Chemother 2003;47(11):3667–71.

[108] Alonso R, Pelaez T, Gonzalez-Abad MJ, et al. In vitro activity of new quinolones against Clostridium difficile. J Antimicrob Chemother 2001;47(2):195–7.

[109] Ackermann G, Tang YJ, Rodloff AC, et al. In vitro activity of sitafloxacin against Clostridium difficile. J Antimicrob Chemother 2001;47(5):722–4.

[110] Wilcox MH, Fawley W, Freeman J, et al. In vitro activity of new generation fluoroquinolones against genotypically distinct and indistinguishable Clostridium difficile isolates. J Antimicrob Chemother 2000;46(4):551–6.

[111] Hoogkamp-Korstanje JA, Roelofs-Willemse J. Comparative in vitro activity of moxifloxacin against gram-positive clinical isolates. J Antimicrob Chemother 2000;45(1):31–9.

[112] Fung-Tomc J, Minassian B, Kolek B, et al. In vitro antibacterial spectrum of a new broad-spectrum 8-methoxy fluoroquinolone, gatifloxacin. J Antimicrob Chemother 2000;45(4): 437–46.

[113] Goldstein EJ, Citron DM, Warren Y, et al. In vitro activity of gemifloxacin (SB 265805) against anaerobes. Antimicrob Agents Chemother 1999;43(9):2231–5.

[114] Goldstein EJ, Citron DM, Vreni Merriam C, et al. Activities of gemifloxacin (SB 265805, LB20304) compared to those of other oral antimicrobial agents against unusual anaerobes. Antimicrob Agents Chemother 1999;43(11):2726–30.

[115] Nord CE. In vitro activity of quinolones and other antimicrobial agents against anaerobic bacteria. Clin Infect Dis 1996;23(Suppl 1):S15–8.

[116] Marks SL, Kather EJ. Antimicrobial susceptibilities of canine Clostridium difficile and Clostridium perfringens isolates to commonly utilized antimicrobial drugs. Vet Microbiol 2003;94(1):39–45.

[117] Marchese A, Salerno A, Pesce A, et al. In vitro activity of rifaximin, metronidazole and vancomycin against Clostridium difficile and the rate of selection of spontaneously resistant mutants against representative anaerobic and aerobic bacteria, including ammonia-producing species. Chemotherapy 2000;46(4):253–66.

[118] Farver DK, Hedge DD, Lee SC. Ramoplanin: a lipoglycodepsipeptide antibiotic. Ann Pharmacother 2005;39(5):863–8 [Epub March 22, 2005].

[119] Pelaez T, Alcala L, Alonso R, et al. In vitro activity of ramoplanin against Clostridium difficile, including strains with reduced susceptibility to vancomycin or with resistance to metronidazole. Antimicrob Agents Chemother 2005;49(3):1157–9.

[120] Goldstein EJ, Citron DM, Merriam CV, et al. In vitro activities of daptomycin, vancomycin, quinupristin–dalfopristin, linezolid, and five other antimicrobials against 307 gram-positive anaerobic and 31 Corynebacterium clinical isolates. Antimicrob Agents Chemother 2003;47(1):337–41.

[121] Chow AW, Cheng N. In vitro activities of daptomycin (LY146032) and paldimycin (U-70,138F) against anaerobic gram-positive bacteria. Antimicrob Agents Chemother 1988;32(5):788–90.

[122] Goldstein EJ, Citron DM, Merriam CV, et al. In vitro activities of the new semisynthetic glycopeptide telavancin (TD-6424), vancomycin, daptomycin, linezolid, and four comparator agents against anaerobic gram-positive species and Corynebacterium spp. Antimicrob Agents Chemother 2004;48(6):2149–52.

[123] Pelaez T, Alonso R, Perez C, et al. In vitro activity of linezolid against Clostridium difficile. Antimicrob Agents Chemother 2002;46(5):1617–8.

[124] Phillips OA, Rotimi VO, Jamal WY, et al. Comparative in vitro activity of PH-027 versus linezolid and other anti-anaerobic antimicrobials against clinical isolates of Clostridium difficile and other anaerobic bacteria. J Chemother 2003;15(2):113–7.

[125] Ackermann G, Adler D, Rodloff AC. In vitro activity of linezolid against Clostridium difficile. J Antimicrob Chemother 2003;51(3):743–5.

[126] McVay CS, Rolfe RD. In vitro and in vivo activities of nitazoxanide against Clostridium difficile. Antimicrob Agents Chemother 2000;44(9):2254–8.

[127] Dubreuil L, Houcke I, Mouton Y, et al. In vitro evaluation of activities of nitazoxanide and tizoxanide against anaerobes and aerobic organisms. Antimicrob Agents Chemother 1996; 40(10):2266–70.

[128] Jang SS, Hansen LM, Breher JE, et al. Antimicrobial susceptibilities of equine isolates of Clostridium difficile and molecular characterization of metronidazole-resistant strains. Clin Infect Dis 1997;25(Suppl 2):S266–7.

[129] Peláez T, Cercenado E, Alcalá L, et al. Heterogeneous resistance to metronidazole in Clostridium difficile isolates from patients with Clostridium difficile associated-diarrhoea. 44th Interscience Conference on Antimicrobial Agents and Chemotherapy. Washington (DC): American Society for Microbiology; 2004.

[130] Olson MM, Shanholtzer CJ, Lee JT Jr, et al. Ten years of prospective Clostridium difficile-associated disease surveillance and treatment at the Minneapolis VA Medical Center, 1982–1991. Infect Control Hosp Epidemiol 1994;15(6):371–81 [see comments].

[131] Teasley DG, Gerding DN, Olson MM, et al. Prospective randomised trial of metronidazole versus vancomycin for Clostridium-difficile-associated diarrhoea and colitis. Lancet 1983; 2(8358):1043–6.

[132] Modena S, Gollamudi S, Friedenberg F. Continuation of antibiotics is associated with failure of metronidazole for Clostridium difficile-associated diarrhea. J Clin Gastroenterol 2006;40(1):49–54.

[133] Wenisch C, Parschalk B, Hasenhundl M, et al. Comparison of vancomycin, teicoplanin, metronidazole, and fusidic acid for the treatment of Clostridium difficile-associated diarrhea. Clin Infect Dis 1996;22(5):813–8.

[134] Bartlett JG. New drugs for Clostridium difficile infection. Clin Infect Dis 2006;43(4):428–31 [Epub July 11, 2006].

[135] Gerding DN. Metronidazole for Clostridium difficile-associated disease: is it okay for mom? Clin Infect Dis 2005;40(11):1598–600 [Epub April 25, 2005].

[136] Fekety R, Shah AB. Diagnosis and treatment of Clostridium difficile colitis. JAMA 1993; 269(1):71–5.

[137] Bricker E, Garg R, Nelson R, et al. Antibiotic treatment for Clostridium difficile-associated diarrhea in adults. Cochrane Database Syst Rev 2005;(1):CD004610.

[138] Young GP, Ward PB, Bayley N, et al. Antibiotic-associated colitis due to Clostridium difficile: double-blind comparison of vancomycin with bacitracin. Gastroenterology 1985; 89(5):1038–45.

[139] Dudley MN, McLaughlin JC, Carrington G, et al. Oral bacitracin vs vancomycin therapy for Clostridium difficile-induced diarrhea. A randomized double-blind trial. Arch Intern Med 1986;146(6):1101–4.

[140] Chang TW, Gorbach SL, Bartlett JG, et al. Bacitracin treatment of antibiotic-associated colitis and diarrhea caused by Clostridium difficile toxin. Gastroenterology 1980;78(6): 1584–6.

[141] de Lalla F, Nicolin R, Rinaldi E, et al. Prospective study of oral teicoplanin versus oral vancomycin for therapy of pseudomembranous colitis and Clostridium difficile-associated diarrhea. Antimicrob Agents Chemother 1992;36(10):2192–6.

[142] de Lalla F, Privitera G, Rinaldi E, et al. Treatment of Clostridium difficile-associated disease with teicoplanin. Antimicrob Agents Chemother 1989;33(7):1125–7.

[143] Wullt M, Odenholt I. A double-blind randomized controlled trial of fusidic acid and metronidazole for treatment of an initial episode of Clostridium difficile-associated diarrhoea. J Antimicrob Chemother 2004;54(1):211–6 [Epub May 26, 2004].

[144] Arya SC. Nitazoxanide as a broad-spectrum antiparasitic agent. J Infect Dis 2002;185(11): 1692.

[145] Cohen SA. Use of nitazoxanide as a new therapeutic option for persistent diarrhea: a pediatric perspective. Curr Med Res Opin 2005;21(7):999–1004.

[146] Musher DM, Logan N, Hamill RJ, et al. Nitazoxanide for the treatment of Clostridium difficile colitis. Clin Infect Dis 2006;43(4):421–7 [Epub July 11, 2006].

[147] Aslam S, Hamill RJ, Musher DM. Treatment of Clostridium difficile-associated disease: old therapies and new strategies. Lancet Infect Dis 2005;5(9):549–57.

[148] Swanson RN, Hardy DJ, Shipkowitz NL, et al. In vitro and in vivo evaluation of tiacumicins B and C against Clostridium difficile. Antimicrob Agents Chemother 1991;35(6):1108–11.

[149] Louie T, Emery J, Krulicky W, et al. PAR-101 is selectively efective against C. difficile in vivo and has minimal effect on the anaerobic fecal flora (Poster LB2–30). In: Microbiology ASf, editor. Proceedings of the 45th Interscience Conference on Antimicrobial Agents and Chemotherapy; Washington (DC): American Society for Microbiology; 2005.

[150] Scarpignato C, Pelosini I. Rifaximin, a poorly absorbed antibiotic: pharmacology and clinical potential. Chemotherapy 2005;51(Suppl 1):36–66.

[151] Ripa S, Mignini F, Prenna M, et al. In vitro antibacterial activity of rifaximin against Clostridium difficile, Campylobacter jejunii and Yersinia spp. Drugs Exp Clin Res 1987;13(8): 483–8.

[152] Trudel JL, Deschenes M, Mayrand S, et al. Toxic megacolon complicating pseudomembranous enterocolitis. Dis Colon Rectum 1995;38(10):1033–8.

[153] Elinav E, Planer D, Gatt ME. Prolonged ileus as a sole manifestation of pseudomembranous enterocolitis. Int J Colorectal Dis 2004;19(3):273–6 [Epub November 15, 2003].

[154] Salcedo J, Keates S, Pothoulakis C, et al. Intravenous immunoglobulin therapy for severe Clostridium difficile colitis. Gut 1997;41(3):366–70.

[155] Wilcox MH. Descriptive study of intravenous immunoglobulin for the treatment of recurrent Clostridium difficile diarrhoea. J Antimicrob Chemother 2004;53(5):882–4 [Epub April 8, 2004].

[156] McPherson S, Rees CJ, Ellis R, et al. Intravenous immunoglobulin for the treatment of severe, refractory, and recurrent Clostridium difficile diarrhea. Dis Colon Rectum 2006;49(5): 640–5.

[157] Kelly CP, Pothoulakis C, Vavva F, et al. Anti-Clostridium difficile bovine immunoglobulin concentrate inhibits cytotoxicity and enterotoxicity of C. difficile toxins. Antimicrob Agents Chemother 1996;40(2):373–9.

[158] Lyerly DM, Bostwick EF, Binion SB, et al. Passive immunization of hamsters against disease caused by Clostridium difficile by use of bovine immunoglobulin G concentrate. Infect Immun 1991;59(6):2215–8.

[159] Kelly CP, Pothoulakis C, Vavva F, et al. Anti-Clostridium difficile bovine immunoglobulin concentrate inhibits cytotoxicity and enterotoxicity of C. difficile toxins. Antimicrob Agents Chemother 1996;40(2):373–9.

[160] van Dissel JT, de Groot N, Hensgens CM, et al. Bovine antibody-enriched whey to aid in the prevention of a relapse of Clostridium difficile-associated diarrhoea: preclinical and preliminary clinical data. J Med Microbiol 2005;54(Pt 2):197–205.

[161] Warny M, Fatimi A, Bostwick EF, et al. Bovine immunoglobulin concentrate-clostridium difficile retains C difficile toxin neutralising activity after passage through the human stomach and small intestine. Gut 1999;44(2):212–7.

[162] Kelly CP, Chetham S, Keates S, et al. Survival of anti-Clostridium difficile bovine immunoglobulin concentrate in the human gastrointestinal tract. Antimicrob Agents Chemother 1997;41(2):236–41.

[163] Banerjee S, Lamont JT. Non-antibiotic therapy for Clostridium difficile infection. Curr Opin Infect Dis 2000;13(3):215–9.

[164] Bartlett JG, Chang TW, Gurwith M, et al. Antibiotic-associated pseudomembranous colitis due to toxin-producing clostridia. N Engl J Med 1978;298:531–4.

[165] Mogg GA, Arabi Y, Youngs D, et al. Therapeutic trials of antibiotic associated colitis. Scand J Infect Dis Suppl 1980;(Suppl 22):41–5.

[166] Mogg GA, George RH, Youngs D, et al. Randomized controlled trial of colestipol in antibiotic-associated colitis. Br J Surg 1982;69(3):137–9.

[167] Taylor NS, Bartlett JG. Binding of Clostridium difficile cytotoxin and vancomycin by anion-exchange resins. J Infect Dis 1980;141(1):92–7.

[168] Cavagnaro C, Berezin S, Medow MS. Corticosteroid treatment of severe, non-responsive Clostridium difficile induced colitis. Arch Dis Child 2003;88(4):342–4.

[169] Lewis S, Burmeister S, Brazier J. Effect of the prebiotic oligofructose on relapse of Clostridium difficile-associated diarrhea: a randomized controlled study. Clin Gastroenterol Hepatol 2005;3(5):442–8.

[170] Lewis S, Burmeister S, Cohen S, et al. Failure of dietary oligofructose to prevent antibiotic-associated diarrhoea. Aliment Pharmacol Ther 2005;21(4):469–77.

[171] Heerze LD, Kelm MA, Talbot JA, et al. Oligosaccharide sequences attached to an inert support (SYNSORB) as potential therapy for antibiotic-associated diarrhea and pseudomembranous colitis. J Infect Dis 1994;169(6):1291–6.

[172] Kurtz CB, Cannon EP, Brezzani A, et al. GT160–246, a toxin binding polymer for treatment of Clostridium difficile colitis. Antimicrob Agents Chemother 2001;45(8):2340–7.

[173] Braunlin W, Xu Q, Hook P, et al. Toxin binding of tolevamer, a polyanionic drug that protects against antibiotic-associated diarrhea. Biophys J 2004;87(1):534–9.

[174] Davidson D, Peppe J, Louie T. A phase 2 study of the toxin binding polymer tolevamer in patients with Clostridium difficile associated diarrhea. First International Clostridium difficile Symposium. Kranjska Gora, Slovenia, May 5–8, 2004.

[175] Davidson D, Peppe J, Louie T., et al. Aphase 2 study of the toxin binding polymer tolevamer in patients with Clostridium difficile associated diarrhea (Abstract P-548). Program

and abstracts of the 14th European Congress of Clinical Microbiology and Infectious Diseases. Prague, Czech Republic, 2004.

[176] Louie TJ, Peppe J, Watt CK, et al. Tolevamer, a novel nonantibiotic polymer, compared with vancomycin in the treatment of mild to moderately severe Clostridium difficile-associated diarrhea. Clin Infect Dis 2006;43(4):411–20 [Epub July 11, 2006].

[177] Koss K, Clark MA, Sanders DS, et al. The outcome of surgery in fulminant Clostridium difficile colitis. Colorectal Dis 2006;8(2):149–54.

[178] Longo WE, Mazuski JE, Virgo KS, et al. Outcome after colectomy for Clostridium difficile colitis. Dis Colon Rectum 2004;47(10):1620–6.

[179] Tjandra JJ, Street A, Thomas RJ, et al. Fatal Clostridium difficile infection of the small bowel after complex colorectal surgery. ANZ J Surg 2001;71(8):500–3.

[180] Duracher C, Mohammedi I, Robert D. Clostridium difficile small intestinal involvement occurring after total colectomy. Ann Fr Anesth Reanim 2002;21(10):826–7.

[181] Freiler JF, Durning SJ, Ender PT. Clostridium difficile small bowel enteritis occurring after total colectomy. Clin Infect Dis 2001;33(8):1429–31 [discussion 32].

[182] Vesoulis Z, Williams G, Matthews B. Pseudomembranous enteritis after proctocolectomy: report of a case. Dis Colon Rectum 2000;43(4):551–4.

[183] Mylonakis E, Ryan ET, Calderwood SB. Clostridium difficile–associated diarrhea: a review. Arch Intern Med 2001;161(4):525–33.

[184] Alonso R, Gros S, Pelaez T, et al. Molecular analysis of relapse vs re-infection in HIV-positive patients suffering from recurrent Clostridium difficile associated diarrhoea. J Hosp Infect 2001;48(2):86–92.

[185] Wilcox MH, Fawley WN, Settle CD, et al. Recurrence of symptoms in Clostridium difficile infection—relapse or reinfection? J Hosp Infect 1998;38(2):93–100.

[186] Bartlett JG. Treatment of antibiotic-associated pseudomembranous colitis. Rev Infect Dis 1984;6(Suppl 1):S235–41.

[187] Nair S, Yadav D, Corpuz M, et al. Clostridium difficile colitis: factors influencing treatment failure and relapse—a prospective evaluation. Am J Gastroenterol 1998;93(10):1873–6.

[188] Silva J Jr, Batts DH, Fekety R, et al. Treatment of Clostridium difficile colitis and diarrhea with vancomycin. Am J Med 1981;71(5):815–22.

[189] Joyce AM, Burns DL. Recurrent Clostridium difficile colitis. Compr Ther 2004;30(3):160–3.

[190] Aas J, Gessert CE, Bakken JS. Recurrent Clostridium difficile colitis: case series involving 18 patients treated with donor stool administered via a nasogastric tube. Clin Infect Dis 2003;36(5):580–5 [Epub February 14, 2003].

[191] Joyce AM, Burns DL. Recurrent Clostridium difficile colitis. Tackling a tenacious nosocomial infection. Postgrad Med 2002;112(5):53–4, 7–8, 65 passim.

[192] Kyne L, Kelly CP. Recurrent Clostridium difficile diarrhoea. Gut 2001;49(1):152–3.

[193] Pepin J, Alary ME, Valiquette L, et al. Increasing risk of relapse after treatment of Clostridium difficile colitis in Quebec, Canada. Clin Infect Dis 2005;40(11):1591–7 [Epub April 25, 2005].

[194] Fernandez A, Anand G, Friedenberg F. Factors associated with failure of metronidazole in Clostridium difficile-associated disease. J Clin Gastroenterol 2004;38(5):414–8.

[195] Modena S, Bearelly D, Swartz K, et al. Clostridium difficile among hospitalized patients receiving antibiotics: a case-control study. Infect Control Hosp Epidemiol 2005;26(8): 685–90.

[196] Noren T, Akerlund T, Back E, et al. Molecular epidemiology of hospital-associated and community-acquired Clostridium difficile infection in a Swedish county. J Clin Microbiol 2004;42(8):3635–43.

[197] Johnson S, Adelmann A, Clabots CR, et al. Recurrences of Clostridium difficile diarrhea not caused by the original infecting organism. J Infect Dis 1989;159(2):340–3.

[198] Tang-Feldman Y, Mayo S, Silva J Jr, et al. Molecular analysis of Clostridium difficile strains isolated from 18 cases of recurrent clostridium difficile-associated diarrhea. J Clin Microbiol 2003;41(7):3413–4.

[199] Alonso R, Martin A, Pelaez T, et al. An improved protocol for pulsed-field gel electropho-resis typing of Clostridium difficile. J Med Microbiol 2005;54(Pt 2):155–7.

[200] McFarland LV, Surawicz CM, Greenberg RN, et al. A randomized placebo-controlled trial of Saccharomyces boulardii in combination with standard antibiotics for Clostridium dif-ficile disease. JAMA 1994;271(24):1913–8.

[201] McFarland LV, Surawicz CM, Rubin M, et al. Recurrent Clostridium difficile disease: epidemiology and clinical characteristics. Infect Control Hosp Epidemiol 1999;20(1): 43–50.

[202] McFarland LV. Alternative treatments for Clostridium difficile disease: what really works? J Med Microbiol 2005;54(Pt 2):101–11.

[203] McFarland LV. Meta-analysis of probiotics for the prevention of antibiotic associated diarrhea and the treatment of Clostridium difficile disease. Am J Gastroenterol 2006; 101(4):812–22.

[204] Surawicz CM, McFarland LV, Greenberg RN, et al. The search for a better treatment for recurrent Clostridium difficile disease: use of high-dose vancomycin combined with Saccha-romyces boulardii. Clin Infect Dis 2000;31(4):1012–7.

[205] Munoz P, Bouza E, Cuenca-Estrella M, et al. Saccharomyces cerevisiae fungemia: an emerging infectious disease. Clin Infect Dis 2005;40(11):1625–34 [Epub April 25, 2005].

[206] Gorbach SL, Chang TW, Goldin B. Successful treatment of relapsing Clostridium difficile colitis with Lactobacillus GG. Lancet 1987;2(8574):1519.

[207] Biller JA, Katz AJ, Flores AF, et al. Treatment of recurrent Clostridium difficile colitis with Lactobacillus GG. J Pediatr Gastroenterol Nutr 1995;21(2):224–6.

[208] Pochapin M. The effect of probiotics on Clostridium difficile diarrhea. Am J Gastroenterol 2000;95(1 Suppl):S11–3.

[209] Wullt M, Hagslatt ML, Odenholt I. Lactobacillus plantarum 299v for the treatment of re-current Clostridium difficile-associated diarrhoea: a double-blind, placebo-controlled trial. Scand J Infect Dis 2003;35(6–7):365–7.

[210] Schwan A, Sjolin S, Trottestam U, et al. Relapsing Clostridium difficile enterocolitis cured by rectal infusion of normal faeces. Scand J Infect Dis 1984;16(2):211–5.

[211] Tvede M, Rask-Madsen J. Bacteriotherapy for chronic relapsing Clostridium difficile diar-rhoea in six patients. Lancet 1989;1(8648):1156–60.

[212] Persky SE, Brandt LJ. Treatment of recurrent Clostridium difficile-associated diarrhea by administration of donated stool directly through a colonoscope. Am J Gastroenterol 2000; 95(11):3283–5.

[213] Borody TJ, Warren EF, Leis SM, et al. Bacteriotherapy using fecal flora: toying with hu-man motions. J Clin Gastroenterol 2004;38(6):475–83.

[214] Pepin J, Valiquette L, Alary ME, et al. Clostridium difficile-associated diarrhea in a region of Quebec from 1991 to 2003: a changing pattern of disease severity. CMAJ 2004;171(5): 466–72.

[215] Eggertson L. C. difficile: by the numbers. CMAJ 2004;171(11):1331–2 [Epub November 2, 2004].

[216] Pindera L. Quebec to report on Clostridium difficile in 2005. CMAJ 2004;171(7):715.

[217] Eggertson L. C. difficile hits Sherbrooke, Que., hospital: 100 deaths. CMAJ 2004;171(5): 436.

[218] Eggertson L. Quebec strikes committee on Clostridium difficile. CMAJ 2004;171(2):123.

[219] Eggertson L, Sibbald B. Hospitals battling outbreaks of C. difficile. CMAJ 2004;171(1): 19–21.

[220] Pepin J, Routhier S, Gagnon S, et al. Management and outcomes of a first recurrence of Clostridium difficile-associated disease in Quebec, Canada. Clin Infect Dis 2006;42(6): 758–64 [Epub February 7, 2006].

[221] Musher DM, Aslam S, Logan N, et al. Relatively poor outcome after treatment of Clostrid-ium difficile colitis with metronidazole. Clin Infect Dis 2005;40(11):1586–90 [Epub April 25, 2005].

[222] Sougioultzis S, Kyne L, Drudy D, et al. Clostridium difficile toxoid vaccine in recurrent C. difficile-associated diarrhea. Gastroenterology 2005;128(3):764–70.

[223] McDonald LC, Killgore GE, Thompson A, et al. Emergence of an epidemic strain of Clostridium difficile in the United States, 2001–4: potential role for virulence factors and antimicobial resistance strains (abstract LB-2). 42nd Annual Meeting of the Infectious Disease Society of America, Boston. Alexandria (VA): Infectious Disease Society of America; 2004. p. 58.

[224] Warny M, Pepin J, Fang A, et al. Increased toxins A and B production in an emerging strain of Clostridium difficile. 15th Annual Scientific Meeting of the Society for Healthcare Epidemiology of America. Los Angeles, April 9–12, 2005.

[225] Eggertson L. C. difficile strain 20 times more virulent. CMAJ 2005;172(10):1279.

[226] Ross E. British authorities probe hospital superbug. New York: ABC News; 2005. Available at: http://www.wjla.com/headlines/0605/234194.html. Accessed September 28, 2006.

[227] Barbut F, Mastrantonio P, Delmée M, et al. European prospective study of Clostridium difficile strrains: phenotypic and genotypic characterization of the isolates from different clinical status: interim results. Program and abstracts of the 16th European Congress of Clinical Microbiology and Infectious Diseases. Nice (France), April 1–4, 2006.

ELSEVIER
SAUNDERS

THE MEDICAL
CLINICS
OF NORTH AMERICA

Med Clin N Am 90 (2006) 1165–1182

Antimicrobial Therapy of Multidrug-Resistant *Streptococcus pneumoniae*, Vancomycin-Resistant Enterococci, and Methicillin-Resistant *Staphylococcus aureus*

Burke A. Cunha, MD[a,b,*]

[a]*State University of New York School of Medicine, Stony Brook, NY, USA*
[b]*Infectious Disease Division, Winthrop-University Hospital, Mineola, NY 11501, USA*

Antibiotic resistance is natural and intrinsic or it is acquired. Intrinsic or natural resistance refers to the inactivity of an antibiotic beyond its usual spectrum of activity (eg, clindamycin has no activity naturally and intrinsically against aerobic gram-negative bacilli). Acquired resistance is limited to relatively few gram-positive and gram-negative organisms. It is uncommon in anaerobic organisms, atypical pulmonary pathogens, *Rickettsiae*, and so on. Among the gram-positive organisms, acquired resistance to some antibiotics has been widespread with *Streptococcus pneumoniae* (eg, macrolides). Vancomycin has increased the prevalence of *Enterococcus faecium*, that is, of vancomycin-resistant enterococci (VRE). Increasing resistance has appeared in methicillin-resistant *Staphylococcus aureus* (MRSA) [1–6].

Acquired resistance may be relative, manifested by an increase in minimal inhibitory concentrations (MICs), particularly in micro-organisms that have three breakpoints. Most organisms have a sensitive resistant breakpoint, but some organisms, such as *S pneumoniae*, have three breakpoints, namely sensitive, intermediate, and resistant. Intermediate resistance may be grouped with the sensitive or the resistant organisms, resulting in great variability among the resistance rates reported in studies. For example, if an administered antibiotic is active against an intermediate

* Infectious Disease Division, Winthrop-University Hospital, 222 Station Plaza North, Suite 432, Mineola, NY 11501.

0025-7125/06/$ - see front matter © 2006 Elsevier Inc. All rights reserved.
doi:10.1016/j.mcna.2006.07.007
medical.theclinics.com

strain of *S pneumoniae*, and the antibiotic achieves therapeutic concentrations in serum/tissue in excess of the intermediate breakpoint, then such organisms should be considered "sensitive" rather than "resistant." Therefore, in organisms that are in the resistant range, resistance may be viewed as being moderate or high. Moderately resistant strains have MICs that are achievable with the commonly used doses of antibiotics against the organism. Highly resistant strains may require antibiotics from a different class [7–10].

Acquired antibiotic resistance

Resistance is not a generalized phenomenon but is limited to relatively few organisms. For example, among streptococci, resistance to penicillin is of concern with *S pneumoniae* but not with others (ie, group A, group B, group C, nonenterococcal group D, and group G streptococci). Acquired resistance may be the result of widespread dissemination of a resistant clone that has occurred because of point mutation. In surveys of antibiotic resistance, the practitioner should be careful to differentiate between an increase in acquired resistance secondary to antibiotic use and an increase in apparent antibiotic resistance secondary to the dissemination of a resistant clone [3,7,8,10].

It is a popular misconception that antibiotic resistance is related to the volume or duration of antimicrobial use and that acquired resistance is inevitable. Although resistance has increased over the past several decades, the problem of acquired antibiotic resistance is not generally related to antibiotic overuse in terms of volume or antibiotic tonnage—that is, there has been no appreciable increase in *S pneumoniae* resistance to doxycycline after decades of extensive worldwide use [11–13]. Doxycycline also illustrates another point. Despite concern about rare strains of *S pneumoniae* highly resistant to doxycycline, doxycycline retains its activity against the other common respiratory pathogens, namely *Hemophilus influenzae* and *Moraxella catarrhalis*, as well as the atypical pulmonary pathogens causing respiratory tract infections [14,15]. Doxycycline has retained its usefulness against the zoonotic pathogens, which have also been implicated in bioterrorist attacks. It retains its activity against all these pathogens without the development of appreciable resistance [16,17].

The antibiotic resistance that occurs with most organisms and antibiotics is acquired resistance. Some antibiotics, such as macrolides, encounter both intrinsic and acquired resistance when used against certain organisms (ie, *S pneumoniae*) [9,11,12]. Approximately 30% of strains of *S pneumoniae* are naturally or intrinsically resistant to macrolides. Intrinsic resistance is not a function of volume of use, but acquired macrolide resistance is a function of volume of use. Therefore, extensive macrolide use results in resistance that is additive. That is, the combined effect of a background of natural resistance superimposed on the component of acquired resistance related to use results in very high levels of macrolide-resistant *S pneumoniae* (MRSP) (ie, approximately 40%) [18–23].

For reasons that are unclear, resistance is largely limited to certain members of various antibiotic classes and is usually relegated to one or two organisms. For example, trimethoprim sulfamethoxazole (TMP-SMX) use is associated with an increase in penicillin-resistant *S pneumoniae* (PRSP) as well as in MRSP. However, the activity of TMP-SMX against strains of methicillin-sensitive *S aureus* (MSSA) remains good. With conventional tetracycline, there has been an increase in resistance in MSSA, but other members of the class (ie, doxycycline and minocycline) maintain their anti-MSSA activity [12,13]. At the present time, doxycycline is even active against community-acquired MRSA (CA-MRSA), and minocycline is highly active against strains of hospital-acquired MRSA (HA-MRSA) [20].

In vitro antibiotic susceptibility and in vivo effectiveness

For the clinician, there are interpretation problems with antimicrobial susceptibility reports. With certain antibiotic organism combinations, a discrepancy may exist between in vitro and in vivo activity. Certain antibiotics may be reported as "sensitive" in vitro to certain organisms, but the drugs are, in fact, ineffective in vivo in clinical experience. All streptococci are reported as being sensitive in vitro to aminoglycosides, but in fact they are all intrinsically resistant to aminoglycosides when used alone. When an aminoglycoside is combined with penicillin, for example, the combination has antienterococcal activity against most strains of *E faecalis*, namely vancomycin-sensitive enterococci (VSE). Discrepancy between in vivo and in vitro sensitivity testing is also a practical problem in treating HA-MRSA. Strains of HA-MRSA are often reported as being "sensitive" in vitro to a wide variety of antibiotics, which usually does not correlate with in vivo effectiveness. In treating MRSA infections, it is prudent to disregard susceptibility testing and select a drug for empiric therapy with proven clinical effectiveness against HA-MRSA (ie, vancomycin, quinupristin-dalfopristin, minocycline, linezolid, daptomycin, tigecycline) [20,23,24].

Interestingly, strains of CA-MRSA resemble MSSA in susceptibility testing as well as in their clinical expression. CA-MRSA strains without the Panton-Valentine leukocidin gene cause the same spectrum of disease as does MSSA. Strains of CA-MSSA (SCC$_{mec}$ IV) are sensitive to antibiotics that are not effective in treating HA-MRSA (ie, clindamycin, TMP-SMX, doxycycline). Clinicians should know when to rely on in vitro susceptibility testing to guide therapy and when to rely on clinical experience [20,25].

Prolonged or extensive use of an antibiotic does not, per se, result in an increase in resistance. The example of doxycycline has been given in regard to respiratory pathogens, but the same may be said of first-, second-, and third-generation cephalosporins in regard to *S pneumoniae*. With prerespiratory quinolones, *S pneumoniae* resistance was a problem. But, after decades of intensive worldwide use of ceftriaxone, there has been no increase in resistance in *S pneumoniae* [11–13]. Among enterococci, ampicillin remains highly active. The same is true for vancomycin, considering its volume of use. The increase in VRE has resulted in but was not caused by widespread vancomycin usage. Enterococci are part of the normal fecal flora. Approximately 95% of fecal enterococci are of the *E faecalis* variety. Because virtually all strains of *E faecalis* are sensitive to vancomycin, *E faecalis* is essentially synonymous with VSE. When vancomycin is given, the VSE component of the fecal flora is diminished. The naturally or intrinsically resistant *E faecium* strains (ie, VRE) then become the predominant part of the fecal flora. As a result, VRE have become more prevalent but not more resistant per se [5,6]. This is a good example of how increased antibiotic use may have an indirect effect on antibiotic resistance, not by increasing acquired resistance but by permitting the emergence of an uncommon organism in the fecal flora, which is given a selective advantage as vancomycin increases its numbers. For this and other reasons, VRE has emerged as a highly resistant gram-positive pathogen without becoming more resistant to vancomycin [26–29].

Because antibiotic resistance is complex, clinicians should become familiar with the nuances of resistance terminology and the factors that affect resistance. Clinicians should also be familiar with differentiation between colonization and infection, because colonization is ordinarily not treated, whereas infection is. Furthermore, clinicians should be familiar with the differences between vitro sensitivity testing and in vivo effectiveness, so that effective empiric therapy may be selected when treatment of resistant organisms is necessary [9,11–13,20,30].

Antibiotic-resistant *Streptococcus pneumoniae*

Because *S pneumoniae* is the most important bacterial pathogen in upper and lower respiratory tract infections, there is concern about increased antibiotic resistance in *S pneumoniae*. "Penicillin resistance," particularly of the intermediate variety, has limited clinical significance [8]. As mentioned earlier, when β-lactams are given in the usual dose appropriate for the anatomic location of the respiratory tract infection due to *S pneumoniae*, these strains are, in fact, responsive and clinically susceptible to β-lactam antibiotics. Overuse of β-lactam antibiotics per se has not resulted in an increase in *S pneumoniae* resistance [9,11–13]. An increase in the MICs (ie, "MIC drift") has occurred with some β-lactams, but the achievable blood/tissue levels of β-lactams in non–central nervous system infections are sufficiently high that these strains are easily eliminated [7,8,10].

Because β-lactam antibiotics obey time-dependent kinetics, any concentration in excess of the MIC will eliminate the organism if the concentration is maintained for about three quarters of the dosing interval. Pharmacokinetic and pharmacodynamic information readily explains this phenomenon. The breakpoints for penicillin for *S pneumoniae* are as follows: less than 1 μg/mL is sensitive, between 1–2 μg/mL is intermediate, and 2 μg/mL or greater is reported. With intermediate or even resistant strains, with MICs of 6–10 μg/mL, empiric therapy with ceftriaxone, for example, provides serum levels far in excess of 6 μg/mL (ie, after a 1-g intravenous dose, achievable serum levels are approximately 150 μg/mL). Even when one uses oral antimicrobial therapy for infections except those of the central nervous system (CNS), concentrations in sinus fluid, middle ear fluid, bronchial fluid, and lung parenchyma are readily achieved with usual full doses of orally administered β-lactams. The only therapeutic concern regarding PRSP involves the treatment of CNS infections. Even in CNS infections, as long as therapeutic concentrations are achieved in the cerebrospinal fluid, PRSP meningitis is not a major therapeutic problem [20,31,32].

Acquired resistance to "high-resistance-potential" antibiotics is related to volume of antibiotic use. Overuse of TMP-SMX and macrolides for the treatment of respiratory tract infections has led to problems with PRSP and MRSP worldwide. TMP-SMX predisposes to PRSP and MRSP as well as to multidrug-resistant *S pneumoniae* (MDRSP). The use of TMP-SMX should be avoided when possible in respiratory tract infections. TMP-SMX does not predispose to resistance in other organisms and continues to be useful in nonpneumococcal infections (ie, aerobic gram-negative bacillary infections, MSSA). Overuse of macrolides in particular has resulted in the emergence of MDRSP because of the macrolide-induced PRSP and MRSP. Like TMP-SMX, macrolides should be avoided if possible in the treatment of respiratory tract infections [9–12,18–23]. Other antibiotics with the appropriate spectrum and a "low resistance potential" should be used preferentially. "Macrolide-sparing" antibiotics include doxycycline, telithromycin, and respiratory quinolones [11,13,20]. Telithromycin and the respiratory quinolones are effective against PRSP, MRSP, and MDRSP [33–39]. From an antibiotic resistance perspective, it is preferable to use antibiotics with a "low resistance potential," such as doxycycline, telithromycin, and respiratory quinolones, to treat respiratory tract infections. Using these agents preferentially both treats and prevents further pneumococcal resistance (Table 1) [7–9,11–13].

Vancomycin-resistant enterococci

VSE and VRE are part of the normal fecal flora. The relative proportions of VSE and VRE may be modified by antimicrobial therapy or prolonged hospitalization. As part of the normal fecal flora, enterococci commonly

Table 1
Clinical comparison of *Streptococcus pneumoniae* antibiotics

	Usual adult dose	Side effects	Advantages	Disadvantages
PRSP/MRSP	Amoxicillin 1 g (PO) q 8 h	Drug fever/rash	Inexpensive Well tolerated Excellent bioavailability (90%)	No IV formulation Inactive against atypical respiratory pathogens
	Doxycycline 100–200 mg (IV/PO) q 12 h	Nausea/vomiting (if taken without food)	Low resistance potential Excellent bioavailability (93%) IV/PO formulation Active against typical and atypical respiratory pathogens	None
	Ceftriaxone 1 g (IV) q 24 h	Non–*C difficile* diarrhea Drug fever/rash	Low resistance potential After 1 g (IV) serum concentrations ~150 µg/mL exceed MICs of even highly resistant strains (MICs 6–10 µg/mL) May be given IM (with lidocaine)	No PO formulation Inactive against atypical respiratory pathogens
MDRSP	Levofloxacin 750 mg (IV/PO) q 24 h	Nausea/vomiting/diarrhea ↑ QTc	Low resistance potential IV/PO formulation Excellent bioavailability (99%) Active against typical and atypical respiratory pathogens	None
	Moxifloxacin 400 mg (IV/PO) q 24 h	Nausea/vomiting/diarrhea ↑ QTc	Low resistance potential IV/PO formulation Excellent bioavailability (90%) Active against typical and atypical respiratory pathogens	None

Drug/dose	Side effects	Comments	Notes
Gatifloxacin 400 mg (IV/PO) q 24 h	Nausea/vomiting/diarrhea ↑ QTc	Low resistance potential IV/PO formulation Excellent bioavailability (96%) Active against typical and atypical respiratory pathogens	Avoid in diabetics
Gemifloxacin 320 mg (PO) q 24 h	Nausea/vomiting/diarrhea ↑ QTc	Low resistance potential Good bioavailability (71%) Active against typical and atypical respiratory pathogens	No IV formulation
Telithromycin 800 mg (PO) q 24 h	Nausea/vomiting/diarrhea ↑ QTc	Low resistance potential Good bioavailability (57%) Active against typical and atypical respiratory pathogens	No IV formulation
Tigecycline 100 mg (IV) × 1 dose, then 50 mg (IV) q 24 h	Nausea/vomiting/diarrhea ↑ QTc	Low resistance potential	No PO formulation
Ertapenem 1 g (IV) q 24 h	None	Low resistance potential Once daily dosing May be given IM (with lidocaine)	No PO formulation Inactive against atypical pathogens
Meropenem 500 mg (IV) q 8 h	None	Low resistance potential	No PO formulation

Abbreviations: IM, intramuscular; IV, intravenous; PO, oral.
Adapted from Cunha BA. Antibiotic essentials. 5th edition. Royal Oak (MI): Physicians' Press; 2006.

colonize the perirectal area as well as the skin of the lower extremities. Enterococci are not highly invasive organisms, and colonization represents the majority of strains isolated in the hospital setting. In general, infections, not colonization, should be treated with antimicrobial therapy. Because of the proximity to the rectum, enterococci commonly colonize wounds of the abdomen, lower extremities, and urine. Enterococci may occasionally contaminate the blood culture contaminants in blood samples drawn from the antecubital fossa. In patients whose skin below the waist is colonized with enterococci and who are turning in bed, it is easy to understand how the antecubital fossa could be colonized with enterococci and contaminate blood cultures during venipuncture [5,6].

Enterococci should be viewed as permissive pathogens, capable of causing infection in selected situations. Enterococci are common single pathogens in biliary tract and urinary tract infections. They are uncommon causes of intravenous-line infection. Enterococci also cause bacterial endocarditis. They are the most common organisms associated with bacterial endocarditis with the focus of infection below the waist (ie, the gastrointestinal or the genitourinary tract). Enterococci are not important pulmonary or neuropathogens. They may be pathogens in complicated skin and soft tissue infections below the waist. Enterococci alone are incapable of intra-abdominal infection. In intra-abdominal infections (ie, between the urinary bladder and the gallbladder), enterococci are permissive pathogens, that is, they cause infection only in concert with another pathogen [5,6,40].

The spectrum of enterococcal infections is the same for VSE and VRE. The only difference between VSE and VRE is related to the therapeutic approach [41]. Virtually all strains of VSE remain susceptible to ampicillin and antipseudomonal penicillins, that is, ticarcillin, azlocillin, mezlocillin, piperacillin, and vancomycin. An example of the difference between in vitro susceptibility and in vivo activity is that of penicillin with regard to enterococci [20]. Enterococci are usually reported as being sensitive to penicillin, but penicillin monotherapy is ineffective in treating enterococcal infections. Penicillin combined with an aminoglycoside, such as gentamicin, is active against VSE because of synergy. Clinicians should be aware that, with the exception of the third-generation cephalosporins, cefoperazone, cephalosporins have no anti-VSE activity. Although the MIC_{90} of cefoperazone to VSE is 32 µg/mL and is considerably higher than with ampicillin, serum concentrations of less than 32 µg/mL are readily achieved after 2 g of cefoperazone (intravenous) with resultant serum levels of approximately 240 µg/mL [20]. Quinupristin/dalfopristin is active against VRE but inactive against *E faecalis*, that is, VSE [42–47]. Quinolones have variable anti-VSE activity and should be used in VSE infections with a demonstrated susceptibility to quinolones [5,6].

Strains of VRE are by definition vancomycin resistant and are also resistant to the usual antibiotics that are active against VSE. Fortunately, in vitro susceptibility testing is reliable in VRE, by contrast with VSE or MRSA, and susceptibility results may be used to guide antibiotic selection for VRE infections [22–24]. As with VSE, VRE infection, not colonization, should be treated with antibiotics. Antibiotics with proved effectiveness against VRE include quinupristin/dalfopristin, doxycycline, chloramphenicol, linezolid, daptomycin, and tigecycline [5,6,20,40,41,48–63]. Anti-VRE drugs are also effective against VSE with the exception of quinupristin/dalfopristin, which is only effective against VRE. Nitrofurantoin is the preferred oral antibiotic for treating VRE cystitis or catheter-associated bacteriuria [20]. Oral agents available to treat serious systemic VRE infections include doxycycline, chloramphenicol, and linezolid. High-dose daptomycin should be used for VRE infections (ie, 12 mg/kg intravenously [IV] every 24 hours [with normal renal function]), because the MIC_{90} of VRE is more than double the MIC_{90} for MRSA (ie, 6 mg/kg [IV] every 24 hours) [61–63].

Methicillin-resistant *Staphylococcus aureus*

Staphylococci are part of the normal skin flora. The nares is the primary site of colonization for staphylococci (versus the feces for VSE and VRE). Because staphylococcal colonization of the skin is so common, MSSA/MRSA as well as Coagulase Negative Staphylococci (CoNS) are common blood culture contaminants: the skin organisms are commonly introduced during venipuncture. Colonization is common in respiratory secretions of intubated patients, on broad-spectrum antimicrobial therapy, in nonpurulent surgical wounds, draining body fluids (chest tube or abdominal drainage), and urine in catheterized or instrumented patients. As with enterococci, staphylococcal colonization should not be treated; treatment should be reserved for infection. The spectrum of infection with MSSA resembles that of MRSA with some important differences. Staphylococci are the most common cause of suppurative wound infections, are important causes of IV-line infection, and are now the most common cause of acute bacterial endocarditis (ABE) (Table 2) [20,64].

Antibiotics traditionally effective against MSSA include antistaphylococcal penicillins, such as oxacillin, nafcillin, first-, second-, and third-generation cephalosporins (excluding ceftazidime), TMP-SMX, clindamycin, doxycycline, gentamicin, vancomycin, piperacillin/tazobactam, and cefepime. The preferred antibiotics to use for MSSA infections include antistaphylococcal penicillins, antistaphylococcal cephalosporins, and cefepime [20]. The preferred oral agents commonly used to treat MSSA infections include TMP-SMX, clindamycin, and oral first-generation cephalosporins. Oral antipseudomonal penicillins are erratically absorbed and are frequently associated with gastrointestinal upset. If a β-lactam is selected, first-generation cephalosporins are preferred as oral anti-MSSA therapy [20].

Susceptibility testing with MRSA presents interpretation difficulties because there is often a discrepancy between in vitro susceptibility and in

Table 2
Clinical comparison of enterococcal (vancomycin-resistant enterococci) and staphylococcal (methicillin-sensitive *Staphylococcus aureus*/methicillin-resistant *Staphylococcus aureus*) antibiotics

Antistaphylococcal agent	Usual adult dose[a]	Side effects	Advantages	Disadvantages
Daptomycin	Complicated skin/soft tissue infections 4 mg/kg (IV) q 24 h Bacteremias 6 mg/kg (IV) q 24 h (q 24 h dosing CrCl > 30 mL/min; q 48 h dosing CrCl ≤30 mL/min)	None	Most effective/rapidly bactericidal MSSA/MRSA antibiotic No ↑ VRE prevalence Also useful for VISA/VRSA Once daily dosing	No PO formulation Potential cytochrome P450 interactions
Linezolid	600 mg (IV/PO) q 12 h	Transient/reversible thrombocytopenia	PO formulation (excellent bioavailability) Excellent CNS penetrations (70%) Also useful for VISA/VRSA	Potential cytochrome P450 interactions Serotonin syndrome
Quinupristin/ dalfopristin	7.5 mg/kg (IV) q 8 h	Painful myalgias (rare)	Proven effectiveness	No PO formulation Q 8 h dosing Ineffective against VSE Poor CNS penetration (<10%) Limited VRE experience
Minocycline	100–200 mg (IV/PO) q 12 h	Skin discoloration with prolonged use	PO formulation (excellent bioavailability) Excellent CNS penetration (50%) Inexpensive	

Drug	Dose	Adverse effects	Advantages	Disadvantages
Vancomycin	1 g (IV) q 12 h	Neutropenia "Red Man" syndrome	Proven effectiveness No nephrotoxicity (vancomycin levels unnecessary; dose ~ CrCl) Poor CNS penetration (15%)	↑ MICs/resistance (VISA/VRSA) No PO formulation for MRSA/VSE ↑ VRE prevalence Slow resolution of MSSA/MRSA infections ↑ Therapeutic failures Total cost of IV vancomycin more expensive than PO linezolid
Tigecycline	100 mg (IV) × 1 dose, then 50 mg (IV) q 12 h	None	No side effects No ↑ VRE prevalence No potential cytochrome P450 interactions	No PO formulation

All may be used in penicillin-allergic patients.

Abbreviations: CrCl, creatinine clearance; PO, oral; VISA, vancomycin-intermediate *S aureus*; VRSA, vancomycin-resistant *S aureus*.

[a] Normal renal/hepatic function.

Adapted from Cunha BA. Antibiotic essentials. 5th edition. Royal Oak (MI): Physicians' Press; 2006.

vivo effectiveness [23,24]. Many antibiotics appear to be sensitive against strains of HA-MRSA by in vitro susceptibility testing but are inconsistently reliable clinically, and other agents should be used. Antibiotics with demonstrated MRSA activity include vancomycin, quinupristin-dalfopristin, minocycline, linezolid, daptomycin, and tigecycline [64–90]. The only oral agents available to treat MRSA infections are minocycline and linezolid [20,58].

Community-acquired methicillin-resistant *Staphylococcus aureus* and hospital-acquired methicillin-resistant *Staphylococcus aureus*

Recently, there has been an increase in reports of CA-MRSA. For decades, MRSA was primarily a hospital organism (ie, HA-MRSA), but over the years, strains also originated from the community that were related genetically to hospital strains. Currently, CA-MRSA implies not only origin in the community but also a different genetic strain of MRSA. CA-MRSA differs from HA-MRSA in its spectrum and antibiotic susceptibility.

CA-MRSA strains are of the $SCC_{mec}IV$ type. CA-MRSA strains may carry the Panton-Valentine leukocidin (PVL) gene. PVL is a potent toxin which causes tissue necrosis. PVL-positive CA-MRSA strains are highly virulent and are the cause of severe pyodermas/necrotizing fasciitis as well as necrotizing community-acquired pneumonia (CAP). PVL-negative CA-MRSA strains are less virulent and resemble clinically the spectrum of infection caused by MSSA. Patients presenting with otherwise unexplained, unusually severe necrotizing fasciitis/pyomyositis should be suspected of having PVL-positive CA-MRSA until proven otherwise. To date, virtually all of the cases of severe/necrotizing MRSA CAP have been due to PVL-positive CA-MRSA following viral influenza. MSSA/MRSA is a rare cause of CAP. MSSA/MRSA CAP is rare even in diabetics commonly colonized with staphylococci. Essentially, all staphylococcal CAP occurs in the postviral influenza setting. Extremely severe necrotic MRSA CAP may occur after viral influenza in patients infected with PVL-positive CA-MRSA strains (Table 3) [91–105].

Strains of HA-MRSA are usually pen-resistant and are susceptible and responsive to only a small number of antibiotics, such as vancomycin, minocycline, quinupristin-dalfopristin, linezolid, daptomycin, and tigecycline. Antibiotics with known effectiveness against HA-MRSA are also effective against CA-MRSA. CA-MRSA strains are pauci-resistant to antistaphylococcal antibiotics and are sensitive to some of the agents active against MSSA strains. For this reason, CA-MRSA strains may be treated with clindamycin, doxycycline, or TMP-SMX [20,104,105]. However, serious or fulminant infections due to CA-MRSA PVL-positive strains should be treated with antibiotics known to be effective against HA-MRSA.

Table 3
Comparative clinical features of community-acquired methicillin-resistant *Staphylococcus aureus* and hospital-acquired methicillin-resistant *Staphylococcus aureus* infections

MRSA clinical and laboratory features	CA-MRSA	HA-MRSA
Epidemiology	Young adults	Older adults/elderly
	Community origin	Hospital origin
Cassette chromosome type	SCC_{mec} IV	SCC_{mec} I, II, III
Toxins	PVL±	PVL−
Susceptibility testing	In vitro Susceptibility = In vivo Effectiveness	In vitro Susceptibility ≠ In vivo Effectiveness
Antibiotic susceptibility pattern	Pauci-resistant (susceptible to many antibiotics)	Multidrug resistant (not susceptible to most antibiotics)
Clinical features	Severe necrotizing CAP Postviral influenza with PVL+ strains	Bacteremias
	Nonsevere CAP with PVL− strains	Nosocomial ABE
	Severe pyomyositis/fasciitis with PVL+ strains	Skin/soft tissue infections
	Nonsevere cSSSI with PVL− strains	Respiratory secretions colonization common in ventilator patients
		MRSA VAP uncommon
Empiric antibiotic therapy	Clindamycin	Daptomycin[a]
	Doxycycline	Linezolid[a]
	TMP-SMX	Tigecycline[a]
		Minocycline[a]
		Quinupristin/dalfopristin[a]
		Vancomycin[a]

Abbreviations: cSSSI, complicated skin/soft tissue infection; SCC, staphylococcal casette chromosome; VAP, ventilator-associated pneumonia.

[a] Also effective against CA-MRSA.

Adapted from Cunha BA. Clinical manifestations and antimicrobial therapy of methicillin-resistant *Staphylococcus aureus* (MRSA). Clin Microbiol Infect 2005;11:33–42; Arshad S, Brown RB. Community-acquired methicillin-resistant *Staphylococcus aureus* (CA-MRSA). Infectious Disease Practice 2006;30:479–83; Cunha BA. Antibiotic essentials. 5th edition. Royal Oak (MI): Physicians' Press; 2006.

References

[1] Bassetti M, Melica G, Cenderello G, et al. Gram-positive bacterial resistance. A challenge for the next millennium. Panminerva Med 2002;44:179–84.

[2] Pallares R, Fenoll A, Linares J, et al. The epidemiology of antibiotic resistance in *Streptococcus pneumoniae* and the clinical relevance of resistance to cephalosporins, macrolides and quinolones. Int J Antimicrob Agents 2003;22(Suppl 1):S15–24.

[3] Cunha BA. Antibiotic resistance. Drugs for Today 1998;31:691–8.

[4] Boneca IG, Chiosis G. Vancomycin resistance: occurrence, mechanisms and strategies to combat it. Expert Opin Ther Targets 2003;7:311–28.

[5] Bonten MJ, Willems R, Weinstein RA. Vancomycin-resistant enterococci. Clin Infect Dis 2000;31:1058–65.

[6] Cetinkaya Y, Falk P, Mayhall CG. Vancomycin-resistant enterococci. Clin Microbiol Rev 2000;13:686–707.

[7] Cunha BA. Penicillin-resistant pneumococci. Postgrad Med 2003;113:42–54.

[8] Feldman C. Clinical relevance of antimicrobial resistance in the management of pneumococcal community-acquired pneumonia. J Lab Clin Med 2004;143:269–83.

[9] Lynch JP 3rd, Zhanel GG. Escalation of antimicrobial resistance among *Streptococcus pneumoniae*: implications for therapy. Semin Respir Crit Care Med 2005;26:575–16.

[10] Cunha BA. Penicillin resistant *Streptococcus pneumoniae*. Drugs Today 1998;31:31–5.

[11] Cunha BA. Antibiotic resistance: control strategies. Crit Care Clin 1998;8:309–28.

[12] Cunha BA. Strategies to control antibiotic resistance. Semin Respir Crit Care Med 2000;21:3–8.

[13] Cunha BA. Effective antibiotic resistance and control strategies. Lancet 2001;3570:1307–8.

[14] Shea KW, Ueno Y, Abumustafa F, et al. Doxycycline activity against *Streptococcus pneumoniae*. Chest 1995;107:1775–6.

[15] Lederman ER, Gleeson TD, Driscoll T, et al. Doxycycline sensitivity of *S. pneumoniae* isolates. Clin Infect Dis 2003;36:1091.

[16] Jones RN, Sader HS, Fritsche TR. Doxycycline use for community-acquired pneumonia: contemporary in vitro spectrum of activity against *Streptococcus pneumoniae* (1999–2002). Diagn Microbiol Infect Dis 2004;(49):147–9.

[17] Johnson JR. Doxycycline for treatment of community-acquired pneumonia. Clin Infect Dis 2002;35:632–3.

[18] Klugman KP, Lonks JR. Hidden epidemic of macrolide-resistant pneumococci. Emerg Infect Dis 2005;11:802–7.

[19] Pihlajamaki M, Kotilainen P, Kaurila T, et al. Macrolide-resistant *Streptococcus pneumoniae* and use of antimicrobial agents. Clin Infect Dis 2001;33:483–8.

[20] Cunha BA, editor. Antibiotic essentials. 5th edition. Royal Oak (MI): Physicians' Press; 2006.

[21] Lonks JR, Garau J, Medeiros AA. Implications of antimicrobial resistance in the empirical treatment of community-acquired respiratory tract infections: the case of macrolides. J Antimicrob Chemother 2002;50(Suppl S2):87–92.

[22] Rzeszutek M, Wierzbowski A, Hoban DJ, et al. A review of clinical failures associated with macrolide-resistant *Streptococcus pneumoniae*. Int J Antimicrob Agents 2004;24:95–104.

[23] Cunha BA. The significance of antibiotic false sensitivity testing with in vitro testing. J Chemother 1997;9:25–35.

[24] Cunha BA. MRSA & VRE: in vitro susceptibility versus in vivo efficacy. A cause of skin and soft tissue infections. Ann Intern Med 2006;144:309–17.

[25] Schito GC. The importance of the development of antibiotic resistance in *Staphylococcus aureus*. Clin Microbiol Infect 2006;12(Suppl 1):3–8.

[26] Hayden MK. Insights into the epidemiology and control of infection with vancomycin-resistant enterococci: why are they here, and where do they come from? Lancet Infect Dis 2000;31:1058–65.

[27] Chavers LS, Moser SA, Benjamin WH, et al. Vancomycin-resistant enterococci: 15 years and counting. J Hosp Infect 2003;53:159–71.

[28] Patel R. Clinical impact of vancomycin-sresistant enterococci. J Antimicrob Chemother 2003;51(Suppl 3):iii3–21.

[29] Donskey CJ, Hoyen CK, Das SM, et al. Recurrence of vancomycin-resistant *Enterococcus* stool colonization during antibiotic therapy. Infect Control Hosp Epidemiol 2002;23: 436–40.

[30] Lautenbach E, LaRosa LA, Marr AM, et al. Changes in the prevalence of vancomycin-resistant enterococci in response to antimicrobial formulary interventions: impact of progressive restrictions on use of vancomycin and third-generation cephalosporins. Clin Infect Dis 2003;36:440–6.

[31] Cunha BA. Clinical relevance of penicillin resistant *Streptococcus pneumoniae*. Semin Respir Infect 2002;17:204–14.

[32] Fuller JD, McGeer A, Low DE. Drug-resistant pneumococcal pneumonia: clinical relevance and approach to management. Eur J Clin Microbiol Infect Dis 2005;24:780–8.

[33] Zhanel GG, Hisanaga T, Nichol K, et al. Ketolides: an emerging treatment for macrolide-resistant respiratory infections, focusing on *S. pneumoniae*. Expert Opin Emerg Drugs 2003; 8:297–321.

[34] Craig WA. Overview of newer antimicrobial formulations for overcoming pneumococcal resistance. Am J Med 2004;117(Suppl 3A):16S–22S.

[35] Ortega M, Marco F, Almela M, et al. Activity of telithromycin against erythromycin-susceptible and resistant *Streptococcus pneumoniae* is from adults with invasive infections. Int J Antimicrob Agents 2004;24:616–8.

[36] Quintiliani R. Clinical management of respiratory tract infections in the community: experience with telithromycin. Infection 2001;(Suppl 2):16–22.

[37] Low DE, Felmingham D, Brown SD, et al. Activity of telithromycin against key pathogens associated with community-acquired respiratory tract infections. J Infect 2004;49: 115–25.

[38] Reinert RR. Clinical efficacy of ketolides in the treatment of respiratory tract infections. J Antimicrob Chemother 2004;53:918–27.

[39] van Rensburg DJ, Fogarty C, Kohno S, et al. Efficacy of telithromycin in community-acquired pneumonia caused by pneumococci with reduced susceptibility to penicillin and/or erythromycin. Chemotherapy 2005;51:186–92.

[40] Mascini EM, Bonten MJ. Vancomycin-resistant enterococci: consequences for therapy and infection control. Clin Microbiol Infect 2005;11(Suppl 4):43–56.

[41] Linden PK. Treatment options for vancomycin-resistant enterococcal infections. Drugs 2002;62:425–41.

[42] Chant C, Ryback MH. Quinupristin/dalfopristin (RP 59500): a new streptogramin antibiotic. Ann Pharmacother 1995;29:1022–7.

[43] Bryson HM, Spencer CM. Quinupristin/dalfopristin. Drugs 1996;52:406–15.

[44] Griswold MW, Lomaestro BM, Briceland LL. Quinupristin-dalfopristin (RP 59500): an injectable streptogramin combination. Am J Health Syst Pharm 1996;53:2045–53.

[45] Kim MK, Nicolau DP, Nightingale CH, et al. Quinupristin/dalfopristin: a treatment option for vancomycin-resistant enterococci. Conn Med 2000;64:209–12.

[46] Goff DA, Sierawski SJ. Clinical experience of quinupristin-dalfopristin for the treatment of antimicrobial-resistant gram-positive infections. Pharmacotherapy 2002;22:748–58.

[47] Blondeau JM, Sanche SE. Quinupristin/dalfopristin. Expert Opin Pharmacother 2002;3: 1341–64.

[48] Gould CV, Fishman NO, Nachamkin I, et al. Chloramphenicol resistance in vancomycin-resistant enterococcal bacteremia: impact of prior fluoroquinolone use? Infect Control Hosp Epidemiol 2004;25:138–45.

[49] Kauffman CA. Therapeutic and preventative options for the management of vancomycin-resistant enterococcal infections. J Antimicrob Chemother 2003;51(Suppl 3):iii23–30.

[50] Zirakzadeh A, Patel R. Vancomycin-resistant enterococci: colonization, infection, detection, and treatment. Mayo Clin Proc 2006;81:529–36.

[51] Tigecycline. Med Lett Drugs Ther 2005;47:73–4.

[52] Sader HS, Jones RN, Dowzicky MJ, et al. Antimicrobial activity of tigecycline tested against nosocomial bacterial pathogens from patients hospitalized in the intensive care unit. Diagn Microbiol Infect Dis 2005;52:203–8.

[53] Frampton JE, Curran MP. Tigecycline. Drugs 2005;65:2623–35.

[54] Felmingham D. Tigecycline: an expanded broad-spectrum intravenous antibiotic. Preface and summary. J Chemother 2005;17(Suppl 1):3–4.

[55] Livermore DM. Tigecycline: what is it, and where should it be used? J Antimicrob Chemother 2005;56:611–4.

[56] Zhanel GG, Karlowsky JA, Rubinstein E, et al. Tigecycline: a novel glycylcycline antibiotic. Expert Rev Anti Infect Ther 2006;4:9–25.

[57] Jones CH, Petersen PJ. Tigecycline: a review of preclinical and clinical studies of the first-in-class glycylcycline antibiotic. Drugs Today (Barc) 2005;41:637–69.

[58] Clemett D, Markham A. Linezolid. Drugs 2000;59:815–27.

[59] Wilcox MH. Efficacy of linezolid versus comparator therapies in gram-positive infections. J Antimicrob Chemother 2003;51(Suppl 2):ii27–35.

[60] Carpenter CF, Chambers HF. Daptomycin: another novel agent for treating infections due to drug-resistant gram-positive pathogens. Clin Infect Dis 2004;38:994–1000.

[61] Fenton C, Keating GM, Curran MP. Daptomycin. Drugs 2004;64:445–55.

[62] Cha R, Grucz RG Jr, Rybak MJ. Daptomycin dose-effect relationship against resistant gram-positive organisms. Antimicrob Agents Chemother 2003;47:1598–603.

[63] Dvorchik BH, Brazier D, DeBruin MF, et al. Daptomycin pharmacokinetics and safety following administration of escalating doses once daily to healthy subjects. Antimicrob Agents Chemother 2003;47:1318–23.

[64] Cunha BA. Methicillin-resistant Staphylococcus aureus: clinical manifestations and antimicrobial therapy. Clin Microbiol Infect 2005;11(Suppl 4):33–42.

[65] Anstead GM, Owens AD. Recent advances in the treatment of infections due to resistant Staphylococcus aureus. Curr Opin Infect Dis 2004;17:549–55.

[66] Mounzer KC, DiNubile MJ. Clinical presentation and management of methicillin-resistant Staphylococcus aureus (MRSA) infections. Antibiotics Clinicians 1998;2:15–20.

[67] Paradisi F, Corti G, Messeri D. Antistaphylococcal (MSSA, MRSA, MSSE, MRSE) antibiotics. Med Clin North Am 2001;85:1–17.

[68] Turnidge J, Grayson ML. Optimum treatment of staphylococcal infections. Drugs 1993;45:353–66.

[69] Segreti J. Efficacy of current agents used in the treatment of gram-positive infections and the consequences of resistance. Clin Microbiol Infect 2005;11(Suppl 3):29–35.

[70] Eliopoulos GM. Antimicrobial agents for treatment of serious infections caused by resistant Staphylococcus aureus and enterococci. Eur J Clin Microbiol Infect Dis 2005;24:826–31.

[71] Alder JD. Daptomycin: a new drug class for the treatment of gram-positive infections. Drugs Today (Barc) 2005;41:81–90.

[72] Rybak MJ. The efficacy and safety of daptomycin: first in a new class of antibiotics for gram-positive bacteria. Clin Microbiol Infect 2006;12(Suppl 1):24–32.

[73] Tally FP, Zeckel M, Wasilewski MM, et al. Daptomycin: a novel agent for gram-positive infections. Expert Opin Investig Drugs 1999;8:1223–38.

[74] Eisenstein BI. Lipopeptides, focusing on daptomycin, for the treatment of gram-positive infections. Expert Opin Investig Drugs 2004;13:1159–69.

[75] Sader HS, Streit JM, Fritsche TR, et al. Antimicrobial activity of daptomycin against multidrug-resistant gram-positive strains collected worldwide. Diagn Microbiol Infect Dis 2004;50:201–4.

[76] Tedesco KL, Rybak MJ. Daptomycin. Pharmacotherapy 2004;24:41–57.

[77] Wilcox MH. Tigecycline and the need for a new broad-spectrum antibiotic class. Surg Infect (Larchmt) 2006;7:69–80.
[78] Menichetti F. Current and emerging serious gram-positive infections. Clin Microbiol Infect 2005;11(Suppl 3):22–8.
[79] LaPlante KL, Rybak MJ. Clinical glycopeptide-intermediate staphylococcal tested against arbekacin, daptomycin, and tigecycline. Diagn Microbiol Infect Dis 2004;50:125–30.
[80] Stevens DL, Herr D, Lampiris H, et al. Linezolid versus vancomycin for the treatment of methicillin-resistant *Staphylococcal aureus* infections. Clin Infect Dis 2002;34:1481–90.
[81] Hill EE, Herijgers P, Herregods M-C, et al. Infective endocarditis treated with linezolid: case report and literature review. Eur J Clin Microbiol Infect Dis 2006;25:202–4.
[82] Itani KM, Weigelt J, Li JZ, et al. Linezolid reduces length of stay and duration of intravenous treatment compared with vancomycin for complicated skin and soft tissue infections due to suspected or proven methicillin-resistant *Staphylococcus aureus* (MRSA). Int J Antimicrob Agents 2005;26:442–8.
[83] Souli M, Pontikis K, Chryssouli Z, et al. Successful treatment of right-sided prosthetic valve endocarditis due to methicillin-resistant teicoplanin-heteroresistant *Staphylococcus aureus* with linezolid. Eur J Clin Microbiol Infect Dis 2005;24:760–2.
[84] Pankey GA, Sabath LD. Clinical relevance of bacteriostatic versus bactericidal mechanisms of action in the treatment of gram-positive bacterial infections. Clin Infect Dis 2004;38:864–70.
[85] Jonas M, Cunha BA. Minocycline. Ther Drug Monit 1982;4:137–45.
[86] Clumeck N, Marcelis L, Amiri-Lamraski MH, et al. Treatment of severe staphylococcal infections with rifampin-minocycline association. J Antimicrob Chemother 1984;13:71–2.
[87] Lawler MT, Sullivan MC, Levitz RE, et al. Treatment of prosthetic valve endocarditis due to methicillin-resistant *Staphylococcus aureus* with minocycline. J Infect Dis 1990;161:812–4.
[88] Lewis S, Lewis B. Minocycline therapy of resistant *Staphylococcus aureus* infections. Infect Control Hosp Epidemiol 1993;14:423.
[89] Yuk JH, Dignani MC, Harris RL, et al. Minocycline as an alternative antistaphylococcal agent. Rev Infect Dis 1991;13:1023.
[90] Cunha BA. Oral antibiotics to treat MRSA infections. J Hosp Infect 2005;60:88–90.
[91] Padmanabhan RA, Fraser TC. The emergence of methicillin-resistant *Staphylococcus aureus* in the community. Cleve Clin J Med 2005;72:235–41.
[92] Chini V, Petinaki E, Foka A, et al. Spread of *Staphylococcus aureus* clinical isolates carrying Panton-Valentine leukocidin genes during a 3-year period in Greece. Clin Microbiol Infect 2006;12:29–34.
[93] Kluytmans-Vandenbergh MF, Kluytmans JA. Community-acquired, methicillin-resistant *Staphylococcus aureus*: current perspectives. Clin Microbiol Infect 2006;12(Suppl 1):9–15.
[94] Diederen BMW, Kluytmans JAJW. The emergence of infections with community-associated methicillin-resistant *Staphylococcus aureus*. J Infect 2006;52:157–68.
[95] Tenover FC. Community-associated methicillin-resistant *Staphylococcus aureus*: it's not just in communities anymore. Clin Microbiol Newsl 2005;28:33–5.
[96] Rybak MJ, LaPlante KL. Community-associated methicillin-resistant *Staphylococcus aureus*: a review. Pharmacotherapy 2005;25:74–85.
[97] Maltezou HC, Giamarellou H. Community-acquired methicillin-resistant *Staphylococcus aureus* infections. Int J Antimicrob Agents 2006;27:87–96.
[98] King MD, Humphrey BJ, Wang YF, et al. Emergence of community-acquired methicillin-resistant *Staphylococcus aureus* WSA 300 clone as the predominant cause of skin and soft-tissue infections. Ann Intern Med 2006;144(5):309–17.
[99] Miller LG, Perdreau-Remington F, Rieg G, et al. Necrotizing fasciitis caused by community-associated methicillin-resistant *Staphylococcus aureus* in Los Angeles. N Engl J Med 2005;352:1445–53.

[100] Francis JS, Doherty MC, Lopatin U, et al. Severe community-onset pneumonia in healthy adults caused by methicillin-resistant *Staphylococcus aureus* carrying the Panton-Valentine leukocidin genes. Clin Infect Dis 2005;40:100–7.

[101] Gillet Y, Issartel B, Vanhems P, et al. Association between *Staphylococcus aureus* strains carrying genes for Panton-Valentine leukocidin and highly lethal necrotizing pneumonia in young immunocompetent patients. Lancet 2002;359:753–9.

[102] Alonso-Tarrés C, Villegas ML, de Gispert FJ, et al. Favorable outcome of pneumonia due to Panton-Valentine leukocidin–producing *Staphylococcus aureus* associated with hematogenous origin and absence of flu-like illness. Eur J Clin Microbiol Infect Dis 2005;24:756–9.

[103] Shopsin B, Zhao X, Kreiswirth BN, et al. Are the new quinolones appropriate treatment for community-acquired methicillin-resistant *Staphylococcus aureus*? Int J Antimicrob Agents 2004;24:32–4.

[104] Moellering RC Jr. The growing menace of community-acquired methicillin-resistant *Staphylococcus aureus*. Ann Intern Med 2006;144:368–70.

[105] Arshad S, Brown RB. Community-acquired methicillin-resistant *Staphylococcus aureus* (CA-MRSA). Infectious Disease Practice 2006;30:479–83.

THE MEDICAL
CLINICS
OF NORTH AMERICA

Med Clin N Am 90 (2006) 1183–1195

Monotherapy Versus Combination Therapy

Shilpa M. Patel, MD[a],*,
Louis D. Saravolatz, MD, MACP[b]

[a]Division of Infectious Diseases, Department of Internal Medicine, St. John Hospital and
Medical Center, 19251 Mack Avenue, Suite 340, Grosse Pointe Woods, MI 48236, USA
[b]Department of Medicine, St. John Hospital and Medical Center, 19251 Mack Avenue,
Suite 335, Grosse Pointe Woods, MI 48236, USA

The science of antibiotic therapy for infectious diseases continues to evolve. In many instances where empiric coverage is necessary, treatment with more than one agent is considered prudent. If an etiology is identified, antibiotics are modified based on culture and susceptibility data. Even when the organism is known, more than one antibiotic may be needed for effective treatment. Decisions about antibiotics should be made after assessments of pertinent clinical information, laboratory and microbiology information, ease of administration, patient compliance, potential adverse effects, cost, and available evidence supporting various treatment options. Clinicians also need to consider synergy and local resistance patterns in selecting therapeutic options. In this article, the authors outline current therapies for several common infectious diseases, describing both monotherapy and combination therapy options.

Cellulitis

Cellulitis is a common infectious disease managed by physicians in both primary care and specialty practices, and in inpatient and outpatient settings alike. Because scientific data describing therapeutic trials remain limited, clinical experience has guided treatment. Antibiotic therapy should initially be directed at gram-positive organisms, such as staphylococci and streptococci, as these are the most common organisms responsible for causing

---

* Corresponding author.
E-mail address: shilpa.patel@stjohn.org (S.M. Patel).

cellulitis. If, however, the patient's history suggests any other potential causative organisms, these should be treated as well.

Classically, cellulitis involves erythema, warmth, tenderness, and swelling that is usually localized. Many patients present with symptoms as outpatients. These individuals may be managed in the outpatient setting as clinical judgment warrants. The decision to hospitalize patients should be based on signs of systemic toxicity, ability of the patient to follow through with therapeutic measures, and ease of follow-up.

If the patient appears nontoxic, is reliable to present for frequent visits to assure close monitoring, and is able to tolerate oral antibiotics, treating the cellulitis with an oral agent is appropriate. The cephalosporins are commonly used as first-line agents because they offer adequate coverage for staphylococci and streptococci and are generally well tolerated and effective. Cephalexin (500 mg by mouth every 6 to 12 hours) is a common regimen, and, if the patient does not have erysipelas, then dicloxacillin (500 mg by mouth every 6 hours) can also be used. Both of these agents can be used as monotherapy in the setting of uncomplicated cellulitis with no other known exposures. If *Haemophilus influenzae* is a potential pathogen, cefuroxime axetil (500 mg by mouth every 12 hours) can be used.

In cases of cellulitis that may involve gram-negative organisms, treatment with a fluoroquinolone may be warranted. Levofloxacin, gatifloxacin, and moxifloxacin have been approved for the treatment of uncomplicated cellulitis as they all have increased gram-positive activity. However only levofloxacin is approved for the treatment of complicated skin infections. If other quinolones are selected for treatment, then clindamycin should be added for additional gram-positive coverage, especially in situations where treatment is empiric.

Clindamycin (300 mg by mouth every 6 hours) may be given, though there is an increased risk of diarrhea with this agent. Macrolides, such as erythromycin, azithromycin, and clarithromycin, can also be used. However, resistance to these agents among streptococci is increasing and, therefore, these drugs may be less effective. In the setting of serious penicillin allergies, clindamycin or levofloxacin are reasonable alternative choices for treatment. With the increase in community-acquired methicillin-resistant *Staphylococcus aureus* (MRSA) being reported throughout the United States, oral agents effective against these strains are limited to trimethoprim–sulfamethoxazole, clindamycin, and linezolid. Linezolid is significantly more expensive and may be associated with thrombocytopenia if prolonged therapy is required.

In cases where oral antibiotics may not be used or when individuals are hospitalized for treatment, intravenous antibiotics should be initiated. Because the specific pathogen may not be identified at the initial presentation of acute cellulitis, empiric antibiotics are reasonable. Again, unless there is concern for unusual exposures that may involve other organisms, the antibiotic chosen should cover gram-positive organisms well, especially staphylococci and streptococci.

The 2005 Infectious Diseases Society of America (IDSA) guidelines [1] recommend initial empiric therapy with a penicillinase-resistant penicillin, such as nafcillin or oxacillin, or a first-generation cephalosporin, such as cefazolin. If patients have a serious allergy to penicillin, clindamycin or vancomycin can be used. In settings where MRSA is considered a causative organism, initial therapy should include vancomycin. In one study that compared tigecycline, a new glycylcycline agent with activity against gram-positive cocci, with the combination of vancomycin and aztreonam, clinical cure rates were not found to be significantly different [2].

If the patient has erysipelas, aqueous crystalline penicillin G or cefazolin may be used. Once patients show clinical improvement, they can be switched to oral therapy to complete the remaining treatment course.

In most cases of cellulitis, monotherapy may suffice. However, if there is concern for unusual exposures or if broader coverage may be needed (eg, in the setting of immunosuppression or resistant pathogens), then antibiotic coverage may be broadened to include gram-negative organisms and anaerobes.

Osteomyelitis

Osteomyelitis is associated with significant morbidity. Diabetics are at increased risk of developing ulcers and subsequent osteomyelitis because of motor and sensory neuropathy, peripheral vascular disease, and impaired neutrophil function and host defenses due to hyperglycemia. Osteomyelitis can occur as a result of trauma or hematogenous spread of infection. Ideally, treatment involves organism-specific antimicrobial therapy in conjunction with surgery or debridement if necessary.

In the setting of osteomyelitis without any known etiologic agent, a bone biopsy is the definitive method for diagnosis. If ulceration is present, superficial swabs do not reflect the pathogens responsible for deeper infection with the exception of *S aureus*. These specimens should not guide therapy. In these situations, deep cultures obtained from debridement are more useful.

Therapy is often empiric. If the patient has an ulcer related to diabetes and is not hospitalized and the infection is not limb threatening, oral therapy with cephalexin or clindamycin may be tried [3]. These agents may not lead to clinical improvement if the causative agent is MRSA, and so local epidemiologic factors must be considered. If gram-negatives are strongly suspected, oral ciprofloxacin (750 mg by mouth twice a day) may be used.

In limb-threatening infections and osteomyelitis, parenteral therapy is advised. Therapy should ideally be based on culture results as well. However, empiric therapy is often initiated while a workup ensues. Per the IDSA guidelines [4], if there is a mild soft tissue infection, therapy should be directed toward gram-positive organisms. Monotherapy with a first-generation cephalosporin, trimethoprim–sulfamethoxazole, or clindamycin may be attempted in the antibiotic-naïve patient. If patients have already been treated with antibiotics or failed an agent above, therapy should be broadened to include gram-negative coverage. Ciprofloxacin, levofloxacin, or amoxicillin–clavulanate may be added. If MRSA is suspected and the patient is not responding to clindamycin or trimethoprim–sulfamethoxazole, linezolid, daptomycin, or vancomycin may be used. Treatment in these situations may be continued for approximately 2 weeks. For moderate infections, antibiotic therapy should be broad spectrum from the start; monotherapy with levofloxacin or amoxicillin–clavulanate or combination therapy with ciprofloxacin plus clindamycin may be used. If patients exhibit signs of systemic toxicity and need to be admitted, parenteral antibiotics should be given. Ideally culture results should guide treatment, however, initial antibiotic choices can include ciprofloxacin plus clindamycin, ampicillin–sulbactam, or piperacillin–tazobactam. MRSA coverage with trimethoprim–sulfamethoxazole, linezolid, daptomycin, or vancomycin may be added. Gram-negative coverage and anaerobic coverage with metronidazole may be added as well, given the clinical picture. Those patients with severe soft tissue infections should receive intravenous antibiotics with the above agents in combination, to provide adequate coverage for gram-positive, gram-negative, and anaerobic infections.

For patients with documented osteomyelitis, intravenous therapy is generally considered more effective than oral therapy. However, oral therapy may be used if the pathogen is known and susceptible to the agent, the infection is not limb threatening, and the patient will be compliant with the treatment. According to the IDSA guidelines, 4 to 6 weeks of treatment are necessary. Debridement is often necessary, and vasculopaths often need their vascular issues addressed before adequate healing can take place. Antibacterial therapy is similar to the above recommendations. Monotherapy is preferred given the need for long-term therapy, given both the cost and convenience of treatment, but decisions should be based on epidemiologic factors, culture data, and clinical responses whenever possible.

Neutropenic fever

Patients who develop neutropenia complicated by fever need broad antibiotic coverage for gram-positive, gram-negative, and anaerobic organisms until an infectious agent can be identified. In many of these situations, initial combination therapy may be appropriate.

If the individual is considered low-risk and oral therapy is considered, treatment with ciprofloxacin plus amoxicillin–clavulanate is recommended. This regimen can provide adequate coverage for most common pathogens. If the patient is hospitalized, then intravenous therapy is indicated. If there is no suspicion for MRSA, monotherapy with the cephalosporin ceftazidime or cefepime, or a carbapenem, such as imipenem or meropenem, may be used [5]. If there is suspicion of a gram-negative pathogen, including *Pseudomonas aeruginosa* infection, an antipseudomonal penicillin or cephalosporin, such as ceftazidime or cefepime, may be used in conjunction with an aminoglycoside. Monotherapy with a carbapenem in this case may be used, but this approach may be associated with the selection of resistant gram-negative organisms more often than combination therapy. In settings where MRSA is a consideration, vancomycin should also be added to the treatment regimen. These patients should undergo an extensive workup looking for potential causes of fever, and antibiotic therapy should be reassessed every 48 to 72 hours, depending on clinical response, persistence of fevers, and diagnostic data. Eventually, if fever and neutropenia continue for 3 to 5 days despite aggressive therapy with multiple antibacterials, addition of antifungal therapy should be considered.

Initial antibiotic therapy should be selected with consideration of local resistance patterns and concern for potential adverse effects of antimicrobials, given the patients' probable exposure to other toxic agents. Patients may also have been receiving prophylaxis with antibiotics as outpatients as well. In the setting of neutropenic fever, combination therapy offers the advantage of effective, if not synergistic, broad coverage of many gram-negative organisms and it can minimize the emergence of resistant organisms. Nevertheless, there is the potential for missing some gram-positive organisms and inducing nephrotoxicity or ototoxicity with the use of aminoglycosides. Drug levels and clinical status should be monitored frequently. Fluoroquinolones may be used if these agents were not used as prophylaxis before. A recent randomized prospective trial compared piperacillin–tazobactam with ceftazidime for treatment of neutropenic fever in patients with acute leukemia or after autologous bone marrow transplantation. The trial found that monotherapy with piperacillin–tazobactam was as effective with equivalent direct and indirect costs as monotherapy with ceftazidime [6].

Endocarditis

Before antibiotic therapy became widely available, endocarditis was considered uniformly fatal. Although the prognosis of patients with endocarditis remains guarded, about 80% of patients today survive with appropriate timely antibiotic therapy. The causative organism, once isolated, guides antibiotic choices. It is important to choose bactericidal, not bacteriostatic therapy, to effectively treat endocarditis.

Staphylococcus

Methicillin-sensitive *S aureus* (MSSA) and MRSA remain as two of the most common causative pathogens for native-valve endocarditis.

Staphylococcal endocarditis is usually left-sided in the general population. In the population of intravenous drug users (IVDUs) Staphylococcal endocarditis is often right-sided. However, a recent study has suggested that in the IVDU population, left-sided endocarditis is still more common than right-sided endocarditis [7]. This information helps guide the length of antibiotic therapy, as shorter courses of treatment are needed to successfully treat uncomplicated right-sided native-valve endocarditis.

For MSSA native-valve left-sided endocarditis, therapy with a parenteral β-lactam, such as nafcillin or oxacillin (2 g intravenous every 4 hours) in conjunction with gentamicin (dosed 2 to 3 times daily), is appropriate. Because of issues with nephrotoxicity, gentamicin should be discontinued after 3 to 5 days of therapy if bacteremia has cleared. Evidence is insufficient to support or refute the use of an aminoglycoside in this situation beyond that duration of time [8]. Based on a multicenter study, nafcillin plus gentamicin is associated with a more rapid clearing of bacteremia when compared with using nafcillin alone [9]. Therapy should be continued for a total of 6 weeks for all left-sided endocarditis and in those right-sided cases complicated by valvular abscess or septic emboli; 2 weeks of therapy should be sufficient for uncomplicated right-sided endocarditis. For patients with penicillin allergies, desensitization should be considered. If that is not a viable option, then patients with a nonanaphylactoid reaction to penicillin can use a first-generation cephalosporin for treatment, whereas those with anaphylactoid reactions to penicillin may be treated with vancomycin. There are some reports of using oral therapy to treat endocarditis, especially for IVDUs. In a study in 44 IVDUs, the use of rifampin with ciprofloxacin was compared with parenteral treatment. The study showed no significant difference in treatment failures. Therefore oral therapy involving rifampin with ciprofloxacin may be considered as a therapeutic option [10].

For patients with documented endocarditis due to MRSA, vancomycin is the mainstay of treatment, and this should continue for at least 4 to 6 weeks. If patients are intolerant to vancomycin or seem to be failing therapy with this agent, then antimicrobials, such as daptomycin, linezolid, or quinupristin–dalfopristin, may be tried though randomized controlled trials are lacking to support this approach.

For MSSA endocarditis, combination antibiotic therapy is useful for the first 3 to 5 days of therapy. However, in endocarditis caused by MRSA, monotherapy should suffice. Patients should be treated for a sufficient length of time to ensure clearing of bacteremia and clinical improvement.

Viridans and other streptococci

Viridans and other streptococci commonly cause native-valve endocarditis seen in clinical practice. They are usually susceptible to penicillin. If the organism is proven to have a minimum inhibitory concentration (MIC) of

<0.12 µg/mL to penicillin showing that it is sensitive, monotherapy with an intravenous β-lactam agent for 4 to 6 weeks is advised. In cases where the organism has a higher MIC to penicillin and shows intermediate susceptibility, an intravenous β-lactam agent for 4 to 6 weeks should be combined with an aminoglycoside (given for the first 2 weeks of treatment) for effective therapy. Patients with nonanaphylactoid penicillin allergy may be treated with ceftriaxone as once-daily monotherapy for 4 to 6 weeks. Patients with more serious allergies may be given vancomycin or desensitization to penicillin may be considered.

Intravenous penicillin G remains the treatment of choice for penicillin-sensitive *Streptococcus pneumoniae* and *Streptococcus pyogenes* endocarditis. In cases where penicillin cannot be given, whether due to resistance, intolerance, or allergy, vancomycin may be used.

Enterococci

The enterococci generally have a low-level resistance to penicillin and, as such, ampicillin or vancomycin should be the mainstay treatment. Most cases of enterococcal endocarditis are caused by *Enterococcus faecalis*, which are sensitive to ampicillin. These patients should be treated with ampicillin and gentamicin. Vancomycin should be considered for those patients with a resistant organism or penicillin allergy, in which case desensitization may be considered. Treatment is recommended for at least 4 weeks, and if vancomycin is used, treatment is recommended for 6 weeks because vancomycin intrinsically has decreased activity against the enterococci. Occasionally, these organisms exhibit high-level aminoglycoside, penicillin, or vancomycin resistance, in which case other agents may be used, after consultation with an infectious-disease specialist.

Coagulase-negative staphylococci

Most cases of prosthetic-valve endocarditis are caused by coagulase-negative staphylococci, and these are usually methicillin-resistant. Antibiotic treatment of endocarditis due to these organisms is identical to the treatment of endocarditis caused by MRSA. These cases often need to be treated for a longer duration than native-valve endocarditis. In prosthetic-valve endocarditis, surgical consultation is of critical importance because these infections (unlike uncomplicated native-valve endocarditis) cannot be successfully treated with antibiotics alone.

Rifampin can be added in the setting of prosthetic-valve endocarditis because data suggest that this agent kills staphylococci that are adherent to foreign material. The β-lactam or vancomycin and aminoglycoside should ideally be in place for 3 to 5 days before the rifampin is begun to minimize the development of resistance.

HACEK organisms

The HACEK organisms include *Haemophilus influenzae*, *Haemophilus parainfluenzae*, *Actinobacillus actinomycetemcomitans*, *Cardiobacterium hominis*, *Eikenella corrodens*, and *Kingella kingae*. These are fastidious gram-negative bacilli that cause approximately 5% to 10% of all native-valve endocarditis in non-IVDUs. If automated blood-culture detection methods are used, then longer incubation of blood cultures is not necessary. Many of these organisms now produce ß-lactamase but remain quite sensitive to third-generation cephalosporins. Therapeutic options per the American Heart Association (AHA) guidelines [11] include monotherapy with ceftriaxone, ampicillin–sulbactam, or even ciprofloxacin for 4 weeks.

If other causes of traditionally "culture-negative" endocarditis are being considered, empiric therapy should be given with a combination of agents that cover both gram-positive and gram-negative organisms. Suggestions per the AHA guidelines include using ampicillin–sulbactam plus gentamicin, or vancomycin plus ciprofloxacin for 4 to 6 weeks while a workup ensues. If endocarditis due to a gram-negative organism is confirmed, combination therapy with a synergistic regimen should be used.

In summary, the causative organism, once isolated, should guide endocarditis therapy (Table 1). Treatment should be sufficient to ensure clearing of bacteremia and clinical improvement. If aminoglycoside is used for synergy and combination therapy, patients should be monitored for clinical signs of nephrotoxicity and levels should be followed, with doses adjusted accordingly. Based on a meta-analysis done of comparator studies, limited evidence supports the addition of an aminoglycoside to a β-lactam for treatment of endocarditis caused by gram-positive cocci [12]. Followup or

Table 1
Summary recommendations for endocarditis therapy

Organism	First-line antibiotics	Duration
Methicillin-sensitive S aureus	Nafcillin plus gentamicin; or oxacillin plus gentamicin	6 weeks[a] with gentamicin for the first 3–5 days
Methicillin-resistant S aureus	Vancomycin	4–6 weeks
Viridans streptococci and other streptococci	Intravenous β-lactam with or without aminoglycoside	4–6 weeks; if aminoglycoside used, give for first 2 weeks of therapy
Enterococci	Ampicillin plus gentamicin	4–6 weeks
Coagulase-negative staphylococci	Vancomycin	6 weeks[a] with gentamicin for the first 3–5 days
HACEK organisms	Ceftriaxone; or ampicillin–sulbactam	4 weeks
"Culture-negative"	Ampicillin–sulbactam plus gentamicin; or vancomycin plus ciprofloxacin	4–6 weeks

[a] Treat for 2 weeks if uncomplicated right-sided endocarditis.

surveillance blood cultures should be done periodically while on antibiotic therapy. Patients should be monitored for signs of clinical deterioration with prompt surgical evaluation as necessary.

Diverticulitis

Diverticulitis involves microscopic or larger perforation of a diverticulum in the intestine. Most cases are uncomplicated and respond well to medical therapy alone. However, sometimes cases of diverticulitis are complicated by perforation, obstruction, abscess, or fistula. Most of these patients require surgical intervention in addition to antibiotic therapy for effective treatment.

If patients with uncomplicated diverticulitis are reliable and able to tolerate oral medications, oral antibiotic therapy is reasonable. Antibiotic choices should have activity against gastrointestinal flora, namely gram-negative and anaerobic organisms, as first priority. Appropriate agents in this setting include a fluoroquinolone with metronidazole, or amoxicillin–clavulanate, or trimethoprim–sulfamethoxazole with metronidazole. Seven to 10 days of therapy should suffice. If, however, patients require hospitalization or have complicated disease, parenteral coverage becomes important. The same causative organisms need to be targeted. Monotherapy with piperacillin–tazobactam or the use of imipenem–cilastatin may be given, but the combination of ampicillin, gentamicin, and metronidazole can also be effective [13]. A regimen should be chosen and started empirically in these situations, as microbiologic data often cannot be obtained. Monotherapy with moxifloxacin may be considered [14]. Tigecycline is also a novel agent currently approved for the treatment of intra-abdominal infections [15].

Pneumonia

Community-acquired pneumonia (CAP) is a common infectious process that is a significant cause of morbidity. Primary-care and specialty physicians alike encounter patients with CAP. A variety of different pathogens may be responsible for the clinical syndrome. Thus, management issues are also different for each case. Therapy is often empiric, as clinical presentation and radiographic findings may not identify a specific etiology of infection.

If the patient shows no signs of systemic toxicity, is able to maintain adequate oral intake, has good functional status, and will be compliant with medications and follow-up, outpatient management with oral antibiotics can be considered. The patient's clinical presentation and prior antibiotic therapies should be assessed before making therapeutic commitments. Patients who exhibit signs of more advanced illness should be hospitalized and treated with parenteral antibiotics.

Outpatients who are otherwise healthy can be treated with a macrolide, such as erythromycin, azithromycin, or clarithromycin, as monotherapy, or doxycycline. Those who have had recent antibiotic exposure may be offered a fluoroquinolone alone (levofloxacin, moxifloxacin, or gatifloxacin), or amoxicillin–clavulanate, or the combinations of azithromycin or clarithromycin plus high-dose amoxicillin. Although the fluoroquinolones offer convenient once-daily dosing, there are issues with increasing resistance among isolates to this class of agents. If the patient has comorbidities that put him or her at risk for infection with other organisms, antibiotics with broader coverage should be given. For example, if there is no history of prior antibiotic exposures, monotherapy with azithromycin or clarithromycin, or a fluoroquinolone may be offered. If there is history of prior antibiotic therapy, then azithromycin or clarithromycin plus a β-lactam should be offered, although, again, monotherapy with a fluoroquinolone remains an option here as well. If an aspiration component is suspected, therapy should include either amoxicillin–clavulanate or clindamycin [16].

Inpatients who are not admitted to the intensive care unit requiring treatment of CAP should be offered azithromycin or clarithromycin plus a β-lactam agent. Respiratory fluoroquinolones may be offered as monotherapy also, though concern over resistance has limited this approach. If patients are in the intensive are unit and pseudomonas infection is a concern, then an antipseudomonal agent plus ciprofloxacin, or an antipseudomonal agent plus an aminoglycoside plus a respiratory fluoroquinolone or a macrolide may be used. In this setting, if the patient has a serious allergy to β-lactams, either aztreonam plus levofloxacin, or aztreonam plus moxifloxacin or gatifloxacin, with or without an aminoglycoside, may be used. If pseudomonas infection is not an issue, the antibiotic regimens described earlier can be offered. If the patient has a serious β-lactam allergy in this situation, a respiratory fluoroquinolone plus clindamycin may be used. Patients who have been exposed to a nursing home should be treated following the same guidelines. However, in these patients, amoxicillin–clavulanate plus a macrolide (or a respiratory fluoroquinolone alone) is an appropriate alternative.

Efforts should be made at obtaining a microbiologic diagnosis either with sputum cultures, blood cultures, or other more invasive measures if necessary, depending on the clinical course, so that antibiotic management can be pathogen directed. Drug-resistant organisms, especially drug-resistant pneumococcus, are a concern. Therefore careful assessment is necessary to ensure optimal treatment. Telithromycin, a new agent in the ketolide class, may be used in the treatment of resistant pneumococcal pneumonia. However, concerns regarding widespread use of this drug mirror those regarding the extensive use of fluoroquinolones, in that resistant strains may emerge, limiting future treatment options. Reports of potential hepatotoxicity related to telithromycin may be another concern.

Meningitis

Bacterial meningitis is a medical emergency that can be rapidly fatal. Swift diagnosis and initiation of broad, empiric treatment remain the keys to survival.

Once the diagnosis is suspected and proper history, physical examination, and diagnostic workup, including lumbar puncture, have been initiated, empiric antibiotic therapy must be given. Ideally, a Gram stain of cerebrospinal fluid is available to help guide therapy. In many cases, however, this useful information is not readily available. Nonetheless, antibiotic therapy should be started without delay once initial microbiology samples are obtained. The antibiotics chosen should be bactericidal and able to cross the blood–brain barrier to enter the cerebrospinal fluid.

Empiric therapy should cover most of the common causes of bacterial meningitis. Third-generation cephalosporins, such as cefotaxime (2 g intravenous every 6 hours) and ceftriaxone (2 g intravenous twice daily) have become the mainstay of initial therapy for bacterial meningitis. These agents treat many of the common culprit organisms with the exception of *Listeria monocytogenes*. If this organism is suspected, then penicillin G (4 million units intravenous every 4 hours) or ampicillin (2 g intravenous every 4 hours) plus gentamicin for synergy must be added for appropriate coverage. Because of the increase in penicillin-resistant *S pneumoniae* cases, vancomycin is often added to empiric therapy until identification and susceptibility of the causative organism is available [17]. Vancomycin does not have reliable cerebrospinal fluid penetration and is generally not recommended as monotherapy for pneumococcal meningitis. In most cases of bacterial meningitis, initial combination therapy is recommended, with modifications in the antibiotic regimen once further culture information becomes available. Meningitis due to gram-negative organisms is rare in the community setting but occurs more commonly in nosocomial cases. When this occurs, organism-directed therapy employing combination agents or even intrathecal gentamicin may be needed.

Summary

In summary, several treatment options are available for patients with these common infectious diseases (Table 2). When empiric treatment is needed, combination therapy is often advised, with subsequent modification of antibiotic therapy once further information becomes available. In all cases, the potential risk/benefit of combination therapy versus monotherapy must be considered. If hospitalized patients are treated with parenteral antibiotics, they should be switched to an oral regimen once clinical improvement occurs, if appropriate. Regimens should be simple and cost-effective, with consideration given to the diagnosis, clinical response, patient

Table 2
Summary recommendations for common infections

Disease	First-line antibiotics
Cellulitis	
Outpatient	Cephalexin
Erysipelas	Cephalexin
Gram-negative pathogen	Levofloxacin; gatifloxacin; or moxifloxacin
Methicillin-resistant *S aureus*	Trimethoprim–sulfamethoxazole; clindamycin; or vancomycin
Hospitalized	Cefazolin
Osteomyelitis	
Empiric, not limb threatening	Cephalexin; clindamycin; or ciprofloxacin
Empiric, limb threatening	Ciprofloxacin plus clindamycin; ampicillin–sulbactam; or piperacillin–tazobactam
Methicillin-resistant *S aureus*	Vancomycin
Neutropenic fever	
Outpatient empiric therapy	Amoxicillin–clavulanate plus ciprofloxacin
Initial inpatient empiric therapy	Cefepime; or ceftazidime
Methicillin-resistant *S aureus*	Vancomycin
Fever persisting after 3–5 days; no identified cause of infection	Add antifungal
Confirmed gram-negative pathogen	Consider aminoglycoside
Diverticulitis	
Outpatient, uncomplicated	Amoxicillin–clavulanate; or fluoroquinolone plus metronidazole; or trimethoprim–sulfamethoxazole plus metronidazole
Inpatient, complicated	Piperacillin–tazobactam; or imipenem–cilastatin; or ampicillin plus gentamicin plus metronidazole
Pneumonia	
Outpatient	Macrolide; or fluoroquinolone
Inpatient	Macrolide plus β-lactam
Nursing home patient	May use fluoroquinolone; or amoxicillin–clavulanate
Meningitis	
Initial empiric therapy	Ceftriaxone
Penicillin-resistant *S pneumoniae* or methicillin-resistant *S aureus*	Vancomycin
Listeria monocytogenes	Ampicilllin

compliance, and ease of administration. The topic of combination therapy versus monotherapy continues to evolve.

References

[1] Stevens DL, Bisno AL, Chamber HF, et al. Practice guidelines from the Infectious Diseases Society of America. Clin Infect Dis 2005. Available at: http://www.journals.uchicago.edu/IDSA/guidelines/. Accessed March 22, 2006.
[2] Ellis-Grosse EJ, Babinchak T, Dartois N, et al. The efficacy and safety of tigecycline in the treatment of skin and skin-structure infections: results of 2 double-blind phase 3 comparison studies with vancomycin-aztreonam. Clin Infect Dis 2005;41(Suppl 5):S341.

[3] Lipsky BA, Pecoraro RE, Larson SA, et al. Outpatient management of uncomplicated lower-extremity infections in diabetic patients. Arch Intern Med 1990;150:790.

[4] Lipsky BA, Berendt AR, Deery HG, et al. Diagnosis and treatment of diabetic foot infections. Clin Infect Dis 2004;39:885–910.

[5] Hughes WT, Armstrong D, Bodey GP, et al. 2002 guidelines for the use of antimicrobial agents in neutropenic patients with cancer. Clin Infect Dis 2002;34:730–51.

[6] Harter C, Schulze B, Goldschmidt H, et al. Piperacillin/tazobactam vs ceftazidime in the treatment of neutropenic fever in patients with acute leukemia or following autologous peripheral blood stem cell transplantation: a prospective randomized trial. Bone Marrow Transplant 2006;37(4):373–9.

[7] Carozza A, DeSanto LS, Romano G, et al. Infective endocarditis in intravenous drug abusers: patterns of presentation and long-term outcomes of surgical treatment. J Heart Valve Dis 2006;15(1):125–31.

[8] Le T, Bayer AS. Combination antibiotic therapy for infective endocarditis. Clin Infect Dis 2003;36:615–21.

[9] Korzeniowski O, Sande MA. National Collaborative Endocarditis Study Group. Combination antimicrobial therapy for Staphylococcus aureus endocarditis in patients addicted to parenteral drugs and in nonaddicts: a prospective study. Ann Intern Med 1982;97:496.

[10] Heldman AW, Hartert TV, Ray SC, et al. Oral antibiotic treatment of right-sided staphylococcal endocarditis in injection drug users: prospective randomized comparison with parenteral therapy. Am J Med 1996;101:68.

[11] Baddour LM, Wilson WR, Bayer AS, et al. Infective endocarditis diagnosis, antimicrobial therapy, and management of complications: a statement for healthcare professionals from the Committee on Rheumatic Fever, Endocarditis, and Kawasaki Disease, Council on Cardiovascular Disease in the Young, and Councils on Clinical Cardiology, Stroke, and Cardiovascular Surgery and Anesthesia, American Heart Association: endorsed by the Infectious Diseases Society of America. Circulation 2005;111:e394–434. Available at: http://circ.ahajournals.org/cgi/content/full/111/23/e394. Accessed March 24, 2006.

[12] Falagas ME, Matthaiou DK, Bliziotis IA. The role of aminoglycosides in combination with a beta-lactam for the treatment of bacterial endocarditis: a meta-analysis of comparative trials. J Antimicrob Chemother 2006;57(4):639–47.

[13] Solomkin JS, Mazuski JE, Baron EJ, et al. Guidelines for the selection of anti-infective agents for complicated intra-abdominal infections. Clin Infect Dis 2003;37:997–1005.

[14] Goldstein EJ, Citron DM, Warren YA, et al. In vitro activity of moxifloxacin against 923 anaerobes isolated from human intra-abdominal infections. Antimicrob Agents Chemother 2006;50(1):148–55.

[15] Olivia ME, Rekha A, Yellin A, et al. A multicenter trial of the efficacy and safety of tigecycline versus imipenem/cilastatin in patients with complicated intra-abdominal infections. BMC Infect Dis 2005;5:88.

[16] Mandell LA, Bartlett JG, Dowell SF, et al. Update of practice guidelines for the management of community-acquired pneumonia in immunocompetent adults. Clin Infect Dis 2003;37:1405–33.

[17] Tunkel AR, Hartman BJ, Kaplan SL, et al. Practice guidelines for the management of bacterial meningitis. Clin Infect Dis 2004;39:1267–84.

ELSEVIER
SAUNDERS

THE MEDICAL
CLINICS
OF NORTH AMERICA

Med Clin N Am 90 (2006) 1197–1222

Oral Antibiotic Therapy of Serious Systemic Infections

Burke A. Cunha, MD

Infectious Disease Division, Winthrop-University Hospital, Mineola, NY 11501, USA

Antimicrobial therapy for serious systemic infections has been treated via the parenteral or oral route. Traditionally, serious systemic infections have been treated initially with intravenous antibiotics. Intravenously (IV) administered antibiotics rapidly achieve therapeutic blood/tissue concentrations, desirable in individuals with serious systemic infection. For serious systemic infections, the intramuscular (IM) route of antibiotic administration may result in lower but prolonged peak serum/tissue concentrations. Patients in shock due to a systemic infection have an increased in splanchnic blood flow at the expense of peripheral perfusion. IM administration of antibiotics in patients in shock therefore may be suboptimal. For these reasons, IV administration of an antibiotic for septic shock is the preferred route of antibiotic administration.

Because parenteral antibiotics have traditionally been viewed as more rapid/more potent than their oral counterparts, IV antibiotic therapy for serious and nonlife-threatening infections became common practice. Early in the development of antimicrobials, there were relatively few oral antibiotics available for serious systemic infections, for example, chloramphenicol. In the early decades of antibiotic use, the spectrum of activity, determination of therapeutic dose/dosing interval, and side effect profile were the main concerns in antibiotic therapy. Early in the 1960s, pharmacokinetic (PK) considerations, and more recently, pharmacodynamic (PD) considerations have been helpful in optimizing antimicrobial therapy. Bioavailability, that is, the percentage of drug absorbed became an important PK parameter, particularly for antibiotics with IV and oral (PO) formulations [1–3].

medical.theclinics.com

Overview of oral antibiotic therapy

Antibiotic bioavailability

Bioavailability is a key determinant in selecting an antibiotic for oral therapy. Orally administered antibiotics may be divided into three categories based upon their oral bioavailability. In the first category are antibiotics that are not well absorbed and have low bioavailability, making them unsuitable oral agents for use in serious systemic infections. Some of these antimicrobials are not well absorbed orally, and concentrate in particular compartments/body fluids, making them useful for selected indications, that is, methenamine salts and nitrofurantoin are only available orally, are not present in the serum, achieve no systemic therapeutically useful concentrations, but concentrate in the urine of the lower urinary tract. The second category of oral antibiotics are those that have an acceptably good oral bioavailability, such that although blood and tissue concentrations are not equal using their IV counterparts, therapeutic concentrations well in excess of that needed for therapeutic effectiveness are readily achieved, for example, use of oral cephalexin versus cefazolin for skin/soft tissue infections. The third category of orally available antibiotics are those with high bioavailability, that is, $\geq 90\%$ absorption when administered orally. These agents are ideal for oral antimicrobial therapy for the treatment of nonlife-threatening and serious systemic infections due to susceptible organisms, for example, trimethoprim-sulfamethoxazole (TMP-SMX), quinolones, doxycycline, minocycline, chloramphenicol, linezolid. Oral antibiotics suitable for the treatment of serious systemic infections are those that have acceptably good or excellent bioavailability, and a spectrum appropriate for the infection and target site being treated [4–6].

Oral absorption in the critically ill

Even in critically ill patients, oral antibiotics with good/excellent bioavailability are rapidly/well absorbed and achieve blood/target tissue levels, within an hour after administration. Even in patients with diabetes mellitus, with glycosylated capillaries/gastric paresis, absorption is approximately the same as in normal individuals [7,8]. Unless a patient presents in septic shock, oral therapy may be used in place of intravenous therapy if an oral antibiotic with an appropriate spectrum for the presumed pathogens of the infection is available and can be administered orally, that is, per os, per nasogastric tube, or per percutaneous enteroscopic gastroscopy tube. When oral antibiotics with good/excellent bioavailability and the appropriate spectrum are used for serious systemic infections, it is important to realize that blood/target tissue levels are approximately the same as their IV counterpart, that is, levofloxacin or moxifloxacin administered orally achieve the same blood/target tissue levels as the same dose when administered intravenously at the same dose [9–15].

Oral/intravenous therapeutic equivalence

There is no advantage to using antibiotics IV that are available PO and have high bioavailability, because the blood/target tissue concentrations are the same with either the IV or PO formulation, for example, doxycycline, minocycline, TMP-SMX. Except for patients *in extremis* that are critically ill, nearly all patients capable of oral absorption may be treated with PO antibiotics if a PO antibiotic provides the suitable spectrum/tissue penetration appropriate for the infection being treated is available. Patients should no longer be admitted "for IV therapy," which presumes that IV therapy is more effective than well-chosen equivalent PO antibiotic therapy. Except for patients in shock or with impaired gastrointestinal absorption, there is no advantage to use IV therapy if an appropriate oral agent is available suitable to treat the infection [1–3,6,16] (Box 1).

Intravenous → oral switch therapy

Physicians are creatures of habit, and old habits die hard. Because IV therapy was first used for serious systemic infections, and many infections susceptible to IV antibiotics, intravenously administered antibiotics became the preferred mode of antibiotic administration. As pharmacokinetic

---

Box 1. Requirements of an oral antibiotic for serious systemic infections

Antibiotic Factors
- Select an oral antibiotic formulation that has a *high degree of activity against presumed/known pathogens.*
- Select an oral antibiotic *with high bioavailability that approximates intravenous serum/tissue concentrations.*
- Select an oral antibiotic therapy with a *"low resistance" potential* against the presumed/known pathogens.
- Select an oral antibiotic that is *well tolerated* with a *good safety profile.*

Host Factors
- Patients with serious systemic infections may be treated with an oral antibiotic *when therapeutic effect desired in >1 hour.* (If therapeutic effect needed in <1 hour, begin therapy IV.)
- Patient able to *sufficiently absorb an oral antibiotic* (absorption approximately normal in critically ill patients).
- Avoid in patients with impaired gastrointestinal absorption.

Adapted from Cunha BA. Antibiotic essentials. 5th edition. Royal Oak (MI): Physicians' Press; 2006.

parameters became known and accepted, physicians began to use PO antibiotic therapy as part of the antibiotic regimen. The past 2 decades there has been a dramatic increase in "transitional antibiotic therapy," also known as "IV to PO switch therapy" to treat a wide variety of infectious diseases [4,17]. As experience and confidence using IV to PO switch programs has increased, IV to PO switch therapy has become accepted to treat infectious diseases. The efficacy of IV to PO switch therapy was well shown in a landmark study of community-acquired pneumonia (CAP). In this study, patients were divided into groups with different durations of IV therapy for CAP. CAP was treated for 2 weeks; 14 days of IV therapy was comparable to patients treated initially for 2 to 3 days IV and completed with 11 days PO. Not surprisingly, the CAP results/outcomes were exactly the same. Importantly, nearly all of antimicrobial therapy could be given PO with no sacrifice of therapeutic efficacy [18].

As more antibiotics have become available with appropriate spectrum to treat serious systemic infections, IV to PO switch therapy is used for many infectious diseases at the present time. Astute clinicians realized if using equivalent IV and PO antibiotics (1/7 IV and 6/7 PO) for the duration of therapy, why not use oral only antibiotic therapy for the full duration of therapy? If 11 to 12 days of PO therapy plus 2 to 3 days of IV therapy is equivalent to 14 days of IV therapy, then 14 days of oral therapy, not different, are essentially the same [1,6,16,18] (Box 2).

Advantages of oral antibiotic therapy

The use of entirely oral antibiotic therapy for serious systemic infections has increased slowly over time. Some physicians still have difficulty conceptually switching from IV therapy to IV to PO switch therapy. Expectedly, if one is not an infectious disease clinician with expertise in antimicrobial therapy, there remains some reluctance to rely solely on PO therapy for therapy of serious systemic infections. Over time, as familiarity and experience has been accrued, there has been a gradual acceptance in using oral therapy for serious infections.

The use of PO therapy or as part of IV to PO switch therapy for the entire duration of antimicrobial therapy has several important advantages over IV therapy [4,17]. First, PO therapy is less expensive than its IV equivalent. For all antibiotics that are available IV and PO, the PO formulation, at the same dose, is always much less expensive than the IV formulation. Oral therapy is always less expensive than its IV equivalent in terms of acquisition cost. IV administered antibiotics also have an IV administration fee, which nationally averages approximately $10 per IV dose. With some antibiotics, the cost of administration can exceed the cost of the antibiotic itself. There are other advantages to PO antimicrobial therapy, which includes decreasing hospital length of stay (LOS) [4,6]. In the era of managed health care, LOS is an important economic consideration. Two different antibiotics

---

Box 2. Oral antibiotic therapy for serious systemic infections

Oral Antibiotic Therapy
Preferred in all patients *except:*
- *Critically ill patients when therapeutic serum/tissue concentrations are needed in <1 hour* of antibiotic administration
- Patients with *impaired gastrointestinal absorption*
- Patients *unable to take oral medications*

Intravenous antibiotic therapy
- Preferred in patients with *life-threatening infections or septic shock*
- For patients *NPO/without NG/PEG tube*
- For patients with *impaired GI absorption*
- *No oral antibiotic equivalent available*

IV → PO switch therapy
- *Any infectious disease treated initially with intravenous antibiotics followed by oral antibiotics* (IV → PO antibiotic switch therapy) *may be treated entirely via the oral route for the duration of therapy* (unless as listed above under intravenous therapy).

Abbreviations: GI, gastrointestinal; NG, nasogastric; NPO, nil per orum; PEG, percutaneous endoscopic gastrostomy.
Adapted from Cunha BA. Antibiotic essentials. 5th edition. Royal Oak (MI): Physicians' Press; 2006.

---

may be used to treat a specific infectious disease, and one is associated with a shorter length of stay; then that antibiotic may be preferable purely from an administration/economic perspective. Another advantage of PO antimicrobial therapy is the obvious elimination of phlebitis and IV-line infections. Obviously, PO-administered antibiotics are not complicated by IV lines, decreasing not only IV-related complications, but also those related to a prolonged hospital stay sometimes uses the justification for IV therapy. Well selected oral antimicrobial therapy for selected serious systemic infections can largely eliminate the need for home-administered antibiotics via peripherally inserted central catheters (PICC lines) [4,6,17] (Table 1).

Serious infections traditionally treated with oral antibiotics

Because there is virtually no difference between PO and IV therapy, there are important pharmacoeconomic and clinical reasons to rely more on PO therapy for most infectious diseases including serious systemic infections.

Table 1
Clinical and pharmacoeconomic advantages of oral antibiotic therapy

	Advantages	Disadvantages
Oral antibiotic therapy	• Lower *antibiotic acquisition cost* • *No IV antibiotic administration costs* • *Rapid gastrointestinal absorption* (~1 h) even in critically ill patients • *Eliminates IV-line infections* • *Decreased length of hospital stay* (LOS) • *Earlier discharge*	• Should *not* be used in those with impaired gastrointestinal absorption • *If therapeutic effect is <1 h* (patient in shock), begin therapy intravenously (IV)

Adapted from Cunha BA. Antibiotic essentials. 5th edition. Royal Oak, (MI): Physicians' Press; 2006.

The serious systemic infectious diseases that readily lend themselves to treatment entirely via the oral route, or less desirably but acceptably as part of an IV to PO switch regimen, include febrile neutropenia, severe CAP requiring hospitalization, nosocomial/ventilator-associated pneumonia (NP/VAP), *S viridans* subacute bacterial endocarditis (SBE), and *Staphylococcus aureus* acute bacterial endocarditis (ABE) [1,3,6]. Other serious systemic infectious diseases have been being treated via the oral route, for example, osteomyelitis, anthrax, plague, enteric fevers [16,19–27] (Table 2).

This is the era of oral antimicrobial therapy. Nearly all infectious diseases may be treated with appropriate antibiotics entirely via the oral route or orally for most of an IV to PO switch program [1–3,6]. Except in patients in shock where initial IV therapy is preferred, oral antimicrobial therapy will increasingly be the mainstay of antimicrobial prescribing worldwide, and in those who are NPO or who have impaired GI absorption [6,9–15].

Oral antibiotic selection of serious systemic infections

Factors in oral antibiotic selection

Therapeutically, the selection of an oral antibiotic may conveniently be considered as being in two categories, that is, in those where equivalent IV and PO formulations exist that have a high bioavailability and an appropriate spectrum for the treatment of infection, and the other group of all antibiotics that have good bioavailability and are equivalent in spectrum to IV antibiotics that have no PO formulation. For these patients, the clinician must select and IV equivalent PO antibiotic usually from a different antibiotic class than the IV antibiotic, to achieve comparable therapeutic equivalence [1,5,6,17].

There are many important antibiotics that are used for serious systemic infections that have no currently available oral formulation, for example, imipenem, ertapenem, meropenem, quinupristin/dalfopristin, tigecycline,

Table 2
Traditional oral antibiotic therapy of some serious systemic infectious diseases

Acute infections	Subacute/chronic infections
Anthrax	Q fever
Plague	Brucellosis
Tularemia	Leptospirosis
Rocky Mountain spotted fever (RMSF)	Nocardia
Typhoid fever	Actinomycosis
Legionnaires' disease	Melioidosis
Diphtheria	Bartonella
Vibrio vulnificus	Lung abscesses
Cholera	Liver abscesses
Clostridium difficile	Intraabdominal abscesses
Pneumocystis (jiroveci) carinii pneumonia (PCP)	Pelvic abscesses
Malaria	Renal abscesses
	Sinusitis
	Pyelonephritis
	Prostatitis
	Complicated skin/soft tissue infections (cSSSI)
	Osteomyelitis
	Pulmonary and extrapulmonary TB

Abbreviation: TB, tuberculosis.
Adapted from Cunha BA. Antibiotic essentials. 5th edition. Royal Oak (MI): Physicians' Press; 2006.

daptomycin. Excluding feropenem, there are no oral carbapenems, mono-bactams, or aminoglycosides currently available, depending on the pathogen in a particular infection; oral quinolones have good bioavailability and are effective against many of the organisms effectively covered by carbapenems and aminoglycosides. Quinupristin/dalfopristin, tigecycline, and daptomy-cin are primarily used to treat infections due to resistant Gram-positive cocci, that is, methicillin-resistant *S aureus* (MRSA) or most strains of van-comycin-resistant enterococci (VRE) [2,3,6].

The oral equivalents that may be used to treat MRSA infections initially with one of these antibiotics are linezolid and minocycline [28,29]. The oral equivalents of these antibiotics to treat VRE infections include doxycycline, chloramphenicol, and linezolid. Some antibiotics have an IV and PO formu-lation, but for systemic infections being treated, the PO formulation is inad-equately absorbed, and therefore is unsuitable for IV to PO switch or the only PO treatment of serious infections, for example, vancomycin formula-tions, are available IV/PO, but only IV vancomycin is useful for systemic in-fections, and PO vancomycin use is confined to the treatment of *Clostridium difficile* diarrhea [1,6]. Obviously, because carefully selected PO antibiotic therapy is therapeutically equivalent to IV antibiotic therapy, the duration of therapy for PO and IV therapy for any given infection are the same (Table 3).

Table 3
Intravenous and equivalent oral counterparts

IV antibiotic (usual dose)	Target pathogen	Oral antibiotic (usual dose)	Oral bioavailability	Peak serum concentration
Penicillins				
Penicillin G	S. viridans, nongroup D streptococci	Amoxicillin	90%	16 µg/mL
10 MU (IV) q4h				
Ampicillin	VSE	1 g (PO) q8h		
2 g (IV) q4h				
Antistaphylococcal penicillins				
Nafcillin	MSSA	Cephalexin 1 g (PO) q6h	99%	36 µg/mL
2 g (IV) q4h		Moxifloxacin 400 mg (PO) q24h	90%	4.5 µg/mL
Oxacillin		Levofloxacin 750 mg (PO) q24h	99%	8 µg/mL
2 g (IV) q4h		Gatifloxacin 400 mg (PO) q24h	96%	4.2 µg/mL
		Telithromycin 800 mg (PO) q24h	57%	2.2 µg/mL
Aminoglycosides				
Gentamicin	P aeruginosa, GNB	Levofloxacin 750 mg (PO) q24h	70%	2.9 µg/mL
240 mg (IV) q24h				
Tobramycin	P aeruginosa, GNB	Ciprofloxacin 750 mg (PO) q12h	90%	8 µg/mL
240 mg (IV) q24h				
Amikacin	P aeruginosa, GNB			
1 g (IV) q24h				
1st generation cephalosporin				
Cefazolin	MSSA, Klebsiella	Cephalexin 1 g (PO) q6h	99%	36 µg/mL
1 g (IV) q8h				

IV drug	Usual organisms	Oral switch	%	Serum conc.
2nd generation cephalosporin				
Cefuroxime 1.5 g (IV) q8h	MSSA, Klebsiella, H influenzae	Cefprozil 500 mg (PO) q12h	95%	10 μg/mL
3rd generation cephalosporins				
Ceftriaxone 1–2 g (IV) q12–24h				
Cefotaxime 2 g (IV) q6h	MSSA, GNB	TMP-SMX 1 ss tablet (PO) q6h	99%	8 μg/mL
		Levofloxacin 750 mg (PO) q24h	99%	8 μg/mL
Ceftizoxime 2 g (IV) q8h	MSSA, GNB, B fragilis	Moxifloxacin 400 mg (PO) q24h	90%	4.5 μg/mL
Cefoperazone 2 g (IV) q12h				
4th generation cephalosporin				
Cefepime 2 g (IV) q12h	P aeruginosa, GNB	Levofloxacin 750 mg (PO) q24h	99%	9 μg/mL
		Ciprofloxacin 750 mg (PO) q12h	70%	2.9 μg/mL
Monobactam				
Aztreonam 2 g (IV) q8h	P aeruginosa, GNB	Levofloxacin 750 mg (PO) q12h	99%	9 μg/mL
		Ciprofloxacin 750 mg (PO) q24h	70%	2.9 μg/mL
Carbapenems				
Meropenem 500 mg (IV) q8h	P aeruginosa, GNB	Levofloxacin 750 mg (PO) q24h	70%	8 μg/mL
		Ciprofloxacin 750 mg (PO) q12h	90%	2.9 μg/mL
	MSSA, VSE, B fragilis	Moxifloxacin 400 mg (PO) q24h	99%	4.5 μg/mL

(continued on next page)

Table 3 (*continued*)

IV antibiotic (usual dose)	Target pathogen	Oral antibiotic (usual dose)	Oral bioavailability	Peak serum concentration
Imipenem 500 mg (IV) q6h	MSSA, VSE, GNB, *B fragilis*	Moxifloxacin 400 mg (PO) q24h	90%	4.5 µg/mL
Ertapenem 1 g (IV) q24h	MSSA, VSE, GNB, *B fragilis*	Moxifloxacin 400 mg (PO) q24h	90%	4.5 µg/mL
MRSA antibiotics				
Vancomycin 1 g (IV) 12h	MSSA, MRSA, VSE, VRE	Minocycline 100 mg (PO) q12h	95%	4 µg/mL
Quinupristin/dalfopristin 7.5 mg/kg (IV) q8h	MSSA, MRSA, VRE	Linezolid 600 mg (PO) q12h	100%	20 µg/mL
Daptomycin 6 mg/kg (IV) q24h	MSSA, MRSA, VSE, VRE			
Tigecycline 100 mg (IV) x 1 dose then 50 mg (IV) q12h	MSSA, MRSA, VSE, VRE			
Antipseudomonal Penicillins				
Ticarcillin 3 g (IV) q6h	*P aeruginosa*	Levofloxacin 750 mg (PO) q24h	99%	8 µg/mL
Piperacillin 4 g (IV) q4h	*P aeruginosa*	Ciprofloxacin 750 mg (PO) q12h	70%	2.9 µg/mL
VRE Antibiotics				
Quinupristin/dalfopristin 7.5 mg/kg (IV) q8h	VRE	Doxycycline 100 mg (PO) q12h	70%	2.9 µg/mL
Daptomycin 12 mg/kg (IV) q24h	VRE	Chloramphenicol 500 mg (PO) q6h	90%	9 µg/mL
Tigecycline 100 mg (IV) x 1 dose then 50 mg (IV) q12h	VRE	Linezolid 600 mg (PO) q12h	100%	20 µg/mL

IV dose	Spectrum	PO dose	%	Serum level
Linezolid 600 mg (IV) q12h	VRE			
Tetracyclines				
Doxycycline 100 mg (IV) q12h	CAP pathogens, CA-MRSA, VRE, *B fragilis*	Doxycycline 100 mg (PO) q12h	93%	4 µg/mL
Minocycline 100 mg (IV) q12h	MSSA, HA-MRSA *B fragilis*	Minocycline 100 mg (IV) q12h	100%	4 µg/mL
Quinolones				
Ciprofloxacin 400 (IV) q12h	*P aeruginosa*, GNB, VSE	Ciprofloxacin 750 mg (PO) q12h	70%	4.6 µg/mL
Levofloxacin 750 mg (IV) q24h	MDRSP, MSSA, VSE, *P aeruginosa*, GNB	Levofloxacin 750 mg (PO) q24h	99%	8 µg/mL
Moxifloxacin 450 mg (IV) q24h	MDRSP, MSSA, VSE, GNB, *B fragilis*	Moxifloxacin 400 mg (PO) q24h	90%	4.5µg/mL
Other				
Clindamycin 600 mg (IV) q8h	MSSA, *B fragilis*	Clindamycin 300 mg (PO) q8h	90%	2.5 µg/mL
Metronidazole 1 g (IV) q24h	*B fragilis, C. difficile*	Metronidazole 500 mg (PO) q12h	100%	12 µg/mL
TMP-SMX 2.5 mg/kg (IV) q6h	MSSA, GNB	TMP-SMX 1 ss tablet (PO) q6h	98%	8 µg/mL
Chloramphenicol 500 mg (IV) q6h	MSSA, GNB, VSE, VRE, *B fragilis*	Chloramphenicol 500 mg (PO) q6h	90%	9 µg/mL

Abbreviations: CAP, Community-acquired pneumonia; CA-MRSA, community-acquired methicillin-resistant *S aureus*; GNB, Aerobic Gram-negative bacilli (excluding *P aeruginosa*); HA-MRSA, hospital-acquired methicillin-resistant *S aureus*; MDRSP, Multidrug resistant *S pneumoniae*; MRSA, Methicillin-resistant *S aureus*; MSSA, Methicillin-sensitive *S aureus*; VRE, Vancomycin-resistant enterococci; VSE, Vancomycin-sensitive enterococci.

Adapted from Cunha BA. Antibiotic Essentials, 5th edition, Royal Oak, (MI): Physicians' Press, 2006.

Febrile neutropenia

Febrile neutropenia predisposes patients to Gram-negative bacillary bacteremias, and if prolonged to infection due to *Candida* or *Aspergillus* [1,3]. Ordinarily, empiric antimicrobial therapy primarily is directed against *Pseudomonae aeruginosa*, which will also be effective against other aerobic Gram-negative bacilli, is given until the patient's neutropenia has resolved. Traditionally, antimicrobial therapy for febrile neutropenia has been via the IV route because the number of oral agents highly effective against *P aeruginosa* is limited [2,3]. The only two oral antibiotics with a high degree of systemic anti-*P aeruginosa* activity are ciprofloxacin and levofloxacin [2,3]. Taking into account pharmokinetic/pharmacodynamic considerations, the anti-*P aeruginosa* activity of levofloxacin, 750 mg (IV/PO) every 24 hours is comparable to ciprofloxacin [30,31]. For oral therapy of febrile neutropenia, levofloxacin or ciprofloxacin are suitable candidates on the basis of spectrum, *P aeruginosa* activity, and excellent bioavailability [6]. Gram-positive coccal infections have increased in recent years in patients with febrile neutropenia. Febrile neutropenia does not predispose, per se, to staphylococcal infections. In a series reporting an increase in staphylococcal infections in febrile neutropenic patients, it should be noted that staphylococcal infections are virtually always associated with a semipermanent intravenous device, for example, Hickman or Broviac central line catheters [1–3]. Febrile neutropenia, excluding those complicated by IV-line infections, has been treated with levofloxacin [32]. Levofloxacin, in addition to significant anti-*P aeruginosa* activity, possesses both good anti-*P aeruginosa* and antistaphylococcal activity. As with nonneutropenic patients, the optimal treatment of IV-line infections is primarily by IV catheter removal and secondarily with appropriate antistaphylococcal therapy. PO antibiotic therapy of febrile neutropenia has the added advantage of eliminating the need for an IV line (if unnecessary for other reasons), which would have the effect of decreasing the incidence of staphylococcal IV line infections in patients with febrile neutropenia [30,32] (Table 4).

Table 4
Oral antibiotic therapy of serious systemic infections: febrile neutropenia

Febrile neutropenia	Usual pathogens	Preferred oral antibiotic
Initial/early febrile neutropenia (neutropenia <1 week)	*P aeruginosa*	• Levofloxacin 750 mg (PO) q24h (until neutropenia resolved) • Ciprofloxacin 750 mg (PO) q12h (until neutropenia resolved)

Adapted from Cunha BA. Antibiotic essentials. 5th edition. Royal Oak (MI): Physicians' Press; 2006.

Severe community-acquired pneumonia

CAP may be caused by typical or atypical pulmonary pathogens. The most common typical pulmonary pathogens causing CAP are *Streptococcus pneumoniae, Hemophilus influenza*, or *Moraxella catarrhalis*. The usually encountered CAP pathogens include *Mycoplasma pneumoniae, Chlamydia pneumoniae*, or *Legionella* species. Atypical CAP pathogens predominate in ambulatory patients, whereas typical pathogens predominate in patients hospitalized with CAP. Severe CAP that required hospitalization, with or without admission to an intensive care unit (ICU), is most likely to be due to typical pathogens in patients with severe cardiopulmonary disease or impaired B-cell (humoral) immunity. In these patients with borderline cardiac/pulmonary function, even a relatively avirulent pathogen, for example, *M catarrhalis*, may cause sufficient additional cardiopulmonary dysfunction to require ventilatory support and present as severe CAP.

Severe CAP requiring hospitalization is more common with certain pathogens, particularly with Legionnaires' disease. Uncommonly, *M pneumoniae* or *C pneumoniae* may present as severe CAP in the elderly or those with compromised host defenses [6,33–37].

IV to PO switch programs have been used most extensively in the treatment of severe CAP, but entirely oral therapy may be used as well [38,39]. Antibiotics active against both typical and atypical pathogens which may be administered entirely via the oral route include respiratory quinolones, for example, levofloxacin [40–43], moxifloxacin [44–48], doxycycline [49–54], or telithromycin [55–62]. Macrolides should not be used as monotherapy for CAP patients who are moderately/severely ill on the basis of pharmacokinetic and resistance considerations. Therapeutic failures with macrolide monotherapy have been increasingly reported in the treatment of CAP. Approximately 20% to 25% of *S pneumoniae* strains are naturally resistant to all macrolides. Extensive macrolide usage has resulted in acquired resistance, which when added to the background of intrinsic/natural resistance, has resulted in widespread macrolide resistant *S pneumoniae* (MRSP) with a penicillinase of 30% to 40% prevalence. Although penicillin-resistant *S pneumoniae* (PRSP) is of concern, nearly all PRSP strains remain effectively treated with β-lactam antibiotics in the usually recommended doses. In contrast, overuse of macrolides has resulted in high levels worldwide of MRSP. Acquired macrolide resistance also has been associated with penicillin resistance. For this reason, overuse of macrolides has resulted in both an increase in PRSP and MRSP strains, and macrolides along with TMP-SMX are largely responsible for most multidrug-resistant *S pneumoniae* (MDRSP) seen at the present time [63–66]. Pharmacokinetically, macrolides are not optimal agents to treat severe CAP. Spectrum/activity and resistance issues aside, macrolides are not optimally absorbed and therapeutic serum levels are often inadequate against *S pneumoniae*. For these reasons, macrolide monotherapy is suboptimal for moderate/severe CAP

[63–67]. Macrolides have been used in "double-drug" therapy regimens for CAP to provide coverage against atypical organisms, for example, ceftriaxone plus azithromycin. This popular double drug regimen for CAP has several disadvantages including higher cost than equivalent monotherapy, the compounded effect of two drugs on side effects, the increased cost of two agents, and the difficulty in transitioning from IV ceftriaxone/azithromycin to PO azithromycin may not be optimal if the pathogen is *S pneumoniae* with unknown susceptibility. Because there is no oral formulation of ceftriaxone, physicians often use an expensive oral third-generation cephalosporin in combination with an oral macrolide to complete the course of IV initiated therapy for CAP. "Double-drug" oral therapy has many of the same disadvantages of double-drug parenteral antibiotic therapy [68,69].

Well-selected oral monotherapy has several advantages, that is, fewer drugs for the patient, less potential for adverse events or drug–drug interactions, and less cost. Monotherapy with respiratory quinolones, doxycycline, or telithromycin is optimal for mild to moderate and severe CAP [68,69]. These drugs are active against nearly all strains of PRSP, MRSP, and excluding doxycycline for MDRSP. Double drug offers no convincing advantage over monotherapy, and may have disadvantages in the therapy of severe CAP [6,38,69] (Table 5).

Nosocomial/ventilator-associated pneumonias

The usual pathogens in NP/VAP are aerobic Gram-negative bacilli (GNB). Although *P aeruginosa* is not the most common NP/VAP pathogen, it is the most virulent NP/VAP pathogen. Gram-positive/Gram-negative anaerobic organisms aspirated during hospitalization have not been shown to

Table 5
Oral antibiotic therapy of serious systemic infections: severe community-acquired pneumonia

Severe community-acquired pneumonia (CAP)	Usual pathogens	Preferred oral antibiotic
Hospitalized severe CAP	*S pneumoniae* *H influenzae*[a] *M catarrhalis*[a] *Legionella* sp.	• Respiratory quinolone Levofloxacin 750 mg (PO) q24h × 1–2 weeks Moxifloxacin 400 mg (PO) q24h × 1–2 weeks Gatifloxacin[b] 400 mg (PO) q24h × 1–2 weeks • Doxycycline 200 mg (PO) q12h x 72 h, then 100 mg (PO) q12h to complete 1–2 weeks.

[a] Only with pre-CAP borderline cardiopulmonary function.
[b] Contraindicated in diabetics.
Adapted from Cunha BA. Antibiotic essentials. 5th edition. Royal Oak, (MI): Physicians' Press; 2006.

be important pathogens in NP/VAP. Antianaerobic coverage is unnecessary in the treatment of NP/VAP. For these reasons, optimal empiric therapy for NP/VAP is directed primarily against *P aeruginosa*, which is also effective against other GNB [70–75].

In patients with hospital-acquired pneumonia, that is, NP/VAP, hospital-ization itself and selective pressure from broad spectrum anti-GNB antibiotics permit the emergence of methicillin sensitive *S aureus* (MSSA)/MRSA in the patient's respiratory secretions. The majority of MSSA/MRSA isolates of recovered from body fluids in hospitalized patients represent colonization rather than infection. Staphylococci colonize the nares/skin, respiratory secretions, and urine in hospitalized patients. Data collected by the National Nosocomial Infections Study survey collect hospital bacteriologic data based on respiratory secretions cultures of patients who are intubated, with fever, leukocytosis, and pulmonary infiltrates with presumed VAP. The difficulty in clinically diagnosing VAP in ICUs is well known. The diagnosis of VAP is difficult, and should be based upon a tissue diagnosis and not on respiratory secretion cultures in patients with fever, leukocytosis, and pulmonary infiltrates, which are often on a noninfectious basis. Practically, patients are often empirically treated for presumed VAP because invasive tissue specimens cannot be obtained for a variety of clinical reasons [70,71,73].

MSSA CAP is uncommon, and occurs virtually only in the postviral influenza setting in hospitalized patients. Presently, strains of community-acquired MRSA (CA-MRSA) have been reported as a cause of severe necrotizing CAP. Analysis of these cases of CA-MRSA CAP reveals that they follow influenza or an influenza-like illness. There are few, if any, cases of severe/necrotizing CA-MRSA CAP that occur in the nonpostviral influenza circumstance. Fortunately, CA-MRSA is susceptible to antibiotics that are not normally active against hospital-acquired MRSA (HA-MRSA) strains, that is, doxycycline, clindamycin, TMP-SMX. However, HA-MRSA, is uncommon in hospitalized patients. The clinical presentation of staphylococcal pneumonia is characteristic and impressive. Patients with MSSA/MRSA pneumonia are acutely ill with high spiking fevers, marked leukocytosis, and rapidly develop cavitary lung lesions within 72 hours. Necrotizing MSSA/MRSA pneumonia is often followed by cyanosis and vascular collapse. This is very different than the usual infectious disease consultation in the ICU, which asks, does this patient have *S aureus* pneumonia (fever, leukocytosis, and pulmonary infiltrates with MSSA/MRSAs has been cultured from the respiratory secretions)? Without the clinical findings characteristic of staphylococcal pneumonia, it is readily apparent that this patient is colonized with MSSA/MRSA but does not have MSSA/MRSA NP/VAP [76–82].

For these reasons, IV or PO therapy should be primarily directed against *P aeruginosa*, which also provides coverage against the aerobic GNB, the most common pathogens of NP/VAP. As with the therapy of CAP, monotherapy is optimal for nosocomial pneumonia [6,83]. Useful oral agents for the oral therapy of nosocomial pneumonia, or as part of an IV to PO switch regimen, are those that have a high degree of anti-*P aeruginosa* activity, that is, ciprofloxacin or levofloxacin. Therapy for NP/VAP is ordinarily continued for 2 weeks, the same total duration of therapy as with IV or IV to PO switch regimens [6,70–72] (Table 6).

S. viridans *subacute and acute bacterial endocarditis*

Most cases of SBE are due to the viridans group of streptococci. Viridans streptococci are relatively avirulent pathogens and require damaged/abnormal valve/endothelial surface to initiate the infectious process. The relative pathogenicity of various *S viridans* strains relates to their ability to produce capital material, that is, strains that have the greatest amount of capsule production are predictably those that most frequently cause SBE. In the laboratory, if their capsules are removed, *S viridans* strains are incapable of causing endocarditis, even on damaged heart valves. In addition to appropriate spectrum, there is another important consideration in treating SBE.

The antibiotics selected, either IV or PO, must be active against the *S viridans* group, and in addition, must penetrate the vegetation sufficiently to eradicate the organism. Traditionally, *S viridans* SBE has been treated for 2 to 4 weeks. Sterilization of the blood is rapidly achieved, but sterilization of the vegetation requires more time. Because of the economic and clinical difficulties associated with parenteral therapy, attempts have been made to shorten the duration of therapy for SBE. The relapse rate for uncomplicated cases of SBE is inversely proportional to duration of therapy. To prevent relapses of SBE, gentamicin was added. It is possible to treat uncomplicated *S viridans* SBE with 2 weeks of IV/PO therapy [84–86].

Table 6
Oral antibiotic therapy of serious systemic infections: nosocomial pneumonia (NP) and ventilator-associated pneumonia (VAP)

NP and VAP	Pathogens	Preferred oral antibiotics
Hospital-acquired pneumonias: NP VAP	Usual pathogens *P. aeruginosa* Gram-negative bacilli Unusual pathogens:[a] *S. aureus*	• Levofloxacin 750 mg (PO) q24h × 2 weeks • Ciprofloxacin 750 mg (PO) q12h × 2 weeks • Linezolid 600 mg (PO) q12h × 2 weeks

[a] *S. aureus* (MSSA/MRSA) pneumonia suggested by rapid cavitation (<72 h on CXR), cyanosis, and MSSA/MRSA bacteremia of lung origin.

Abbreviations: MRSA, methicillin-resistant *S aureus*; MSSA, methicillin-sensitive *S aureus*.

Adapted from Cunha BA. Antibiotic essentials. 5th edition. Royal Oak (MI): Physicians' Press; 2006.

Using full doses of an oral cephalosporin, that is, cephalexin 1 g (PO) every 6 hours, is comparable to parenteral cephalosporin therapy or *S viridans* SBE. There is a growing experience in treating uncomplicated *S viridans* SBE entirely via the oral route or as part of an IV to PO switch program. There is no PK/PD or clinical reason for not using entirely oral therapy with a variety of antibiotics, for example, high-dose amoxicillin, cephalexin, linezolid, or quinolones [87–89].

Acute bacterial endocarditis

The most common cause of acute bacterial endocarditis is *S aureus*, which may be of the MSSA or MRSA variety. Unlike *S viridans*, MSSA/MRSA is capable of attacking normal as well as damaged heart valves. The diagnosis of staphylococcal ABE may be simplified using two clinical criteria, that is, otherwise unexplained high grades/persistent *S aureus* bacteremia in a patient with a cardiac vegetation on a normal heart valve. Patients who have vegetation without a continuous high grade, that is, three of four or four of four positive blood cultures for MSSA/MRSA, have marantic not infectious endocarditis. Patients with MSSA/MRSA bacteremias without demonstrable cardiac vegetation by echocardiography, have a bacteremia from a noncardiac source and do not have MSSA/MRSA ABE. In normal hosts with MSSA/MRSA ABE, the source of infection is usually a central IV line (not associated with peripheral IV lines), cardiac instrumentation, or a distant endovascular or extravascular focus, that is, infected graft, abscess [90].

Treatment for MSSA ABE has been with any antibiotic that has a high degree of activity against MSSA and penetrates cardiac vegetations. The antibiotics most commonly used to treat MSSA ABE include antistaphylococcal penicillins, for example oxacillin, nafcillin, first-generation cephalosporins, for example, cefazolin. Oral antibiotics with a high degree of anti-MSSA activity, good bioavailability, and able to penetrate heart valves include TMP-SMX, cephalexin, minocycline, linezolid. Alternately, antibiotics that are useful to treat MRSA may also be used to treat MSSA if the patient has clinical reasons not to use the usual anti-MSSA drugs, that is, hepatic/renal insufficiency, drug allergy, is intolerant or has antibiotic intolerance/side effects. The parenteral agents available to treat MRSA endocarditis include vancomycin, quinupristin/dalfopristin, minocycline, linezolid, and daptomycin. The oral drugs to treat MRSA ABE are limited to minocycline and linezolid [1–3,6,91–95].

The oral therapy of methicillin sensitive S aureus/methicillin-resistant S aureus acute bacterial endocarditis

Experience has been most extensive but underrepresented in the literature with oral minocycline. Minocycline has been used for decades to treat MSSA/MRSA ABE in intravenous drug abusers (IVDAs). It is well known that IVDAs with MSSA/MRSA ABE are clinically less ill and have more benign course than in normal hosts with *S aureus* endocarditis. Necessarily, most IVDAs with MSSA/MRSA ABE have right-sided ABE primarily involving the tricuspid valve. The clinical presentation of right-sided ABE is that of septic pulmonary emboli because the tricuspid valve is frequently involved. Oral therapy has also been used to treat *S aureus* ABE with minocycline [96–102] and linezolid [103–105]. As experience and confidence are gained, more clinicians will opt for oral therapy for part or all of their therapy. Certainly there is no difference in efficacy/outcome when using IV versus PO linezolid, which has 100% bioavailability. It has been suggested that linezolid is not sufficiently bactericidal, rending it less useful in ABE, but being bactericidal is not essential in treating endocarditis, as many "bacteristatic" antibiotics have been successfully used to treat endocarditis due to a wide variety of organisms for which no bactericidal agent exists [1,3,6,106–110] (Table 7).

Summary

As more experience and confidence is gained in using oral antimicrobial therapy in a wide variety of infections particularly in those with serious systemic infectious diseases, the relative use of parenteral antibiotic therapy will continue to decline. IV antibiotic therapy will continue to have an important role in the initial therapy of critically ill patients, in those with inadequate proximal gastrointestinal absorptive capability, and in those for which no oral equivalent antibiotic is available. For PO therapy to be comparable to IV therapy, the antibiotics selected should have the same spectrum and

Table 7
Oral therapy of serious systemic infections: bacterial endocarditis

Bacterial endocarditis	Usual pathogens	Preferred oral antibiotics

Subacute bacterial endocarditis [a]	*S viridans*	• Amoxicillin
		  1 g (PO) q8h × 2 weeks
		• Cephalexin
		  1 g (PO) q6h × 2 weeks
		• Linezolid
		  600 mg (PO) q12h × 2 weeks

Acute bacterial endocardits	*S aureus* (MSSA)	• Cephalexin
		  1 g (PO) q6h × 2 weeks
		• Minocycline
		  100 mg (PO) q12h × 4–6weeks

	S aureus (MRSA)	• Minocycline
		  100 mg (PO) q12h × 4–6 weeks
		• Linezolid
		  600 mg (PO) q12h × 4–6 weeks

[a] Uncomplicated.
Adapted from Cunha BA. Antibiotic essentials. 5th edition. Royal Oak, (MI): Physicians' Press; 2006.

Table 8
Oral antibiotics useful in selected serious systemic infections

Systemic infection	Oral pathogens	IV antibiotic	PO antibiotic	Oral bioavailability	Peak serum concentration
Febrile neutropenia	P aeruginosa	• Meropenem • Cefepime • Antipseudomonal penicillins (APPs) (ticarcillin, piperacillin)	Ciprofloxacin 750 mg (PO) q12h	70%	2.9 μg/mL
			Levofloxacin 750 mg (PO) q24h	99%	8 μg/mL
Severe CAP	S pneumoniae Legionella	• Respiratory quinolone	Levofloxacin 750 mg (PO) q24h	99%	8 μg/mL
			Moxifloxacin 400 mg (PO) q24h	90%	4.5 μg/mL
			Gatifloxacin 400 mg (PO) q24h	96%	4.2 μg/mL
		• Doxycycline	Doxycycline 200mg (PO) q12h	93%	4 ug/mL
NP/VAP	P aeruginosa	• Meropenem • Cefepime • Antipseudomonal penicillins (APPs)	Levofloxacin 750 mg (PO) q24h	99%	8 μg/mL
			Ciprofloxacin 750 mg (PO) q12h	70%	2.9 μg/mL

(continued on next page)

Table 8 (*continued*)

Systemic infection	Oral pathogens	IV antibiotic	PO antibiotic	Oral bioavailability	Peak serum concentration
Subacute bacterial endocarditis (SBE)	S viridans	• Penicillin • Cefazolin	Cephalexin 1 g (PO) q6h Amoxicillin 1 g (PO) q8h	99% 90%	36 µg/mL 16 µg/mL
Acute bacterial endocarditis (ABE)	S. aureus (MSSA)	• Nafcillin • Cefazolin	Cephalexin 1 g (PO) q6h Linezolid 600 mg (PO) q12h	99% 100%	36 µg/mL 20 µg/mL
	S. aureus (MRSA)[a]	• Daptomycin • Vancomycin • Quinupristin/dalfopristin • Minocycline • Linezolid	Linezolid 600 mg (PO) q12h Minocycline 100 mg (PO) q12h	100% 95%	20 µg/mL 4 µg/mL

[a] Any antibiotic effective against MRSA also effective against MSSA.

Abbreviations: ABE, acute bacterial endocarditis; CAP, community-acquired pneumonia; NP, nosocomial pneumonia; SBE, subacute bacterial endocarditis; VAP, vent-associated pneumonia.

Adapted from Cunha BA. Antibiotic essentials. 5th edition. Royal Oak, (MI): Physicians' Press; 2006.

high degree of activity as its IV counterpart, and have acceptable/excellent bioavailability. Entirely oral or oral therapy as part of an IV to PO regimen has many important clinical and pharmacoeconomic advantages. At any given dose, PO antibiotic therapy is less expensive in terms of acquisition cost than its IV formulation. Oral therapy is not complicated by the added cost or medical complications associated with phlebitis or IV-line infections. Oral therapy is more acceptable to patients freeing them from their IV access line/devices permitting earlier/easier ambulation and recovery from infection. Importantly, oral antimicrobial therapy decreases hospital LOS, and permits earlier discharge of the patient. The pharmacoeconomic implications of lower antibiotic costs, fewer IV-related complications, and earlier hospital discharge cannot be overestimated. Oral antimicrobial therapy will continue to be used for more infectious diseases as clinicians become more familiar with the PK/PD characteristics of their antibiotic selections. Third-party payers are increasingly recognizing that patients admitted for an infectious disease and begun on a PO antibiotic is more cost effective than if admitted and treated intravenously. Third-party payers will soon grasp the economic savings associated with fewer IV-related complications and a shorter hospital stay. As confidence is gained by experience, clinicians will increasingly opt for oral medications whenever possible in the treatment of most infectious diseases including those that are available for the treatment of serious systemic infections (Table 8).

References

[1] Kucers A, Crowe SM, Grayson ML, et al, editors. The use of antibiotics. 5th edition. Oxford: Butterworth-Heinemann; 1997.
[2] Bryskier A, editor. Antimicrobial agents. Washington (DC): ASM Press; 2005.
[3] O'Grady F, Lambert HP, Finch RG, et al, editors. Antibiotics and chemotherapy. 2nd edition. New York: Churchill Livingstone; 1997.
[4] Cunha BA. Intravenous to oral antibiotic switch therapy. Drugs Today 2001;37:311–9.
[5] McCue JD. Oral antibiotics practical prescribing rules for practitioners. Geriatrics 1992;47: 59–66.
[6] Cunha BA, editor. Antibiotic essentials. 5th edition. Royal Oak (MI): Physicians' Press; 2006.
[7] Altemeier WA, Culbertson WR, Coith RL. The intestinal absorption of oral antibiotics in traumatic shock; an experimental study. Surg Gynecol Obstet 1951;92:707–11.
[8] Power BM, Forbes AM, van Heerden PV, et al. Pharmacokinetics of drugs used in critically ill adults. Clin Pharmacokinet 1998;34:25–56.
[9] Fish DN, Abraham E. Pharmacokinetics of a clarithromycin suspension administered via nasogastric tube to seriously ill patients. Antimicrob Agents Chemother 1999;43:1277–80.
[10] Karjagin J, Pähkla R, Karki T, et al. Distribution of metronidazole in muscle tissue of patients with septic shock and its efficacy against *Bacteroides fragilis in vitro*. J Antimicrob Chemother 2005;55:341–6.
[11] Plaisance KI, Quintiliani R, Nightingale CH. The pharmacokinetics of metronidazole and its metabolites in critically ill patients. J Antimicrob Chemother 1988;21:195–200.
[12] Schrenzel J, Cerruti F, Herrmann M, et al. Single-dose pharmacokinetics of oral fleroxacin in bacteremic patients. Antimicrob Agents Chemother 1994;38:1219–24.

[13] Rebuck JA, Fish DN, Abraham E. Pharmacokinetics of intravenous and oral levofloxacin in critically ill adults in a medical intensive care unit. Pharmacotherapy 2002;22:1216–25.

[14] Pea F, Furlanut M. Levofloxacin PK/PD: from sequential therapy model to high dosage for critical patients. J Chemother 2004;16(Suppl 2):8–10.

[15] Sultan E, Richard C, Pezzano M, et al. Pharmacokinetics of pefloxacin and amikacin administered simultaneously to intensive care patients. Eur J Clin Pharmacol 1988;34:637–43.

[16] Sensakovic JW, Smith LG. Oral antibiotic treatment of infectious diseases. Med Clin North Am 2001;85:115–23.

[17] Quintiliani R, Nightingale CH. Transitional antibiotic therapy. Infect Dis Clin Practice 1994;3(Suppl):161–7.

[18] Siegel RE, Halpern NA, Almenoff PL, et al. A prospective randomized study of inpatient intravenous antibiotics for community-acquired pneumonia: the optimal duration of therapy. Chest 1996;110:965–71.

[19] Borg R, Dotevall L, Hagberg L, et al. Intravenous ceftriaxone compared with oral doxycycline for the treatment of Lyme neuroborreliosis. Scand J Infect Dis 2005;37:449–54.

[20] Cunha BA. Minocycline vs. doxycycline for the antimicrobial therapy of Lyme neuroborreliosis. Clin Infect Dis 2000;30:237–8.

[21] Bryskier A. Bacillus anthracis and antibacterial agents. Clin Microbiol Infect 2002;8:467–78.

[22] Boulanger LL, Ettestad P, Fogarty JD, et al. Gentamicin and tetracyclines for the treatment of human plague review of 75 cases in New Mexico, 1985–1999. Clin Infect Dis 2004;38:663–9.

[23] Mwengee W, Butler T, Mgema S, et al. Treatment of plague with gentamicin or doxycycline in a randomized clinical trial in Tanzania. Clin Infect Dis 2006;42:614–21.

[24] Lyamuya EF, Nyanda P, Mohammedali H, et al. Laboratory studies on Yersinia pestis during the 1991 outbreak of plague in Lushoto, Tanzania. J Trop Med Hyg 1992;95:335–8.

[25] Ratsitorahina M, Chanteau S, Rahalison L, et al. Epidemiological and diagnostic aspects of the outbreak of pneumonic plague in Madagascar. Lancet 2000;355:111–3.

[26] Solera J, Geijo P, Largo J, et al. A randomized, double-blind study to assess the optimal duration of doxycycline treatment for human brucellosis. Clin Infect Dis 2004;39:1776–82.

[27] Newton PN, Chaulet JF, Brockman A, et al. Pharmacokinetics of oral doxycycline during combination treatment of severe falciparum malaria. Antimicrob Agents Chemother 2005;49:1622–5.

[28] Clemett D, Markham A. Linezolid. Drugs 2000;59:815–27.

[29] Jonas M, Cunha BA. Minocycline. Ther Drug Monit 1982;4:137–45.

[30] Marchetti F, Viale P. Current and future perspectives for levofloxacin in severe Pseudomonas aeruginosa infections. J Antimicrob Chemother 2003;15:315–22.

[31] Nightingale CH, Grant EM, Quintiliani R. Pharmacodynamics and pharmacokinetics of levofloxacin. Chemotherapy 2000;46:6–14.

[32] Bucaneve G, Micozzi A, Menichetti F, et al. Levofloxacin to prevent bacterial infection in patients with cancer and neutropenia. N Engl J Med 2005;353:977–87.

[33] Cunha BA. Community-acquired pneumonias: reality revisited. Am J Med 2000;108:436–7.

[34] Cunha BA. Severe community-acquired pneumonia. J Crit Illn 1997;12:711–21.

[35] Cunha BA. Severe community-acquired pneumonia. Crit Care Clin 1998;8:105–17.

[36] Cunha BA. Antibiotic treatment of severe community-acquired pneumonia. Semin Respir Crit Care Med 2000;21:61–9.

[37] Cunha BA. Severe community-acquired pneumonia: determinants of severity and approach to therapy. Infect Med 2005;22:53–8.

[38] Cunha BA. Oral or intravenous-to-oral antibiotic switch therapy for treating patients with community-acquired pneumonia. Am J Med 2001;111:412–3.

[39] Ramirez JA, Bordon J. Early switch from intravenous to oral antibiotics in hospitalized patients with bacteremic community-acquired *Streptococcus pneumoniae* pneumonia. Arch Intern Med 2001;161:848–50.

[40] Furlanut M, Brollo L, Lugatti E, et al. Pharmacokinetic aspects of levofloxacin 500 mg once daily during sequential intravenous/oral therapy in patients with lower respiratory tract infections. J Antimicrob Chemother 2003;51:101–6.

[41] Dunbar LM, Wunderink RG, Habib MP, et al. High-dose, short-course levofloxacin for community-acquired pneumonia: a new treatment paradigm. Clin Infect Dis 2003;37: 752–60.

[42] File TM Jr, Milkovich G, Tennenberg AM, et al. Clinical implications of 750 mg 5-day levofloxacin for the treatment of community-acquired pneumonia. Curr Med Res Opin 2004; 20:1473–81.

[43] Marrie TJ, Lau CY, Wheeler SL, et al. A controlled trial of a critical pathway for treatment of community-acquired pneumonia. CAPITAL study investigators. Community-Acquired Pneumonia Intervention Trial Assessing Levofloxacin. JAMA 2000;283:749–55.

[44] Hoefken G, Talan D, Larsen LS, et al. Efficacy and safety of sequential moxifloxacin for treatment of community-acquired pneumonia associated with atypical pathogens. Eur J Clin Microbiol Infect Dis 2004;23:772–5.

[45] Katz E, Larsen LS, Fogarty CM, et al. Safety and efficacy of sequential IV to PO moxifloxacin versus conventional combination therapies in the treatment of community-acquired pneumonia in patients requiring initial IV therapy. J Emerg Med 2004;27:554–9.

[46] Lode H, Grossman C, Choudhri S, et al. Sequential IV/PO moxifloxacin treatment of patients with severe community-acquired pneumonia. Respir Med 2003;97:1134–42.

[47] Rijnders BJ. Moxifloxacin for community-acquired pneumonia. Antimicrob Agents Chemother 2003;47:444–5.

[48] Torres A, Muir JF, Corris P, et al. Effectiveness of oral moxifloxacin in standard first-line therapy in community-acquired pneumonia in community-acquired pneumonia. Eur Respir J 2003;21:135–43.

[49] Shea KW, Ueno Y, Abumustafa F, et al. Doxycycline activity against *Streptococcus pneumoniae*. Chest 1995;107:1775–6.

[50] Lederman ER, Gleeson TD, Driscoll T, et al. Doxycycline sensitivity of *S. pneumoniae* isolates. Clin Infect Dis 2003;36:1091.

[51] Jones RN, Sader HS, Fritsche TR. Doxycycline use for community-acquired pneumonia: contemporary in vitro spectrum of activity against *Streptococcus pneumoniae* (1999–2002). Diagn Microbiol Infect Dis 2004;49:147–9.

[52] Johnson JR. Doxycycline for treatment of community-acquired pneumonia. Clin Infect Dis 2002;35:632–3.

[53] Cunha BA. Doxycycline re-visited. Arch Intern Med 1999;159:1006–7.

[54] Cunha BA. Doxycycline for community-acquired pneumonia. Clin Infect Dis 2003;37:870.

[55] Carbon C, Moola S, Velancsics I, et al. Telithromycin 800 mg once daily for seven to ten days is an effective and well-tolerated treatment for community-acquired pneumonia. Clin Microbiol Infect 2003;9:691–703.

[56] Hagberg L, Torres A, van Rensburg D, et al. Efficacy and tolerability of once-daily telithromycin compared with high-dose amoxicillin for treatment of community-acquired pneumonia. Infection 2002;30:378–86.

[57] Ortega M, Marco F, Almela M, et al. Activity of telithromycin against erythromycin-susceptible and resistant *Streptococcus pneumoniae* is from adults with invasive infections. Int J Antimicrob Agents 2004;24:616–8.

[58] Pullman J, Champlin J, Vrooman PS. Efficacy and tolerability of once-daily oral therapy with telithromycin compared with trovafloxacin for the treatment of community-acquired pneumonia in adults. Int J Clin Pract 2003;57:377–84.

[59] Tellier G, Niederman MS, Nusrat R, et al. Clinical and bacteriological efficacy and safety of 5 and 7 day regimens of telithromycin once daily compared with a 10-day regimen of

clarithromycin twice daily in patients with mild to moderate community-acquired pneumonia. J Antimicrob Chemother 2004;54:515–23.

[60] Reinert RR. Clinical efficacy of ketolides in the treatment of respiratory tract infections. J Antimicrob Chemother 2004;53:918–27.

[61] van Rensburg DJ, Fogarty C, Kohno S, et al. Efficacy of telithromycin in community-acquired pneumonia caused by pneumococci with reduced susceptibility to penicillin and/or erythromycin. Chemotherapy 2005;51:186–92.

[62] Carbon C, Nusrat R. Efficacy of telithromycin in community-acquired pneumonia caused by *Legionella pneumophila*. Eur J Clin Microbiol Infect Dis 2004;23:650–2.

[63] Low DE, Felmingham D, Brown SD, et al. Activity of telithromycin against key pathogens associated with community-acquired respiratory tract infections. J Infect 2004;49:115–25.

[64] Klugman KP, Lonks JR. Hidden epidemic of macrolide-resistant pneumococci. Emerg Infect Dis 2005;11:802–7.

[65] Pihlajamaki M, Kotilainen P, Kaurila T, et al. Macrolide-resistant *Streptococcus pneumoniae* and use of antimicrobial agents. Clin Infect Dis 2001;33:483–8.

[66] Lonks JR, Garau J, Gomez L, et al. Failure of macrolide antibiotic treatment in patients with bacteremia due to erythromycin-resistant *Streptococcus pneumoniae*. Clin Infect Dis 2002;35:556–64.

[67] Rzeszutek M, Wierzbowski A, Hoban DJ, et al. A review of clinical failures associated with macrolide-resistant *Streptococcus pneumoniae*. Int J Antimicrob Agents 2004;24:95–104.

[68] Cunha BA. Empiric therapy of community-acquired pneumonia: guidelines for the perplexed? Chest 2004;125:1913–9.

[69] Cunha BA. Empiric oral monotherapy for hospitalized patients with community-acquired pneumonia: an idea whose time has come. Eur J Clin Microbiol Infect Dis 2004;23:78–81.

[70] Cunha BA. Nosocomial pneumonia. Diagnostic and therapeutic considerations. Med Clin North Am 2001;85:79–114.

[71] Bartlett JG, O'Keefe P, Tally F, et al. Bacteriology of hospital-acquired pneumonia. Arch Intern Med 1986;146:868–71.

[72] Bonten MJM, Bergmans DCJJ. Nosocomial pneumonia. In: Mayhall CG, editor. Hospital epidemiology and infection control. 2nd edition. Philadelphia (PA): Lippincott Williams & Wilkins; 1999.

[73] Bonten MJM, Gaillard CA, Wouters EF, et al. Problems in diagnosing nosocomial pneumonia in mechanically ventilated patients: a review. Crit Care Med 1994;22:1683–91.

[74] Cunha BA. Fever in the intensive care unit. Intensive Care Med 1999;25:648–51.

[75] Meduri GU, Mauldin GL, Wunderink RG, et al. Causes of fever and pulmonary densities in patients with clinical manifestations of ventilator-associated pneumonia. Chest 1994; 106:221–35.

[76] Francis JS, Doherty MC, Lopatin U, et al. Severe community-onset pneumonia in healthy adults caused by methicillin-resistant *Staphylococcus aureus* carrying the Panton-Valentine leukocidin genes. Clin Infect Dis 2005;40:100–7.

[77] Gillet Y, Issartel B, Vanhems P, et al. Association between *Staphylococcus aureus* strains carrying genes for Panton-Valentine leukocidin and highly lethal necrotizing pneumonia in young immunocompetent patients. Lancet 2002;359:753–9.

[78] Padmanabhan RA, Fraser TC. The emergence of methicillin-resistant *Staphylococcus aureus* in the community. Cleve Clin J Med 2005;72:235–41.

[79] Chini V, Petinaki E, Foka A, et al. Spread of *Staphylococcus aureus* clinical isolates carrying Panton-Valentine leukocidin genes during a 3-year period in Greece. Clin Microbiol Infect 2006;12:29–34.

[80] Alonso-Tarrés C, Villegas ML, de Gispert FJ, et al. Favorable outcome of pneumonia due to Panton-Valentine leukocidin-producing *Staphylococcus aureus* associated with hematogenous origin and absence of flu-like illness. Eur J Clin Microbiol Infect Dis 2005;24:756–9.

[81] Diederen BMW, Kluytmans JAJW. The emergence of infections with community-associated methicillin-resistant *Staphylococcus aureus*. J Infect 2006;52:157–68.

[82] Kluytmans-VandenBergh MFQ, Kluytmans JAJW. Community-acquired methicillin-resistant *Staphylococcus aureus:* current perspectives. Clin Microbiol Infect 2006;12(Suppl 1):9–15.

[83] Cunha BA. Ventilator-associated pneumonia: monotherapy is optimal if chosen wisely. Crit Care 2006;10:141.

[84] Weinstein L, Brusch JL. Infective endocarditis. New York: Oxford University Press; 1966.

[85] Kaye D. Infective endocarditis. 2nd edition. New York: Raven Press; 1992.

[86] Barry J, Gump DW. Endocarditis: an overview. Heart Lung 1982;11:137–45.

[87] Levine DP, Holley HP, Eiseman I, et al. Clinafloxacin for the treatment of bacterial endocarditis. Clin Infect Dis 2004;38:620–31.

[88] Ng KH, Lee S, Yip SF, et al. A case of *Streptococcus mitis* endocarditis successfully treated by linezolid. Hong Kong Med J 2005;11:411–3.

[89] Ravidran V, John J, Kaye GC, et al. Successful use of oral linezolid as a single active agent in endocarditis unresponsive to conventional antibiotic therapy. J Infect 2003;47:164–6.

[90] Cunha BA, Gill MV, Lazar JM. Acute infective endocarditis. Infect Dis Clin North Am 1996;10:811–34.

[91] Yuk JH, Dignani MC, Harris RL, et al. Minocycline as an alternative antistaphylococcal agent. Rev Infect Dis 1991;13:1023.

[92] Steinberg PJ, Clark CC, Hickman BO. Nosocomial and community-acquired *Staphylococcus aureus* bacteremias from 1980 to 1993: impact of intravascular devices and methicillin resistance. Clin Infect Dis 1996;23:255–9.

[93] Mounzer KC, DiNubile MJ. Clinical presentation and management of methicillin-resistant *Staphylococcus aureus* (MRSA) infections. Antibiot Clin 1998;2:15–20.

[94] Paradisi F, Corti G, Messeri D. Antistaphylococcal (MSSA, MRSA, MSSE, MRSE) antibiotics. Med Clin North Am 2001;85:1–17.

[95] Cunha BA. Methicillin-resistant *Staphylococcus aureus:* clinical manifestations and antimicrobial therapy. Clin Microbiol Infect 2005;11(Suppl 4):33–42.

[96] Cunha BA. Oral antibiotics to treat MRSA infections. J Hosp Infect 2005;60:88–90.

[97] Clumeck N, Marcelis L, Amiri-Lamraski MH, et al. Treatment of severe staphylococcal infections with rifampin-minocycline association. J Antimicrob Chemother 1984;13:71–2.

[98] Kuwabara K, Shigeoka H, Ontonari T, et al. Successful treatment with minocycline of 2 cases of endocarditis caused by staphylococcus. Chemotherapy (Tokyo) 1985;33:904.

[99] Lawler MT, Sullivan MC, Levitz RE, et al. Treatment of prosthetic valve endocarditis due to methicillin-resistant *Staphylococcus aureus* with minocycline. J Infect Dis 1990;161:812–4.

[100] Levine DP, Cushing RD, Jui J, et al. Community-acquired methicillin-resistant *Staphylococcus aureus* endocarditis in the Detroit Medical Center. Ann Intern Med 1982;97:330–8.

[101] Lewis S, Lewis B. Minocycline therapy of resistant *Staphylococcus aureus* infections. Infect Control Hosp Epidemiol 1993;14:423.

[102] Safdar A, Bryan CS, Stinson S, et al. Prosthetic valve endocarditis due to vancomycin-resistant *Enterococcus faecium:* treatment with chloramphenicol plus minocycline. Clin Infect Dis 2002;34:E61–3.

[103] de Feiter PW, Jacobs JA, Jacobs JHM, et al. Successful treatment of *Staphylococcus epidermidis* prosthetic valve endocarditis with linezolid after failure of treatment with oxacillin, gentamicin, rifampicin, vancomycin, and fusidic acid regimens. Scan J Infect Dis 2005; 37:173–6.

[104] Hill EE, Herijgers P, Herregods M-C, et al. Infective endocarditis treated with linezolid: case report and literature review. Eur J Clin Microbiol Infect Dis 2006;25:202–4.

[105] Stevens DL, Herr D, Lampiris H, et al. Linezolid versus vancomycin for the treatment of methicillin-resistant *Staphylococcal aureus* infections. Clin Infect Dis 2002;34:1481–90.

[106] Babcock HM, Ritchie DJ, Christiansen E, et al. Successful treatment of vancomycin-resistant *Enterococcus* endocarditis with oral linezolid. Clin Infect Dis 2001;32:1373–5.

[107] Park D, Pugliese A, Cunha BA. Legionella micdadei prosthetic valve endocarditis. Infection 1994;22:213–5.

[108] Rolain JM, Boulos A, Mallet MN, et al. Correlation between ratio of serum doxycycline concentration to MIC and rapid decline of antibody levels during treatment of Q fever endocarditis. Antimicrob Agents Chemother 2005;49:2673–6.

[109] Rolain JM, Mallet MN, Raoult D. Correlation between serum doxycycline concentrations and serologic evolution in patients with *Coxiella burnetii* endocarditis. J Infect Dis 2003; 188:1322–5.

[110] Tompkins LS, Roessler BJ, Redd SC, et al. *Legionella* prosthetic-valve endocarditis. N Engl J Med 1988;318:530–5.

ELSEVIER
SAUNDERS

THE MEDICAL
CLINICS
OF NORTH AMERICA

Med Clin N Am 90 (2006) 1223–1255

Antibiotic Drug Interactions

Manjunath P. Pai, PharmD[a],
Kathryn M. Momary, PharmD[b],
Keith A. Rodvold, PharmD[b,c,*]

[a]University of New Mexico, College of Pharmacy, MSC09 5360,
Albuquerque, NM 87131, USA
[b]University of Illinois at Chicago, College of Pharmacy, Room #164, 833 South Wood Street,
m/c 886, Chicago, IL 60612, USA
[c]University of Illinois at Chicago, College of Medicine, 833 South Wood Street,
m/c 886c, Chicago, IL 60612, USA

The prescribing of safe and effective drug therapy is becoming increasingly complex. More and more patients are receiving multiple drug therapies for acute and chronic conditions or diseases. As the number of medications taken by the individual patient increases, so does the potential for drug–drug interactions that have clinically important consequences. Because of the increasing concern about drug interactions, both the pharmaceutical industry and regulatory agencies have issued guidance papers on the conduct of in vitro and in vivo pharmacokinetic drug interaction studies [1]. In addition, labeling within various sections of the product package insert describes clinically significant drug interactions as well as relevant information about metabolic pathways of a drug.

Recent regulatory actions by the US Food and Drug Administration (FDA) remind us of the potential risk for important drug interactions with anti-infective agents. In the early 1990s, patients experienced serious cardiac toxicity after taking antihistamine or prokinetic drugs in combination with macrolide antibiotics or azole antifungals. It was identified that inhibiting cytochrome P450 (CYP450) 3A isoenzymes resulted in higher plasma drug concentrations. Subsequently, terfenadine, astemizole, and cisapride were withdrawn from the marketplace, in part because of safety concerns about drug interactions [2]. In 2002, the antiviral agent pleconaril was not recommended for FDA approval for the treatment of the common

* Corresponding author. University of Illinois at Chicago, College of Pharmacy, Room #164, 833 South Wood Street, m/c 886, Chicago, IL 60612.
E-mail address: kar@uic.edu (K.A. Rodvold).

cold secondary to the potential for drug–drug interactions [3]. Pleconaril, a known CYP3A inducer, can potentially lower the plasma drug concentrations of CYP3A substrates, including oral contraceptive steroids such as ethinyl estradiol, and reduce their effectiveness.

Drug–drug interactions in the field of infectious diseases continue to expand as new drugs are approved, metabolic enzymes and transporters are identified, and recommendations for coadministration of drugs are revised. This article provides an overview of the principles and mechanisms of drug–drug interactions and describes pharmacokinetic-pharmacodynamic interactions commonly associated with antibacterial therapy, antiviral agents (nonretroviral), and drugs for tuberculosis. Physicochemical and in vitro antimicrobial activity (eg, additive, synergistic, or antagonistic) interactions are not discussed. This review is based on information available in the product package inserts, articles retrieved from PubMed, computer databases of the Micromedex Drugdex System (Thomson Healthcare, Inc., Greenwood Village, Colorado), and current issues of textbooks, including Piscitelli and Rodvold's *Drug Interactions in Infectious Diseases* [4], Hansten and Horn's *Managing Clinically Important Drug Interactions* [5], Tatro's *Drug Interaction Facts* [6], and Baxter and Stockley's *Drug Interactions* [7]. The reader is referred to these resources for further information, detailed reference lists, and specific information about drug–drug interactions associated with antifungal and antiretroviral agents.

Pharmacokinetic-pharmacodynamic drug–drug interactions

A drug interaction is defined as concomitantly administered medications that interfere with one another's efficacy or safety profile. Generally, the object drug is the medication that is affected by the interaction, whereas the precipitant drug is the medication that causes the interaction. In addition, drug interactions may be broken down into two separate groups: those that affect the pharmacokinetic profile of the object drug and those that affect the pharmacodynamic profile of the object drug.

Pharmacokinetic drug interactions are associated with changes in the concentration of a medication in body fluids and tissues. These interactions can occur at any point in the absorption, distribution, metabolism, or elimination of a medication. Absorption interactions generally occur in the gut. The absorption of medications that have pH-dependent dissolution may be affected by antacids, proton pump inhibitors, and histamine H_2-antagonists. This type of interaction can occur with some of the oral cephalosporins. In addition, antacids (ie, calcium carbonate or magnesium oxide) can chelate antibacterials such as tetracyclines or fluoroquinolones in the gastrointestinal (GI) tract, preventing their absorption [4–7]. Another common absorption drug interaction occurs when antibiotics alter the normal GI flora and thus affect the metabolism and absorption of medications such as warfarin and estrogens.

Pharmacokinetic drug interactions can be related to distribution and protein binding of medications. Several transport proteins play a role in the tissue distribution as well as absorption and excretion of medications [8]. One of the most studied transport proteins is P-glycoprotein (PGP). This efflux transporter prevents the absorption of medications from the GI tract. Rifampin is an inducer of PGP that leads to decreased absorption of medications that are substrates for PGP. In addition, PGP and other transport proteins are located throughout the body and transport medications to their sites of action or elimination. This is a growing field of research where many more clinically significant drug interactions are likely to be found. Drug interactions involving protein binding and drug displacement have become less important clinically, because steady-state unbound drug concentrations often redistribute and remain unaltered [9].

Drug metabolism is a site where many pharmacokinetic interactions evolve. Metabolism of medications is divided into two phases. Phase I metabolism increases the polarity of medications through oxidative transformation. Phase I reactions generally go through the CYP450 enzymes in the liver and small intestine. Phase II reactions further increase the polarity of medications by conjugating them with endogenous groups such as glucuronides or sulfates. Drug interactions can occur in both Phase I and II reactions. The precipitant drug can induce, inhibit, or simply be a substrate for these reactions (Table 1). When the precipitant drug inhibits the enzyme, it can do so either competitively or noncompetitively. Competitive inhibition occurs when the metabolism of the precipitant drug by the enzyme prevents the metabolism of the object drug. Noncompetitive inhibition occurs when the precipitant drug binds to the enzyme without being metabolized and prevents the metabolism of the object drug. The onset and dissipation of these interactions is rapid. Specifically, isoniazid both competitively and noncompetitively inhibits several different CYP450 isoenzymes. When isoniazid inhibits the metabolism of object medications, their concentrations are increased almost immediately.

Phase I and II reactions may also be induced. Enzyme induction occurs when the precipitant drug induces the synthesis of the drug-metabolizing enzyme. Because induction requires creation of new enzyme, it occurs more gradually than inhibition. In fact, the full effects of enzyme induction may not be seen for as long as 2 weeks. Rifampin is a classic enzyme inducer and has effects on both Phase I and II metabolism. When rifampin induces the metabolism of object drugs, their concentrations are decreased, and the full effect may not be seen for as long as 2 weeks.

The most common enzymes involved in phase I metabolic reactions are CYP3A4, CYP2D6, CYP1A2, CYP2C8/9, and CYP2C19 (Fig. 1). The FDA has placed emphasis on in vitro and in vivo drug interaction assessment of new medications involved with these enzymes. Such information is commonly included in the product package insert of new compounds to assist the clinician in determining the potential for drug interactions

Table 1
Selected substrates, inhibitors, and inducers of cytochrome P450 enzymes, organic anion transporter–1, and P-glycoprotein

	Substrates	Inhibitors	Inducers
CYP1A2	Theophylline	Erythromycin	Cigarette smoke
CYP2C9	Warfarin	Erythromycin	Carbamazepine
	Phenytoin	Amiodarone	Rifampin
	Dapsone	SMX/TMP	Phenobarb
		Isoniazid	
		Metronidazole	
CYP3A4	Cyclosporine	Erythromycin	...
	Tacrolimus	Amiodarone	
	Simvastatin		
	Diltiazem		
OAT1	Cidofivir	Probenecid	...
	Oseltamivir		
PGP	Quinolones	Cyclosporine	Rifampin
	Itraconazole	Tacrolimus	
	Digoxin		

Abbreviations: OAT-1, organic anion transporter–1; SMX-TMP, trimethoprim-sulfamethoxazole.

involving CYP450 enzymes [1]. Phase II reactions are most commonly mediated by Uridine diphosphate (UDP)-glucuronosyltransferase, sulfotransferase, N-acetyltransferase, and glutathione-S-transferase.

Pharmacokinetic drug interactions can also occur during renal excretion. These interactions are usually competitive interactions that occur rapidly and often involve the active secretion of medications. The organic anion transport proteins (OAT1 and 3) are primarily located in the kidney and facilitate excretion of weakly acidic drugs, such as penicillins and some antiviral agents [8]. Probenecid is an inhibitor of OAT1 and thus leads to decreased renal clearance of OAT1 substrates.

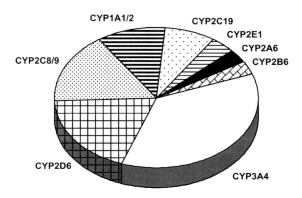

Fig. 1. The relative proportions of clinically used drug metabolized by cytochrome P450 enzymes.

Significant interindividual variability exists in the outcomes of drug interactions. This variability is associated with patient-specific factors such as disease state, other concomitant medications, and genetics. Specifically, there is at least 10-fold interindividual variability in CYP450 content, which is most likely due to a combination of clinical factors and genetics. In addition, certain CYP450 enzymes (eg, CYP2D6, CYP2C9, CYP2C19) exhibit clinically important polymorphisms that contribute to ethnic differences in metabolism as well as drug safety and efficacy. Thus, each interaction in each individual patient must be assessed for clinical relevance.

In addition to pharmacokinetic drug interactions, pharmacodynamic drug interactions may occur. Pharmacodynamic drug interactions are associated with a change in efficacy or safety of the object drug, with or without a change in its pharmacokinetics. Examples of this type of interactions include the additive risk for developing nephrotoxicity with the concurrent administration of aminoglycoside antibiotics and other nephrotoxic agents, such as amphotericin B, cisplatin, cyclosporine, or vancomycin.

Antibacterials

β-lactams

The β-lactams are the oldest class of antibiotics in clinical use and are delineated as penicillins, cephalosporins, carbapenems, and monobactams [10]. These agents exhibit an excellent safety profile, with the rare exception of epileptogenic activity in populations such as those with renal insufficiency, the elderly, and patients who have a history of seizure disorders [11]. The drug interaction profiles of these agents are typically associated with the inhibition of their secretion and specific pharmacodynamic interactions. In addition, β-lactams can alter the GI flora, leading to alteration of drugs dependent on enterohepatic recirculation. Metabolic inhibition and induction are not common mechanisms by which β-lactams interact with other drugs. A summary of potential drug interactions based on the mechanism of interaction is provided in this section.

Gastric acid suppression

Oral penicillins, such as penicillin V, amoxicillin, ampicillin, and amoxicillin/clavulanate, are generally not affected by the use of H_2-antagonists or proton pump inhibitors [7,10]. In contrast, oral cephalosporin prodrugs, such as cefpodoxime proxetil, cefuroxime axetil, and cefditoren pivoxil, have reduced bioavailability (30% to 40% reduction in area under the concentration-time curve [AUC]) when coadministered with H_2-antagonists [6,7,10]. Concomitant antacid use has also been shown to reduce the exposure of cefaclor, cefdinir, cefpodoxime, and cefditoren by 20% to 40% [5,7,10]. These oral cephalosporins should be separated by at least 2 hours if concomitant use with H_2-antagonists or antacids cannot be avoided.

Inhibition of renal tubular secretion

Probenecid inhibits the renal tubular secretion of most β-lactams eliminated by the kidney [7,10]. The AUCs of amoxicillin, ampicillin, ticarcillin, and nafcillin almost double when used with probenecid [7,10]. A similar effect is noted with the use of ceftizoxime, cefoxitin, cefaclor, and cefdinir with probenecid [10]. This effect, however, is minimal with concomitant use of piperacillin/tazobactam, ceftazidime, or ceftriaxone and probenecid. The effect on carbapenems is mixed, with minimal interaction noted with use of either imipenem or ertapenem with probenecid [10]. By contrast, the AUC of meropenem increases by 55% when it is coadministered with probenecid [7,10]. Achieving higher concentrations of these agents may be beneficial for the management of patients who have meningitis and endocarditis. However, the use of probenecid to boost β-lactam concentrations should be avoided in patients who are elderly, have renal dysfunction, or have a history of seizure disorder [11]. Other agents with the potential to inhibit tubular secretion of β-lactams include methotrexate, aspirin, and indomethacin [10]. The clinical relevance of interactions associated with these agents has not been well characterized.

Pharmacodynamic interactions

The pharmacodynamic interactions associated with β-lactams include synergy or antagonism with combined antimicrobial use and an increased risk for select toxicities. Synergy and antagonism are well-defined laboratory phenomena that have a limited number of clinical correlates. These limited few clinical correlates include the combination of ampicillin with aminoglycosides for susceptible *Enterococcus* spp–related endocarditis. The combination of ampicillin and gentamicin for enterococcal endocarditis is associated with fewer relapses compared with ampicillin monotherapy [6,7,10]. Antagonism has been reported with concomitant use of tetracycline and β-lactams in the setting of *Streptococcus (S) pneumoniae*–related meningitis [12]. Although better agents (than tetracycline) are available for meningitis, the poor response noted with these agents supports the idea that use of bactericidal agents with bacteriostatic agents may result in antagonistic outcomes.

Other noteworthy interactions include an increased risk (threefold higher) for rash with the combined use of allopurinol and amoxicillin or ampicillin. The mechanism of this interaction is not known, although patients who have hyperuricemia are noted to be at higher risk for allergic reactions. An increased risk for seizures is possible with the use of ganciclovir and imipenem/cilastatin, so concomitant use of these agents is not recommended [4,7]. Similarly, use of imipenem/cilastatin in transplant recipients receiving cyclosporine has been associated with an increased risk for central nervous system toxicity. An increased risk for seizures has also been noted with use of valproic acid and carbapenems. This interaction is associated with a rapid reduction in valproic acid concentrations, so therapeutic drug monitoring and dosage increment of valproic acid should be performed when concomitant use of a carbapenem is necessary [7,13].

Alteration in gastrointestinal flora

Oral estrogens undergo phase II hepatic metabolism to form glucuronide and sulfate conjugates that are excreted in bile. GI flora hydrolyze these conjugates, allowing for reabsorption of estrogens and maintenance of their pharmacologic effect. Consequently, breakthrough bleeding and pregnancies have been reported with use of oral contraceptives and antibiotics [14]. The estimated likelihood of this interaction is rare (approximately 1%), and the recommendation to counsel patients about the potential for oral contraceptive failure remains controversial [14]. Alteration in gut flora that synthesize vitamin K is also thought to be one of the mechanisms by which β-lactams interact with warfarin. Warfarin exerts its anticoagulant effect by inhibiting the synthesis of vitamin K–dependent clotting factors and has a high potential for drug and food interactions [15]. Reducing endogenous vitamin K production can augment the effect of warfarin. In addition, semisynthetic cephalosporins such as cefamandole, cefoperazone, and cefotetan (which contain an N-methylthiotetrazole side chain) can prolong the prothrombin time [6,7,10]. Use of these agents may increase the risk for bleeding in patients who are receiving warfarin, so patients receiving the combination should be monitored for signs and symptoms of bleeding.

Macrolides, azalides, and ketolides

The macrolides (erythromycin and clarithromycin) and ketolides (telithromycin), with the exception of the azalides (azithromycin), are associated with numerous drug interactions [16,17]. The most common mechanism for these interactions involves inhibition of the CYP450 system and PGP. Erythromycin inhibits CYP450 noncompetitively by forming iron-nitrosoalkane complexes, so onset of its potential drug interaction is rapid [18]. In contrast, telithromycin does not form stable CYP-iron-nitrosoalkane complexes but rather competitively inhibits CYP450 isoenzyme systems [18]. Azithromycin also does not form CYP450 complexes and is considered to have the lowest drug interaction potential of this group of agents [18]. The interaction profile is greatest against orally administered CYP3A substrates, because erythromycin, clarithromycin, and telithromycin can inhibit both intestinal and hepatic CYP3A isoenzymes [16–18]. A profile of clinically relevant drug interactions based on CYP450 isoenzyme and other mechanistic systems is provided in this section.

Inhibition of CYP3A4

Increased concentrations of key CYP3A4 substrates can have harmful effects; these substrates include midazolam, cyclosporine, tacrolimus, lovastatin, simvastatin, and calcium channel blockers, to name a few. A twofold to sixfold increase in the AUC of oral midazolam can occur when it is used with erythromycin, clarithromycin, or telithromycin [5–7,16,17].

Benzodiazepines not metabolized by CYP3A4, such as lorazepam or oxazepam, should be considered as alternatives, especially in the elderly and those sensitive to the effects of benzodiazepines. A twofold to fivefold increase in serum concentrations of cyclosporine and tacrolimus can occur within 2 days of concomitant clarithromycin or erythromycin use [5–7,16]. Although this interaction has not been characterized with telithromycin, a similar interaction profile is expected. Therapeutic drug monitoring is vital for these immunosuppressants, given that nephrotoxicity has been associated with this interaction.

Similarly, elevation in concentrations of statins, such as lovastatin and simvastatin, and development of rhabdomyolysis secondary to CYP3A4 inhibition have occurred. A fourfold to eightfold increase in the AUC of simvastatin occurs when it is coadministered with erythromycin, clarithromycin, or telithromycin [5–7,16,17]. Azithromycin appears to be the safest choice when coadministered with lovastatin or simvastatin [16]. Atorvastatin is less extensively metabolized by CYP3A4; only a 30% increase in AUC is noted when it is administered with erythromycin [5–7,16]. Pravastatin and rovustatin are not metabolized by CYP3A4, and fluvastatin is metabolized by CYP2C9, so these agents are less likely to be affected when used with macrolides and ketolides [17]. Similarly, calcium channel blockers such as nifedipine, felodipine, diltiazem, and verapamil have similar interactions with these CYP3A inhibitors [5–7,16,18]. Patients should be monitored for hypotension, tachycardia, edema, flushing, and dizziness when using calcium channel blockers with erythromycin, clarithromycin, or telithromycin.

Inhibition of CYP3A4 by erythromycin and clarithromycin can lead to fatal drug interactions. The primary causes of these fatalities include QT_c prolongation, leading to torsades de pointes and death. Erythromycin can directly increase the QT_c interval and also increase concentrations of antiarrhythmics such as quinidine, ibulitide, sotalol, dofetilide, amiodarone, and bretylium, to name a few. Tricyclic antidepressants such as amitryptilline and antipsychotic agents such as haloperidol, respiridone, and quetapine can all become elevated and augment the risk for development of torsades de pointes. Key agents, such as cisapride, terfenadine, and astemizole, have been removed from the United States market because of this adverse event. Furthermore, use of CYP3A4 inhibitors such as diltiazem, verapamil, and itraconazole can increase the risk for sudden cardiac death fivefold in patients receiving erythromycin [19]. Similarly, elevation of other CYP3A4 substrates can have serious consequences: priapism (sildenafil), disorientation (clozapine), neutropenia (vinblastine), delirium (fluoxetine), and uveitis (rifabutin) are prime examples [16,20]. The inordinate number of substrates metabolized through the CYP3A4 isoenzyme system requires that one perform a thorough review of potential drug interactions when choosing to use erythromycin, clarithromycin, or telithromycin. Alternative agents should be considered before use of erythromycin in patients who are receiving concomitant CYP3A4 inhibitors [19].

Inhibition of CYP2C9, CYP2C19

Both CYP2C9 and CYP2C19 are encoded by genes associated with significant polymorphisms [18]. Consequently, the pharmacokinetics of drugs metabolized through these enzyme systems exhibits significant population-based variability. Key substrates of these isoenzyme systems include warfarin, phenytoin, and sulfonylureas. Bruising, hematuria, and a rise in the prothrombin time are associated with the use of erythromycin and warfarin [5–7,16]. The potential for this interaction is considerably reduced with the combination of warfarin and clarithromycin or telithromycin [5–7,16,17]. A 10% to 20% increase in the AUC of warfarin is noted when used with telithromycin [17]. Despite this low potential, patients should be advised of the signs and symptoms of hypoprothrombinemia when using the agents together. Therapeutic drug monitoring of phenytoin and counseling of patients on recognizing signs and symptoms of hypoglycemia (with sulfonylureas) are necessary safety measures with concomitant use of macrolides.

Inhibition of CYP1A2

Theophylline is a key CYP1A2 substrate associated with significant cardiotoxicity when coadministered with erythromycin [5–7,16]. The reported consequences have ranged from GI adverse events to more serious effects such as ventricular fibrillation [16,18]. In contrast, a modest elevation (20%) in theophylline concentrations may be expected when used with clarithromycin or telithromycin [6,7,16,17]. Consequently, the significance of this interaction may be more relevant for patients who are maintained on the upper end of the therapeutic range. Caffeine, a methylxanthine like theophylline, is also metabolized by CYP1A2, and increased jitteriness may be noted in some patients who use macrolides and ketolides.

Inhibition of P-glycoprotein

Erythromycin and clarithromycin are also PGP inhibitors [8]. Digoxin is primarily eliminated by the kidneys as unchanged drug by means of PGP-mediated tubular secretion. The combination of digoxin with erythromycin or clarithromycin has resulted in increased oral bioavailability, decreased renal clearance, and increased serum concentrations of digoxin [5–7,21]. Digoxin toxicity has developed in patients simultaneously treated with these macrolides. A recent drug–drug interaction study identified that hospital admissions due to digoxin toxicity were 13 times more likely to occur in elderly patients who had received clarithromycin therapy within the past week [22]. Patients receiving digoxin and macrolide therapy, alone or in combination, should have their renal function monitored and digoxin dosage regimens adjusted based on lean body weight, creatinine clearance estimation, and serum drug concentrations.

The oral bioavailability, metabolism, and excretion of colchicine are altered by clarithromycin and erythromycin [5–7]. The most likely mechanisms of this interaction are macrolide-mediated inhibition of PGP and CY3A4. In a retrospective study of 116 patients, death occurred in nine (10.2%) of the 88 patients who received concurrent colchicine and clarithromycin therapy, compared with one (3.6%) of the 28 patients who received the two agents sequentially [23]. The independent variables associated with death among the 88 patients who had concomitant therapy included the duration of overlapping therapy, renal impairment, and the development of pancytopenia. Extreme caution must be exercised when inhibitors of PGP and CY3A4 are used with colchicine.

Alteration in gastrointestinal flora

The potential drug interaction of oral contraceptive agents with macrolides, azalides, and ketolides is minimal [7,14]. Telithromycin, for example, has not been shown to affect the antiovulatory effects of ethinyl estradiol and levonorgestrel [17]. Pregnancy as a consequence of oral contraceptive failure has not been causally linked to a macrolide, azalide, or ketolide [14]. Conversely, inhibition of *Eubacterium lentum* (normal gut flora) by these agents is the proposed mechanism by which elevated digoxin concentrations are noted to occur in patients managed with macrolides [24]. Approximately 10% of patients who receive digoxin have significant gut metabolism of digoxin performed by *E lentium* [16]. Consequently, elevated digoxin concentrations may be noted with concomitant use of the macrolides and ketolides, as well as of azithromycin.

Fluoroquinolones

Fluoroquinolones are used routinely in outpatients, given their excellent oral bioavailability and safety profile. The oral bioavailability of fluoroquinolones such as ciprofloxacin, levofloxacin, ofloxacin, norfloxacin, gatifloxacin, moxifloxacin, and gemifloxacin can be significantly reduced by cations [5–7,25]. The degree of this interaction is dependent on the cation in question and the relative timing of oral administration. In general, multivalent cations, such as aluminum, magnesium, iron, and zinc, have been noted to have more serious interactions than does calcium [5–7,25]. These interactions are clinically relevant, given that fluoroquinolones have concentration-dependent pharmacodynamics, implying that reductions in maximium concentration (C_{max}) and AUC values can lead to therapeutic failure [25]. The recommended administration schemes for fluoroquinolones and cation-containing products, such as antacids and supplements, have been based on the manufacturer-dependent study designs. Patient populations with delayed gastric emptying time, such as those who have cystic fibrosis, may require additional studies to assess the optimal separation time of fluoroquinolones and cations [26]. Fluoroquinolones have also been associated with fatalities secondary to hypoglycemia in patients receiving medications to manage diabetes [25]. Fluoroquinolones can cause a drug- and dose-dependent prolongation of the QT_c interval by inhibiting outward flow of potassium in myocytes. The relative potency for inhibiting these channels (human ether-a-go-go–related gene, HERG) in animal models is as follows: moxifloxacin equals gatifloxacin, which is greater than levofloxacin, which equals gemifloxacin and ciprofloxacin, which are greater than ofloxacin [25]. As a general rule, patients who have a history of QT_c prolongation or uncorrected electrolyte abnormalities or those receiving antiarrhythmic agents may be at higher risk for developing torsade de pointes. Use of fluoroquinolones in these patient groups should be closely monitored. Other interactions with fluoroquinolones are minimal, with the exception of those with ciprofloxacin and norfloxacin, which can inhibit CYP1A2 [25]. The specific drug interaction profile for each individual systemic fluoroquinolone is provided as follows.

Ciprofloxacin

Chelation-related drug interactions have been evaluated with concomitant use of ciprofloxacin and iron glucanoate, iron sulfate, magnesium/aluminum-containing antacids, sucralafate, zinc, calcium carbonate, calcium acetate, bismuth subsalicylate, and sevelamer. Simultaneous administration of iron, magnesium, aluminum, and zinc can result in 50% to 90% reduction in both the C_{max} and AUC of oral ciprofloxacin [5–7,25]. In contrast, a 30% to 40% reduction in C_{max} and AUC can occur with coadministration of ciprofloxacin and calcium or sevelamer [6,25]. Bismuth interacts minimally (10% reduction in AUC) with ciprofloxacin [25]. Coadministration of these agents 2 hours prior to or 6 hours after the administration of ciprofloxacin reduces this interaction and is the manufacturer-recommended approach [26].

Hypoglycemia requiring urgent management with use of ciprofloxacin in a previously stable patient receiving glyburide has been reported [6,7,25]. To date, the mechanism for this interaction has not been elucidated but does not appear to be pharmacokinetic.

An increase (of approximately 30%) in theophylline concentrations has been reported with use of concomitant ciprofloxacin, leading to symptoms of theophylline toxicity [5–7]. Therapeutic drug monitoring and a dosage reduction in theophylline may be necessary when using ciprofloxacin in these patients. Other CYP1A2 substrates, such as tizanadine, have been noted to exhibit a 10-fold increase in AUC and resultant hypotensive effects in healthy volunteers receiving concomitant ciprofloxacin [5,27].

Levofloxacin/ofloxacin

Levofloxacin and ofloxacin have been studied against a similar range of cations [25]. Simultaneous administration of these agents with iron, magnesium, and aluminum compounds results in a 20% to 40% reduction in the C_{max} and AUC of levofloxacin [5–7,25]. The interaction of levofloxacin with calcium-containing compounds is also considerably lower compared with ciprofloxacin (10% to 20% reduction in AUC). Administration of levofloxacin 2 hours before or 2 hours after these multivalent cation-containing products is recommended to limit this interaction [28]. The risk for hypoglycemia with use of levofloxacin in patients receiving antidiabetic medications is lower than with gatifloxacin. Ofloxacin does not significantly alter the clearance of theophylline [25].

Norfloxacin

Norfloxacin appears to have a greater potential to interact with cations compared with ciprofloxacin. Combined use of norfloxacin with sucralfate, magnesium/aluminum antacids, and iron sulfate results in a greater than 90% reduction in AUC values [5–7,25]. A 60% reduction in exposure is noted with concomitant use of calcium carbonate. Even administration of sucralfate 2 hours before norfloxacin results in a 40% reduction in norfloxacin exposure [5–7,25]. The manufacturer-recommended schedule is to space metal cations and norfloxacin by at least 2 hours. However, use of alternative agents, such as H_2-antagonists (eg, famotidine) or proton pump inhibitors (eg, omeprazole) may be prudent, given the likelihood of a sustained interaction. Theophylline toxicity has been reported in patients receiving norfloxacin therapy, so patients should be monitored for this interaction [5–7].

Gatifloxacin

Gatifloxacin has a similar metal chelate interaction profile to that of levofloxacin during simultaneous administration of these agents. However, the manufacturer-recommended dosing sequence is to administer gatifloxacin 4 hours before the administration of these cation-containing medications [29]. No alteration in the metabolic disposition of concomitantly used medications has been reported with the use of gatifloxacin [29].

The vast majority of reports of fluoroquinolone-associated alteration in glucose homeostasis involve use of gatifloxacin [25]. These have included cases where release of insulin and a resultant drop in glucose concentrations were noted during initiation of therapy. Elderly patients, patients with renal impairment, and patients who are on concomitant glucose-altering medications are at an increased risk for this adverse event [29]. Two population-based case-control studies from Canada [30] and data reported to the FDA indicate that gatifloxacin is most commonly associated with drug interactions leading to dysglycemia [25]. A "Dear Health care Professional" letter was issued on February 15, 2006 concerning labeling changes to the product package insert of gatifloxacin. The update included additions to the existing warning section on hypoglycemia and hyperglycemia and a contraindication to the use of gatifloxacin in diabetic patients.

Moxifloxacin

Moxifloxacin also has a similar cation-interaction profile to levofloxacin and is minimally affected by coadministration with calcium-containing agents. However, the manufacturer recommends administering moxifloxa-cin 4 hours before or 8 hours after these cation-containing agents [31]. The potential for alteration in glucose homeostasis exists with the use of moxifloxacin as well [25]. Moxifloxacin is unique among fluoroquinolones in that it has minimal renal elimination and is almost entirely removed in feces as sulfate and glucuronide conjugates [31]. Despite this disposition profile, it does not alter the CYP system and is not associated with this category of drug interactions.

Gemifloxacin

Gemifloxacin is available as an oral product only and has been studied against calcium carbonate, iron sulfate, magnesium- and aluminum-contain-ing antacids, and sucralfate. These studies indicate that these cations should not be taken within a period 3 hours before or 2 hours after the dose of gem-ifloxacin [6,7,25]. The exception is sucralfate: administration of this agent 3 hours prior resulted in a 50% reduction in the gemifloxacin AUC [25]. How-ever, administration of sucralfate 2 hours after gemifloxacin only resulted in a 10% reduction in AUC. Consequently, the manufacturer recommended the 3-hour before or 2-hour after use of cations with gemifloxacin, with the exception of sucralfate, which should be administered 2 hours after gem-ifloxacin [32]. The specific risk for gemifloxacin alteration of glucose homeo-stasis is not known, but no specific cases have been reported in the literature to date. Gemifloxacin is not known to alter the clearance of other concom-itantly used medications.

Aminoglycosides

The parenteral aminoglycosides (eg, gentamicin, tobramycin, amikacin) have remained important antibacterial agents for the treatment of serious gram-negative infections. These agents are excreted almost completely by the kidneys, primarily by glomerular filtration. The significant adverse events associated with aminoglycoside therapy are nephrotoxicity, ototoxicity, and neuromuscular blockade. As a result, the drug interaction profile for these agents is usually an additive or synergistic risk for these major toxicities.

Numerous reports have documented the increased risk for developing nephrotoxicity with the concurrent administration of aminoglycosides and amphotericin B, cisplatin, cyclosporine, vancomycin, or indomethacin (in neonates with patent ductus arteriosus) [5–7,33–35]. The mechanism appears to be either direct or additive injury to the renal tubule. Patients receiving aminoglycoside therapy should have their renal function moni-tored and dosage regimens adjusted based on body weight, creatinine clearance estimation, or serum drug concentrations. In addition, aminogly-cosides should be avoided or used with caution with the aforementioned agents, as well as with other known nephrotoxic agents, such as foscarnet, intravenous pentamidine, cidofovir, polymyxin B, and colistin.

An increased risk for ototoxicity has been reported with the coadministration of aminoglycosides and loop diuretics [5–7,33]. Ethacrynic acid has been reported to cause hearing loss when administered alone and in conjunction with aminoglycosides such as kanamycin and streptomycin. Furosemide has also been identified as an additive risk factor for the increased rates of nephrotoxicity and ototoxicity with aminoglycosides. Ethacrynic acid, furosemide, urea, and mannitol should be used cautiously at the lowest possible doses in patients receiving concurrent aminoglycoside therapy.

Aminoglycosides may potentiate the effects of neuromuscular blocking agents [5–7,33]. Concurrent administration of these agents has been associated with prolonged respiratory depression and weakness of skeletal muscles. Patients who have myasthenia gravis or severe hypocalcemia or hypomagnesium are particularly susceptible to these adverse effects. The interaction may occur when an aminoglycoside is administered either before or after a neuromuscular blocking agent. Patients should be monitored for prolonged signs of respiratory depression and paralysis during the perioperative and postoperative periods.

Aminoglycosides and β-lactam agents are commonly used in combination for additive or synergistic activity in the treatment of disease caused by gram-positive and gram-negative pathogens [5–7,33]. However, concomitant use of extended-spectrum penicillins (eg, piperacillin, ticarcillin) may produce in vivo inactivation of the aminoglycoside in patients who have severe renal impairment. Administration times of the aminoglycoside should be adjusted to the end of the penicillin dosing interval, and monitoring of aminoglycoside serum concentrations may be warranted in this clinical situation.

Vancomycin

Vancomycin is a glycopeptide antibacterial that has been available since its discovery in 1956. Despite its long history, there are few reported drug interactions of vancomycin with other therapeutic agents. The most notable drug–drug interaction of vancomycin is the potentially increased incidence of nephrotoxicity with the concurrent administration of aminoglycoside antibiotics [5–7,33–35]. The estimated incidence of vancomycin-induced nephrotoxicity is 5% to 7% when it is used alone and 0% to 35% when it is used concurrently with an aminoglycoside. Data from toxicology animal studies provide evidence that vancomycin alone has mild nephrotoxic potential and that concomitant administration of vancomycin and aminoglycosides results in a significant increase in nephrotoxicity over that of either agent alone. A similar trend toward increased nephrotoxicity in patients with the combined use of vancomycin and an aminoglycoside has been observed in numerous studies. However, not all studies have been able to demonstrate a clear association between increased risk for nephrotoxicity and combination therapy. Patients receiving vancomycin and aminoglycoside therapy, alone or in combination, should have their renal function monitored and dosage regimens adjusted based on body weight, creatinine clearance estimation, or serum drug concentrations. Clinicians should attempt to avoid other conditions (hypotension, intravenous contrast media) and risk factors (eg, cumulative doses, other nephrotoxic drugs) that increase the risk for developing nephrotoxicity.

Other drug interactions have included case reports of the possible inactivation of vancomycin by heparin when administered through the same intravenous line, decreased clearance of high-dose methotrexate following recent vancomycin administration, and depression of neuromuscular function after concurrent vecuronium therapy [5–7,33]. Finally, altered disposition (eg, clearance decreased and elimination half-life and apparent volume of distribution increased) of vancomycin has been reported in six neonates who had patent ductus arteriosus and were treated with indomethacin therapy [5,7,33].

Vancomycin may bind to anion-exchange resins such as colestyramine [7].

Daptomycin

Daptomycin is a cyclic lipopeptide that is renally excreted and is not hepatically metabolized. Metabolic drug interactions are unlikely, because in vitro studies have shown that daptomycin neither induces nor inhibits CYP isoforms 1A2, 2A6, 2C9, 2C19, 2D6, 2E1, and 3A4 [36]. In rats, daptomycin decreased aminoglycoside-induced nephrotoxicity when both agents were coadministered. In healthy subjects, a single dose of daptomycin 2 mg/kg, tobramycin 1 mg/kg, or the combination was not associated with a significant change in pharmacokinetic parameters or nephrotoxicity [33,36]. Because both daptomycin and hydroxymethyglutaryl–coenzyme A (HMG-CoA) reductase inhibitors may increase creatinine phosphokinase concentrations or cause rhabdomyolysis, the manufacturer recommends that HMG-CoA reductase inhibitors and other drugs associated with rhabdomyolysis be temporarily discontinued during daptomycin therapy [36].

Linezolid

Linezolid is a novel synthetic antibacterial agent from the oxazolidinone class. The drug interaction profile of this antibiotic class is typically associated with the inhibition of monoamine oxidase (MAO), which results in an increase in serotonin concentrations and the development of the serotonin syndrome [7,33]. Metabolic inhibition is an unlikely mechanism for drug interactions, because in vitro studies have demonstrated that linezolid is not metabolized and does not have activity to inhibit common human CYP isoforms (1A2, 2C9, 2C19, 2D6, 2E1, and 3A4). In addition, studies in rats suggest that linezolid is not an inducer of CYP isoforms [37].

Several case reports have been published regarding the temporal drug interaction relationship between linezolid and selective serotonin reuptake inhibitors such as sertraline, paroxetine, citalopram, and fluoxetine [6,7,33]. In addition, a few case reports have suggested the serotonin noradrenergic reuptake inhibitor venlafaxine [6,7]. Clinicians need to be aware of the possible risk, and, whenever possible, alternative agents should be prescribed. Management of the serotonin syndrome involves discontinuation of the offending agent or agents and, when necessary, administration of the antiserotonin agent cyproheptadine to relieve symptoms.

The reversible MAO inhibitor activity of linezolid also has the potential for drug interactions involving over-the-counter (OTC) cough and cold preparations that contain adrenergic agents such as pseudoephedrine and phenylpropanolamine [7,33]. A controlled clinical study in healthy subjects demonstrated that significant increases in systolic blood pressure (ie, mean maximum increase from baseline: 32 mm Hg and 38 mm Hg) were observed after the coadministration of linezolid and either pseudoephedrine or phenylpropanolamine [38]. No symptoms of serotonin syndrome or changes in blood pressure, heart rate, or temperature were observed when dextromethorphan (a known serotonin reuptake inhibitor) was coadministered with linezolid. Patients need to be counseled regarding their choice of OTC products and given precautionary information regarding the coadministration of linezolid and products containing pseudoephedrine or phenylpropanolamine.

Quinupristin-dalfopristin

Quinupristin-dalfopristin is a streptogramin antibacterial that is administered intravenously in a fixed 30:70 ratio. Quinupristin-dalfopristin is nonenzymatically metabolized and is primarily excreted in the feces and urine. Although they are not metabolized by CYP or glutathione-transferase enzymes, in vitro studies confirm that quinupristin and dalfopristin are significant inhibitors of CYP 3A4 metabolism of cyclosporine, midazolam, nifedipine, docetaxol, tamoxifen, and terfenadine [5,7,39]. Quinupristin-dalfopristin does not affect other common human CYP isoforms (1A2, 2A6, 2C9, 2C19, 2D6, or 2E1) [39]. In pharmacokinetic studies conducted in healthy subjects, quinupristin-dalfopristin increased the plasma concentrations (AUC and C_{max}, respectively) of cyclosporine (63% and 30%), nifedipine (44% and 18%), and midazolam (33% and 14%) [5,39]. A case report also documented a threefold increase in cyclosporine concentrations in a renal transplant patient [7]. Coadministration of quinupristin-dalfopristin with drugs that are well-known substrates of CYP 3A4 can result in a pharmacokinetic interaction that markedly increases their plasma drug concentrations. Agents with a narrow therapeutic index should be either avoided or administered with caution, plus close monitoring for adverse effects. Plasma drug concentrations should be carefully monitored for agents such as cyclosporine or tacrolimus and the dose adjusted accordingly.

Tetracyclines

The commonly used agents in the tetracycline class (eg, tetracycline, minocycline, doxycycline) differ in their major routes of elimination. Tetracycline is excreted almost completely by the kidneys, primarily by glomerular filtration. Minocycline is metabolized by the liver, and approximately 10% is excreted in the kidney. Doxycycline is mainly eliminated in the feces, with the remaining 20% to 30% eliminated in the urine by glomerular filtration.

Most drug interactions of tetracyclines are pharmacokinetic and reflect changes in absorption and elimination of this drug class or other agents (Table 2). The plasma concentrations of tetracyclines are markedly reduced (30% to 90%) with the concurrent administration of products containing divalent and trivalent cations, such as aluminium, magnesium, calcium, iron, or zinc [5–7,33]. The potential mechanisms associated with this interaction include chelation, decreased dissolution, and binding to the antacid. This interaction has been reported to occur with the intravenous administration of doxycycline. Common products containing multivalent cations include antacids, laxatives, antidiarrheals, multivitamins, sucralfate, didanosine tablets or powder, molindone, and quinapril tablets. In addition, other products known to decrease the bioavailability of tetracyclines include colestipol, kaolin-pectin, activated charcoal, and sodium bicarbonate [5–7,33]. When a tetracycline is used with one of these products, the administration of each agent should be staggered by at least 2 hours to minimize the impact of this interaction.

As with the β-lactams discussed earlier in this article, drug–drug interactions have been reported between tetracyclines and warfarin, digoxin, and oral contraceptives [5–7,14,33]. In addition, tetracyclines may increase plasma concentrations of theophyllline, although studies have been inconsistent [6,7,33]. Although these interactions do not occur in all patients, it remains best to monitor for their occurrence and, in selected circumstances, consider alternative therapy or additional precautions (eg, other methods of contraception).

Tetracycline may potentiate the toxicities of lithium, methrotrexate, methoxyflurane, and ergotamine tartrate [5–7,33]. The combination therapy with retinoids (eg, acitretin, isotretinoin) is not recommended because of the additive effects of pseudotumor cerebri (benign intracranial hypertension) [6,7]. The combination of tetracycline and atovaquone should be avoided, because the plasma concentrations of atovaquone were decreased by approximately 40% [7]. In contrast, a twofold increase in plasma concentrations of quinine has been observed when concomitant tetracycline was administered in patients being treated for *Plasmodium falciparum* malaria. Barbiturates, phenytoin, carbamazepine, rifampin, and chronic ingestion of ethanol can decrease the elimination half-life and plasma concentrations of doxycycline but do not appear to affect the pharmacokinetics of other tetracycline products [6,7,33].

Tigecycline

Tigecycline, a semisynthetic derivative of minocycline, is the first agent from the glycylcycline class of antibiotics. The primary routes of tigecycline

Table 2
Drug–drug interactions involving tetracyclines

Interacting drug	Effects	Management recommendations
Antacids	Decreased tetracycline concentration	Space administration by at least 2 hours.
Atovaquone	Decreased (40%) atovaquone concentration	Use alternative therapy when possible.
Barbiturates	Decreased doxycycline concentration	Use other tetracycline products.
Bismuth	Decreased tetracycline concentration	Space administration by at least 2 hours.
Carbamazepine	Decreased doxycycline concentration	Use other tetracycline products.
Colestipol	Decreased tetracycline concentration	Space administration by at least 2 hours.
Digoxin	Increased digoxin concentration and toxicity	Monitor digoxin concentration and adjust dose appropriately.
Ergotamine tartrate	Increased ergotism	Monitor for ergotism; use alternative therapy when possible.
Ethanol, chronic ingestion	Decreased doxycycline concentration	Use other tetracycline products.
Iron	Decreased tetracycline concentration	Space administration by at least 2 hours.
Isotretinoin	Pseudotumor cerebri	Avoid concurrent use.
Kaolin-pectin	Decreased tetracycline concentration	Space administration by at least 2 hours.
Lithium	Increased lithium concentration and toxicity	Monitor lithium concentration and adjust dose appropriately.
Methotrexate	Increased methotrexate concentration and toxicity	Monitor methotrexate concentration and maintain leucovorin rescue as needed.
Methoxyflurane	Risk of nephrotoxicity	Avoid concurrent use.
Oral contraceptives	Reduced contraceptive effectiveness	Counsel patient to use additional forms of contraception.
Phenytoin/ Fosphenytoin	Decreased doxycycline concentration	Use other tetracycline products.
Quinine	Increased quinine concentration	Monitor for quinine toxicity.
Rifampin/ Rifabutin	Decreased doxycycline concentration	Use other tetracycline products.
Sodium bicarbonate	Decreased tetracycline concentration	Space administration by at least 2 hours.
Theophylline	Increased theophylline concentration	Monitor theophylline concentration and adjust dose appropriately.
Warfarin	Enhanced anticoagulation	Monitor prothrombin time/ international normalized ratio and adjust warfarin dose appropriately.
Zinc	Decreased tetracycline concentration	Space administration by at least 2 hours.

elimination include biliary and renal excretion. Metabolic inhibition is an unlikely mechanism for drug interactions, because in vitro studies in human liver microsomes indicate that common human CYP isoforms (1A2, 2C8, 2C9, 2C19, 2D6, and 3A4) are not inhibited by tigecycline [40]. Because tigecycline is not extensively metabolized, drugs that inhibit or induce the activity of these CYP isoforms are unlikely to affect the clearance of tigecycline.

A limited amount of information regarding drug–drug interactions for tigecycline is available. The results of a study in 20 healthy men indicate that the concomitant administration of tigecycline and digoxin does not affect the pharmacokinetic parameters of either agent [40]. In addition, no pharmacodynamic changes were observed on electrocardiogram measurements. It has been recommended that both agents be concurrently administered without dosage adjustments.

The coadministration of tigecycline and a single dose of warfarin 25 mg to healthy subjects resulted in an increase in plasma concentrations (AUC and C_{max}, respectively) of R-warfarin (68% and 38%) and S-warfarin (29% and 43%) [40]. Observed changes in the warfarin pharmacokinetics did not alter INR values. However, the manufacturer recommends that an appropriate anticoagulation test (eg, prothrombin time/international normalized ratio—PT/INR) be monitored when tigecycline is coadministered with warfarin.

Clindamycin

Clindamycin is eliminated primarily by the liver, with only 5% to 10% of the administered dose excreted unchanged in the urine. Drug interactions with clindamycin are usually pharmacodynamic and not associated with changes in pharmacokinetics.

Clindamycin may enhance the effects of neuromuscular blocking agents (eg, d-tubocurarine, pancuronium, vecuronium) and result in a prolonged duration of neuromuscular blockade [6,7,33]. The effects of clindamycin on neuromuscular function are complex, and reversal agents (eg, calcium, neostigmine) are not always effective. Patients receiving concurrent clindamycin and depolarizing or nondepolarizing neuromuscular blocking agents should have the degree of paralysis and duration of respiratory depression closely monitored.

Clindamycin is not considered a nephrotoxin-inducing antibacterial agent. However, several studies have suggested that clindamycin is a potential risk factor for the development of nephrotoxicity when administered concurrently with aminoglycosides [7,33,41]. One study reported the temporal relationship between the coadministration of gentamicin and clindamycin, with the development of acute renal failure in three patients who did not have predisposing risk factors [42]. Case reports also exist of clindamycin and cyclosporine resulting in nephrotoxicity [6,7].

Metronidazole

Metronidazole undergoes hepatic metabolism, and the two principal oxidative products are hydroxy and acetic acid metabolites. The major route of elimination of metronidazole and its metabolites is renal excretion, with as much as 77% of the dose being recovered in the urine as unchanged drug or metabolites.

Metronidazole is structurally similar to disulfiram, and an acute psychotic or confusional state may occur when these two agents are administered together in patients [5–7,43]. Metronidazole produces a disulfiram-like reaction (eg, flushing, palpitation, tachycardia, nausea, vomiting) in some patients who drink ethanol while taking the drug [5–7,43]. This reaction is a result of acetaldehyde accumulation, because metronidazole inhibits aldehyde dehydrogenase and other alcohol-oxidizing enzymes. Patients should be warned about these potential side effects and should not drink ethanol within 2 to 3 days of taking metronidazole. In addition, careful selection of OTC and prescription medication is necessary, because several oral products (eg, cough and cold preparations, ritonavir solution) and intravenous products (eg, diazepam, nitroglycerin, phenytoin, trimethoprim-sulfamethoxazole) contain ethanol. Metronidazole and medications containing a high content of propylene glycol (eg, amprenavir oral solution) should also be avoided or used with caution, because metronidazole inhibits the alcohol and aldehyde dehydrogenase pathway that metabolizes propylene glycol.

Metronidazole increases the hypoprothrombinemic effect of warfarin by increasing the plasma half-life and plasma concentrations of the S-isomer of warfarin [5–7]. For patients receiving both warfarin and metronidazole, it is important to monitor closely the degree of hypoprothrombinemia and to adjust the dosage of warfarin as necessary. Metronidazole has also been reported to decrease total body clearance and increase plasma drug concentrations of lithium, busulfan, cyclosporine, tacrolimus, carbamazepine, and phenytoin [5–7]. Plasma drug concentration monitoring and dosage adjustments may be warranted, because clinical signs of drug toxicity have been reported with these combinations. Toxicities associated with 5-fluorouracil are enhanced by metronidazole, and coadministration of these two agents should be avoided [5,7]. There is a case report of acute dystonia after a single dose of chloroquine was given to a patient on metronidazole therapy who had previously received both drugs alone without any problems [7].

The oral bioavailability of metronidazole has been reduced by 14.5% and 21.3%, respectively, with concurrent administration of aluminium hydroxide and colestyramine [5,7]. No effects have been observed during the concomitant administration of sucralfate or omeprazole [7]. Phenobarbital, phenytoin, rifampin, and prednisone have been reported to increase total body clearance and lower plasma concentrations of metronidazole [5–7]. Doses of metronidazole may need to be increased in selected patients, especially those who are not responding to therapy. There have been equivocal reports about inhibition of metronidazole metabolism by cimetidine [7].

Chloramphenicol

Chloramphenicol is inactivated primarily by the liver, and its succinate and glucoronide metabolites are excreted in the urine. Chloramphenicol has recently been shown to be a potent inhibitor of CYP2C19 and CYP3A4 and a weak inhibitor of CYP2D6 in human liver microsomes [44]. These findings partially support the older literature and drug interaction information from case reports or small series of patients (Table 3). Chloramphenicol has been shown to prolong the elimination half-life or increased serum drug

Table 3
Drug–drug interactions involving chloramphenicol

Interacting drug	Effects	Management recommendations
Acetaminophen	Equivocal changes to chloramphenicol concentration	Monitor chloramphenicol concentration and adjust dose appropriately; use other analgesic or antipyretic agents.
Cimetidine	Bone marrow suppression; increased risk for aplastic anemia	Avoid combination; use other antiulcer medications.
Cyclophosphamide	Decreased effectiveness and reduced metabolism of cyclophosphamide to its active metabolite	Avoid combination.
Cyclosporine	Increased concentrations of cyclosporine	Monitor cyclosporine concentrations and renal function; adjust dose appropriately.
Folic acid, iron, vitamin B_{12}	Delay response of anemias	Avoid combination.
Phenobarbital	Decreased (30%–40%) chloramphenicol concentration Increased (up to 50%) phenobarbital concentrations	Monitor chloramphenicol and phenobarbital concentrations and adjust dose appropriately.
Phenytoin/ fosphenytoin	Increased phenytoin concentration; phenytoin toxicity Decreased or increased chloramphenicol concentration	Monitor phenytoin and chloramphenicol concentration and adjust dose appropriately.
Rifampin/rifabutin	Decreased chloramphenicol concentration	Monitor chloramphenicol concentration and adjust dose appropriately.
Sulfonylurea hypoglycemics	Enhanced hypoglycemia	Monitor blood glucose concentration.
Tacrolimus	Increased tacrolimus concentrations	Monitor tacrolimus concentration and renal function; adjust dose appropriately.
Warfarin	Enhanced anticoagulation	Monitor PT/INR and adjust warfarin dose appropriately.

concentrations of several agents with narrow therapeutic ranges, including cyclosporine, phenobarbital, phenytoin, tolbutamide, tacrolimus, and oral anticoagulants [5–7,33]. In addition, chloramphenicol has reduced the metabolic conversion of cyclophosphamide to its active alkylating metabolite [6,7]. By contrast, potent drug inducers such as barbiturates, phenytoin, and rifampin may decrease serum chloramphenicol concentrations [5–7,33]. The combination of cimetidine with chloramphenicol has been associated with additive bone marrow suppression and increased risk for aplastic anemia [7]. Decreased hematologic responses have also been observed when chloramphenicol was combined with folic acid, iron, or cyanocobalamin [6,7].

Trimethoprim-sulfamethoxazole

Approximately 60% of trimethoprim is excreted unchanged in the urine over 24 hours. Sulfamethoxazole is metabolized primarily by the liver, and approximately 30% is excreted unchanged in the urine. The mechanisms of drug–drug interactions with trimethoprim or sulfamethoxazole (and other sulfonamides) include inhibition of hepatic metabolism, reduced renal tubular secretion, displacement from protein binding sites, and additive pharmacodynamic activity (Table 4).

Trimethoprim is a potent inhibitor of the renal tubular secretion and can increase plasma concentrations of amantadine, dapsone, digoxin, dofetilide, lamuvidine, methotrexate, procainamide, and zidovudine [5–8]. Trimethoprim can also inhibit sodium channels of the renal distal tubules and may cause hyperkalemia with angiotensin-converting enzyme inhibitors, potassium supplements, and potassium-sparing diuretics [5,7]. In addition, hyponatremia has been associated with thiazide diuretics and trimethoprim therapy [7].

Trimethoprim and sulfamethoxazole are selective inhibitors of CYP2C8 and CYP2C9, respectively [45]. Inhibition of these CYP isoenzymes serves as a potential mechanism of drug–drug interactions between trimethoprim-sulfamethoxazole (TMP-SMX) and glipizide, phenytoin, repaglinide, rosiglitazone, and tolbutamide [5–7]. TMP-SMX may accelerate the metabolism of cyclosporine, resulting in lower serum cyclosporine concentrations [6,7].

Sulfonamides can potentially displace sulfonylurea hypoglycemics and methotrexate from plasma protein binding sites, resulting in hypoglycemia and severe bone marrow depression, respectively [5–7]. Additive inhibition of dihydrofolate reductase to azathioprine, methotrexate, or pyrimethamine contributes, in part, to the increased risk for myelotoxicity, pancytopenia, or megaloblastic anemia when these agents are combined with TMP or SMX [5–7].

Antiviral agents (nonretroviral)

The following section reviews the drug–drug interactions associated with antiviral agents that are systemically administered for non-HIV infections.

The individual drugs have been grouped according to their most common clinical use as antiviral agents.

Antiherpesvirus agents

Acyclovir is intracellularly phosphorylated to become an effective inhibitor of viral DNA synthesis in the treatment of herpes simplex virus and varicella-zoster virus. Famciclovir and valacyclovir are prodrugs that rapidly convert to their respective active components, penciclovir and acyclovir. The primary route of elimination of these agents is glomerular filtration and active tubular secretion.

Probenecid inhibits the renal tubular secretion of acyclovir and has resulted in a 40% increase in plasma AUC of acyclovir [6,7,46]. In addition, an overall increase of 49%, 32%, and 78% in the AUC of acyclovir was observed following the administration of valacyclovir with probenecid, cimetidine, and concomitant probenecid-cimetidine, respectively [6,7]. These interactions are perhaps only significant in patients who are receiving high-dose acyclovir therapy or those who require a dose adjustment because of renal impairment or current side effects. Careful consideration is also needed for other therapeutic agents that may compete with acyclovir for active renal tubular secretion. The coadministration of acyclovir and mycophenolate to 12 healthy subjects resulted in an increase in plasma AUC of 11% and 22% of the glucuronide metabolite of mycophenolate and acyclovir, respectively [7]. In addition, a case of neutropenia was observed in a 54-year-old renal transplantation patient following the addition of valacyclovir to mycophenolate mofetil therapy. Patients who have renal impairment should be carefully monitored when mycophenolate and acyclovir or valacyclovir are coadministered. Finally, caution has also been recommended in the use of high-dose intravenous acyclovir with other nephrotoxic agents (eg, aminoglycosides, amphotericin B, cidofovir, foscarnet, cyclosporine, intravenous pentamidine) because of the additive potential of nephrotoxicity [46].

A case report of a 7-year-old boy who had severe epilepsy suggests that serum concentration monitoring and dosage adjustments of phenytoin and valproic acid may be necessary to prevent decreased antiepileptic activity during concurrent therapy with acyclovir [6,7]. Monitoring of theophylline concentrations and appropriate dosage adjustments have also been suggested with concurrent therapy with acyclovir, because a 45% increase in AUC and 30% decreased total body clearance of theophylline have been observed [6,7]. A case report has suggested that profound drowsiness and lethargy can occur with the coadministration of zidovudine and acyclovir. However, no pharmacokinetic interaction has been demonstrated, and this combination has generally been well tolerated during large clinical trials. No clinically significant drug–drug interactions and only minor alterations in pharmacokinetic parameter values have been observed with the

Table 4
Drug–drug interactions involving trimethoprim-sulfamethoxazole

Interacting drug	Effects	Management recommendations
Amantadine	Acute mental confusion	Monitor for central nervous system side effects.
Azathioprine	Leukopenia	Monitor complete blood count.
Cyclosporine	Decreased cyclosporine concentration; azotemia	Monitor cyclosporine concentration and renal function; adjust dose appropriately.
Dapsone	Increased dapsone and trimethoprim concentrations; methemoglobinemia	Monitor methemoglobin concentration.
Digoxin	Increased digoxin concentration	Monitor digoxin concentration.
Dofetilide	Increased dofetilide concentration	Avoid combination therapy.
Enalapril (ACE inhibitors)	Hyperkalemia	Monitor serum potassium level.
Methenamine	Crystallization of sulfonamides in urine	Avoid combination.
Methotrexate	Severe bone marrow suppression	Avoid combination; monitor whole blood count; maintain leucovorin rescue as needed.
Metronidazole	Disulfiram reaction (ethanol in intravenous TMP-SMX)	Use alternative therapy when possible.
Phenytoin/ Fosphenytoin	Increased phenytoin concentration; phenytoin toxicity	Monitor phenytoin concentration and adjust dose appropriately.
Potassium	Hyperkalemia	Monitor serum potassium level.
Potassium-sparing diuretics	Hyperkalemia	Monitor serum potassium level.
Procainamide	Increased procainamide and N-acetylprocainamide (NAPA) concentration; procainamide toxicity	Monitor procainamide and NAPA concentration and adjust dose appropriately.
Procaine, tetracaine	Decreased effect of sulfonamides	Use alternative therapy when possible.
Pyrimethamine	Megaloblastic anemia and pancytopenia	Avoid combination; monitor complete blood count and considering adding leucovorin rescue.
Repaglinide	Increased repaglinide concentration	Monitor serum glucose concentration.
Rifabutin	Increased sulfamethoxazole hydroxylamine concentration	Observe and monitor for SMX toxicity.
Rifampin	Increased rifampin concentration; decreased TMP-SMX concentrations	Observe and monitor for TMP-SMX efficacy.
Rosiglitazone	Increased rosiglitazone concentration; hypoglycemia	Monitor serum glucose concentration and rosiglitazone adverse effects.
Sulfonylurea hypoglycemics	Increased plasma concentration of sulfonylurea agent; increased hypoglycemic effect	Monitor serum glucose concentration.

(continued on next page)

Table 4 (*continued*)

Interacting drug	Effects	Management recommendations
Thiazide diuretics	Hyponatremia	Monitor serum sodium level.
Warfarin	Enhanced anticoagulation	Monitor PT/INR and adjust warfarin dose appropriately.
Zidovudine	Increased zidovudine and glucuronide metabolite concentrations; cytopenias (in hepatic failure)	Monitor complete blood count.

Abbreviations: ACE, angiotensin-converting enzyme; SMX, sulfamethoxatole; TMP, trimethoprim.

coadministration of famciclovir with digoxin, cimetidine, allopurinol, theo-phyllline, or zidovudine [7].

Ganciclovir is a synthetic guanine nucleoside analogue useful in the treatment of cytomegalovirus infections. The prodrug valganciclovir is rapidly converted to ganciclovir by intestinal and hepatic esterases. The major route of elimination for ganciclovir is glomerular filtration and active tubular secretion, and more than 90% of the unchanged drug is recovered in the urine. Drug–drug interactions of ganciclovir involve the risk for overlapping myelosuppressive or central nervous system toxicity or inhibition of renal tubular secretion. The combined use of ganciclovir and zidovudine should be avoided when possible [6,7,46]. In a controlled trial of patients receiving zidovudine and ganciclovir, approximately 80% of patients required a dosage reduction because of hematologic (anemia or neutropenia) or GI toxicity. Ganciclovir can increase the AUC of zidovudine by approximately 20%. When combined therapy is necessary, careful monitoring of hematologic function, modifications in dosage regimens, or the use of alternative antiretroviral agents must be considered. Cautious use and close monitoring for blood dyscrasias are recommended when ganciclovir is combined with agents such as antineoplastics, amphotericin B, dapsone, flucytosine, intravenous pentamidine, primaquine, pyrimethaine, TMP-SMX, and trimetrexate [46]. In addition, caution has been recommended in the use of ganciclovir with other nephrotoxic agents (eg, aminoglycosides, amphotericin B, cidofovir, foscarnet, cyclosporine, intravenous pentamidine) because of the additive potential of nephrotoxicity.

The combined administration of didanosine at 2 hours before oral ganciclovir has resulted in a 111% increase in the AUC of didanosine and a 21% decrease in the AUC of ganciclovir [5,7,46]. When didanosine was administered with intravenous ganciclovir, a 70% increase in the AUC of didanosine and no change in the pharmacokinetics of ganciclovir occurred. No mechanism of this interaction is known, and the combination therapy should be monitored for didanosine toxicity (eg, diarrhea, pancreatitis, peripheral neuropathy) and efficacy of ganciclovir.

Probenecid inhibits the renal tubular secretion of ganciclovir, which has increased the AUC and reduced the renal clearance of ganciclovir by approximately 50% and 22%, respectively [7,46]. Patients should be monitored for increased risk for dose-related ganciclovir toxicities and probenecid-related interactions with other renal tubular–secreted drugs. Seizures have occurred during the concomitant administration of imipenem/cilastatin and ganciclovir [7,46]. No mechanism of this interaction is known, and the combination should be used only when the potential benefits outweigh the risks.

Foscarnet is an inorganic pyrophosphate analogue that is effective for the treatment of cytomegalovirus (CMV) retinitis and infections caused by herpesvirus and varicella-zoster virus. Foscarnet is mostly excreted unchanged in the urine by glomerular filtration and renal tubular secretion. Drug–drug interactions usually involve additive effects of nephrotoxicity and hypocalcemia, the two major dosing-limited adverse events associated with foscarnet. The use of other nephrotoxic agents (eg, aminoglycosides, amphotericin B, cidofovir, cyclosporine, intravenous pentamidine) should be avoided if possible [6,7,46]. Frequent monitoring of serum creatinine and dosage adjustments of both agents are warranted when combination therapy is used. Severe symptomatic hypocalcemia can be increased when foscarnet is combined with intravenous pentamidine [7]. Serum electrolyte, calcium, and magnesium should be carefully monitored in all patients to minimize adverse effects. Tonic-clonic seizures were been reported in two patients receiving the combination of foscarnet and ciprofloxacin, 750 mg twice daily [5–7]. No pharmacokinetic drug–drug interactions were observed between foscarnet and ganciclovir, zalcitabine, or zidovudine. However, the risk for anemia is often higher with the combination of foscarnet and zidovudine [46].

Cidofovir is a nucleoside phosphonate indicated for the treatment of CMV retinitis in HIV-infected patients. More than 90% of cidofovir is eliminated unchanged by renal excretion through glomerular filtration and active tubular secretion. Cidofovir-associated nephrotoxicity is a result of renal cellular uptake by means of OAT1 and drug accumulation in the renal proximal tubules [8]. To minimize the risk for nephrotoxicity, intravenous cidofovir is administered with high-dose probenecid (2 g, 3 hours before and 1 g, 2 and 8 hours after cidofovir infusion). Probenecid, a known OAT1 inhibitor, blocks the tubular transport of cidofovir and reduces its renal clearance to the rate of glomerular filtration [7,8,46]. Although cidofovir does not affect the disposition of other agents, the concurrent administration of probenecid can inhibit renal tubular secretion of other commonly administered agents, such as reverse transcriptase inhibitors (eg, zidovudine, zalcitabine), β-lactams, methotrexate, and nonsteroidal anti-inflammatory drugs (NSAIDs). The use of other nephrotoxic agents (eg, aminoglycosides, amphotericin B, foscarnet, intravenous pentamidine, NSAID, contrast dye) is contraindicated during cidofovir therapy, and the manufacturer recommends waiting at least 7 days between exposure to these agents and administration of cidofovir [46].

Anti-influenza agents

Amantadine and rimantadine are effective antiviral agents for the prevention and treatment of influenza A virus infections. Amantadine is eliminated primarily unchanged in the urine by means of glomerular filtration and active tubular secretion. Additive anticholinergic effects (especially in elderly patients who have Parkinson's disease) or increased central nervous system adverse effects of amantadine may occur with the concomitant administration of anticholinergic agents (eg, benztropine, biperiden, trihexyphenidyl) or sedating antihistamines (eg, chlorpheniramine, phenylpropanolamine) [5–7]. The combined use of amantadine and buproprion has been associated with increased neurotoxicity (eg, restlessness, agitation, gait disturbances, dizziness), including severe reactions requiring hospitalization [5–7]. When any of the aforementioned combinations is used, patients need to be monitored for central nervous system reactions, and dosage adjustment may be required. Triamterene-hydrochlorothiazine, quinidine, quinine, and trimethoprim (alone or in combination with sulfamethoxazole) can reduce the renal tubular secretion of amantadine and cause increased plasma drug concentrations and central nervous system toxicities [5–8].

Rimantadine is metabolized extensively by means of hydroxylation, conjugation, and glucoronidation, then excreted in the urine. The reported drug–drug interactions for rimantadine have only been minor alterations in pharmacokinetic parameters, which are unlikely to be clinically important. For example, the coadministration of rimantadine and cimetidine results in an 18% reduction in the total body clearance and 20% increase in the plasma AUC of rimantadine [6,7]. In addition, acetaminophen and aspirin have been associated with a 10% and 11% decrease, respectively, in the C_{max} and AUC values of rimantadine.

Oseltamivir and zanamivir are neuraminidases that inhibit influenza A and B viruses. Oral oseltamivir phosphate is a prodrug that is hydrolyzed by liver esterases to form an active metabolite, oseltamivir carboxylate, which is then solely eliminated by glomerular filtration and renal tubular secretion. The coadministration of probenecid completely reduces the anionic tubular secretion of oseltamivir carboxylate and results in a 50% decrease in renal clearance, 1.9-fold increase in C_{max}, and 2.5-fold increase in AUC of oseltamivir carboxylate [47]. Despite these changes, no dosage adjustment is recommended, because of the wide margin of safety associated with the active metabolite. In comparison, oseltamivir carboxylate is a weak competitor for the renal organic anionic transport process and is unlikely to inhibit renal secreted organic acids. In addition, the renal and plasma clearance of oseltamivir carboxylate is not altered when it is coadministered with cimetidine, a known inhibitor of renal tubular secretion of basic or cationic drugs and a nonspecific inhibitor of CYP isoenzymes.

Zanamivir is commercially available as a dry powder that is delivered by oral inhalation and eliminated unchanged by the kidneys. In vitro studies demonstrate that oseltamivir and zanamivir are not substrates and do not affect any of the common human CYP isoenzymes [48]. No clinically significant metabolic drug interactions have been reported with either agent.

Agents for tuberculosis

Treatment of tuberculosis encompasses use of four first-line agents, namely isoniazid, rifampin, ethambutol, and pyrazinamide. Induction of multiple CYP isoenzyme systems, as well as PGP, makes rifampin a particularly challenging agent to use [49,50]. Substitution of rifabutin for rifampin is often performed clinically, especially when it is used concomitantly in patients with HIV who are receiving highly active antiretroviral therapy (HAART) [49]. However, rifampin remains a pivotal part of TB management, so the spectrum of its drug interactions profile should be thoroughly appreciated by clinicians. Similarly, isoniazid inhibits CYP isoenzyme systems and MAO and so is associated with some drug interactions [49]. In contrast, ethambutol and pyrazinamide have a limited drug interaction profile [51]; hence the following sections will principally focus on clinically significant drug interactions with use of isoniazid and rifampin. Most important to note is that few drug interaction studies have incorporated the effect of combination antimicrobials: For example, the inhibitory effect of isoniazid on CYP may be negated or overinfluenced by the induction of this system by rifampin. Consequently, therapeutic drug monitoring and thoughtful consideration of the adverse event profiles of concomitantly used agents are critical.

Isoniazid

The metabolism of isoniazid includes acetylation by N-acetyltransferase 2, an enzyme system associated with several allelic variants that broadly define patients as slow or rapid acetylators [50]. Inhibition of CYP2C9, CYP2C19, and CYP3A4 by isoniazid is considered the mechanism of interaction with phenytoin, carbamazepine, diazepam, and warfarin. The potential for this interaction is greater in slow acetylators, who compose 30% to 50% of whites and African Americans [52]. Closely monitoring serum concentrations of phenytoin and carbamazepine is necessary to avoid serious neurologic toxicities, including death. The inhibitory effects of isoniazid on diazepam metabolism are negated with concomitant use of rifampin. The substantial drug interaction profile of warfarin warrants careful monitoring of INR and education of patients about the signs and symptoms of hypoprothrombinemia [15].

An increased risk for hepatotoxicity associated with concomitant isoniazid and acetaminophen use has been reported [19]. The potential for this interaction is dependent on the timing of the acetaminophen and isoniazid doses, with greatest risk for interaction occurring 24 hours after the last dose of isoniazid [19]. Induction of CYP2E1 is thought to contribute to this interaction [19]. Concomitant use of acetaminophen may exacerbate the potential risk for hepatotoxicity and should be avoided if possible. In addition to these effects on the CYP system, isoniazid may also weakly inhibit MAO and histaminase [19]. Flushing, palpitations, and hypertension have been reported with concomitant use of levodopa and isoniazid. Case reports of tyramine-related reactions with consumption of cheese and wine in patients receiving isoniazid support this drug interaction mechanism [19]. Consumption of fish with high histamine content has also resulted in flushing, headache, diarrhea, wheezing, and palpitations in a small percentage of patients receiving isoniazid treatment [19].

Rifampin

Rifampin, as well as other rifamycins such as rifabutin and rifapentine, is a potent inducer of oxidative metabolic systems such as the CYP isoenzyme system [18]. In addition, rifampin can induce transmembrane efflux pumps, such as PGP, and conjugative enzyme systems, such as UDP-glucuronosyltransferase and sulfonyltransferases [18]. Consequently, an extensive drug interaction profile exists for rifampin, which has previously been well reviewed [50]. Given this extensive list of interactions, a summary of select, clinically significant interactions is illustrated in Table 5 and discussed here.

The clinical significance of drug interactions associated with rifampin is dependent on the pharmacodynamic profile of the affected drug, the adverse event profile of induced metabolite formation, or both [18]. In general, rifampin reduces the plasma concentrations of most drugs with which it interacts by inducing their metabolism. Rifampin is also one of the only antimicrobials that is definitively characterized as decreasing the efficacy of oral contraceptives, so patients must be advised to use an alternative method of contraception [14]. The inducing ability of rifampin has not been characterized as dose dependent; in other words, the interaction profile is not greater at 900 mg/d than at 300 mg/d of rifampin [18,50]. The interaction profile is dependent on the route of administration of the interacting drug [18]. For example, rifampin reduces the concentrations of orally administered nifedipine, whereas it has no substantial interaction with the same agent administered intravenously [50]. This reduction in bioavailability is also the primary mechanism by which rifampin reduces protease inhibitor concentrations. Consequently, rifabutin is the recommended rifamycin when one is treating HIV patients receiving HAART [49,50]. Dosage adjustments of protease inhibitors and nonnucleoside reverse transcriptase inhibitors are still required, albeit to a lesser extent than that required with rifampin use.

Therapeutic drug monitoring is not commercially available for the vast majority of agents used in clinical practice. Consequently, alternative agents that are not metabolized should be used concomitantly with rifampin.

Table 5
Drug–drug interactions involving rifampin

Drug	Interaction and management strategy
Anticoagulants	
Warfarin	Increased warfarin clearance. Monitor INR carefully during initiation and especially discontinuation of rifampin.
Anticonvulsants	
Lamotrigine	Increased clearance noted for all three agents. Monitor clinical
Phenytoin	condition; may require 50% increase in dosage. Measurement
Valproic acid	of phenytoin and valproic acid concentrations suggested.
Anti-infectives	
Caspofungin	Trough concentrations reduced by 30%. Maintain adult daily maintenance dose of caspofungin at 70 mg per day.
Chloramphenicol	Potential for higher risk of aplastic anemia. Avoid concomitant use.
Dapsone	Increased clearance of dapsone by 50% and potential higher risk for methemoglobinemia. Dapsone dosage increase is likely to be necessary but is as yet undefined.
Doxycycline	Decreased doxycycline exposure by 50%. A 50% increase in the doxycycline dosage may be necessary.
Fluconazole	Decreased fluconazole exposure by 50%. An increase in the fluconazole dosage may be necessary.
Itraconazole, ketoconazole, voriconazole	Substantial reduction in itraconazole, ketoconazole, and voriconazole concentrations noted. Concomitant use not recommended.
Antiretrovirals	Concomitant use with protease inhibitors or nonnucleoside reverse transcriptase inhibitors is contraindicated for several agents. Rifabutin should be used if a rifamycin is necessary, with appropriate manufacturer-recommended dosage adjustment.
Cardiovascular agents	
Amiodarone	Increased amiodarone metabolism. Avoid concomitant use.
Carvedilol	Reduced carvedilol exposure by 70%. Monitor clinical response and increase carvedilol dose if necessary.
Digoxin	Digoxin dosage adjustment may be necessary.
Diltiazem, verapamil, nifedipine (PO only)	Substantial reduction in diltiazem, verapamil, and nifedipine concentrations. Avoid concomitant use with rifampin.
Lovastatin, simvastatin, fluvastatin	Increased statin metabolism and reduced efficacy. Doubling or tripling the dose may be necessary.
Metoprolol, propranolol, other β-blockers	Decreased exposure and/or increased clearance, resulting in reduced chronotropic effects. Monitor and increase dosage as necessary.
Mexiletine, tocanide	Increased clearance; monitor dysrhythmia control. May require dosage adjustment.
Quinidine	Avoid concomitant use if possible or monitor concentrations.
Contraceptives, oral	Documented clinical failures; use other, nonpharmacologic contraceptive measure.

(continued on next page)

Table 5 (*continued*)

Drug	Interaction and management strategy
Glucocorticoids	
Prednisone, methylprednisone, dexmethasone	A doubling of the glucocorticoid dose is required to achieve clinical response
Immunosuppressants	
Cyclosporin, tacrolimus, sirolimus	Increased doses and therapeutic drug monitoring are critical to ensure that adequate concentrations of these agents are achieved.
Opioids	
Alfentanil	Substantial increased clearance, requiring dosage increase.
Methadone	A doubling or tripling of the methadone dose may be required because narcotic withdrawal has been noted in 70% of patients
Morphine, codeine	Decreased analgesic effect, requiring dosage increment.
Psychotropic agents	
Antidepressants	Loss of antidepressant effect noted with nortryptyline, and serotonin reuptake inhibitor withdrawal noted with sertraline. Monitor for loss of effect.
Antipsychotics	Loss of psychosis control noted with haloperidol and risperidone use with rifampin. Dose increment may be necessary.
Benzodiazepines	Use lorazepam or oxazepam to avoid an interaction.
Zolpidem, zoplicone	A doubling or tripling of the dose may be necessary to maintain psychomotor effects.
Sulfonlureas	Monitor glucose control and increase doses as needed.

Surrogate markers, such as INR (warfarin), heart rate (β-blockers), and cholesterol concentrations (statins), should be monitored closely when one is using rifampin with this class of agents. It is also important to be aware of the time-course of induction by rifampin. Based on a culmination of drug interaction trials, the full induction effect of rifampin takes approximately 7 days, and a return to baseline metabolic activity occurs approximately 14 days after discontinuation of rifampin [50]. As a result, dosage increments made during concomitant use with rifampin will require reduction after the discontinuation of rifampin. Knowledge of the therapeutic window of the interacting drug, availability of therapeutic drug monitoring, surrogate markers, and good clinical judgment are necessary to avoid serious, life-threatening drug interactions with rifampin [50].

References

[1] Reynolds KS. Drug interactions: regulatory perspective. In: Piscitelli SC, Rodvold KA, editors. Drug interactions in infectious diseases. 2nd edition. Totowa (NJ): Humana Press; 2005. p. 83–99.

[2] Lasser KE, Allen PD, Woolhandler SJ, et al. Timing of new black box warnings and withdrawals for prescription medications. JAMA 2002;287(17):2215–20.

[3] Fleischer R, Laessig K. Safety and efficacy evaluation of pleconaril for treatment of the common cold. Clin Infect Dis 2003;37(12):1722.

[4] Piscitelli SC, Rodvold KA, editors. Drug interactions in infectious diseases. 2nd edition. Totowa (NJ): Humana Press; 2005.

[5] Hansten PD, Horn JR. Hansten and Horn's Managing clinically important drug interactions 2005. St. Louis (MO): Facts and Comparisons; 2005.

[6] Tatro DS. Drug interaction facts 2006: the authority on drug interactions. St. Louis (MO): Facts and Comparisons; 2006.

[7] Baxter K, Stockley IH. Stockley's drug interactions. 7th edition. London: Pharmaceutical Press; 2005.

[8] Penzak SR. Mechanisms of drug interactions II: transport proteins. In: Piscitelli SC, Rodvold KA, editors. Drug interactions in infectious diseases. 2nd edition. Totowa (NJ): Humana Press; 2005. p. 41–82.

[9] Rolan PE. Plasma protein binding displacement interactions: why are they still regarded as clinically important? Br J Clin Pharmacol 1994;37(2):125–8.

[10] Neuhauser MM, Danziger LH. β-lactam antibiotics. In: Piscitelli SC, Rodvold KA, editors. Drug interactions in infectious diseases. 2nd edition. Totowa (NJ): Humana Press; 2005. p. 255–87.

[11] Wallace KL. Antibiotic-induced convulsions. Crit Care Clin 1997;13(4):741–62.

[12] Lepper MH, Dowling HP. Treatment of pneumococcic meningitis with penicillin compared with penicillin plus aureomycin: studies including observations on an apparent antagonism between penicillin and aureomycin. Arch Intern Med 1951;88(4):489–94.

[13] Clause D, Decleire PY, Vanbinst R, et al. Pharmacokinetic interaction between valproic acid and meropenem. Intensive Care Med 2005;31(9):1293–4.

[14] Archer JSM, Archer DF. Oral contraceptive efficacy and antibiotic interaction: a myth debunked. J Am Acad Dermatol 2002;46(6):917–23.

[15] Holbrook AM, Pereira JA, Labiris R, et al. Systematic overview of warfarin and its drug and food interactions. Arch Intern Med 2005;165(10):1095–106.

[16] Pai MP, Graci D, Amsden GW. Macrolide drug interactions: an update. Ann Pharmacother 2000;34(4):495–513.

[17] Shi J, Montay G, Bhargava VO. Clinical pharmacokinetics of telithromycin, the first ketolide antibacterial. Clin Pharmacokinet 2005;44(9):915–34.

[18] Petitjean O, Nicolas P, Tod M, et al. Drug interactions during anti-infective treatments. In: Bryskier A, editor. Antimicrobial agents: antibacterials and antifungals. Washington, DC: ASM Press; 2005. p. 1320–52.

[19] Ray WA, Murray KT, Meredith S, et al. Oral erythromycin and the risk of sudden death from cardiac causes. N Engl J Med 2004;351(11):1089–96.

[20] Rashid A. The efficacy and safety of PDE5 inhibitors. Clin Cornerstone 2005;7(1):47–56.

[21] Rengelshausen J, Goggelmann C, Burhenne J, et al. Contribution of increased oral bioavailability and reduced nonglomerular renal clearance of digoxin to the digoxin-clarithromycin interaction. Br J Clin Pharmacol 2003;56(1):32–8.

[22] Juurlink DN, Mamdani M, Kopp A, et al. Drug–drug interactions among elderly patients hospitalized for drug toxicity. JAMA 2003;289(13):1652–8.

[23] Hung IFN, Wu AKL, Cheng VCC, et al. Fatal interaction between clarithromycin and colchicine in patients with renal insufficiency: a retrospective study. Clin Infect Dis 2005;41(3): 291–300.

[24] Saha JR, Butler VP, Neu HC, et al. Digoxin-inactivating bacteria: identification in human gut flora. Science 1983;220(4594):325–7.

[25] Guay DRP. Quinolones. In: Piscitelli SC, Rodvold KA, editors. Drug interactions in infectious diseases. 2nd edition. Totowa (NJ): Humana Press; 2005. p. 215–54.

[26] Pai MP, Allen SE, Amden GW. Altered steady state pharmacokinetics of levofloxacin in adult cystic fibrosis patients receiving calcium carbonate. J Cyst Fibros 2006;5(3):153–7.

[27] Product information: Cipro, ciprofloxacin hydrochloride tablets, ciprofloxacin oral suspension. West Haven (CT): Bayer Pharmaceuticals Co.; 2005.

[28] Product information: Levaquin, levofloxacin. Raritan (NJ): Ortho-McNeil Pharmaceutical; 2005.

[29] Product information: Tequin, gatifloxacin. Princeton (NJ): Bristol-Myers Squibb Co.; 2006.

[30] Park-Wyllie LY, Juurlilnk DN, Kopp A, et al. Outpatient gatifloxacin therapy and dysgly-cemia in older adults. N Engl J Med 2006;354(13):1352–61.

[31] Product information: Avelox, moxifloxacin. West Haven (CT): Bayer Pharmaceuticals Co.; 2005.

[32] Product information: Factive, gemifloxacin mesylate. Waltham (MA): Oscient Pharmaceuticals; 2004.

[33] Susla GM. Miscellaneous antibiotics. In: Piscitelli SC, Rodvold KA, editors. Drug interactions in infectious diseases. 2nd edition. Totowa (NJ): Humana Press; 2005. p. 339–81.

[34] Rybak MJ, Abate BJ, Kang SL, et al. Prospective evaluation of the effect of an aminoglycoside dosing regimen on rates of observed nephrotoxicity and ototoxicity. Antimicrob Agents Chemother 1999;43(7):1549–55.

[35] Rodvold KA, Erdman SM, Pryka RD. Vancomycin. In: Schumacher GE, editor. Therapeutic drug monitoring. Norwalk (CT): Appleton & Lange; 1995. p. 587–632.

[36] Schriever CA, Fernandez C, Rodvold KA, et al. Daptomycin: a novel cyclic lipopeptide antimicrobial. Am J Health Syst Pharm 2005;62(11):1145–58.

[37] Product information: Zyvox, linezolid. New York: Pfizer; 2005.

[38] Hendershot PE, Antal EJ, Welshman IR, et al. Linezolid: pharmacokinetic and pharmacodynamic evaluation of coadministration with pseudoephedrine HCl, phenylpropanolamine HCl, and dextromethorpan HBr. J Clin Pharmacol 2001;41(5):563–72.

[39] Rubinstein E, Prokocimer P, Talbot GH. Safety and tolerability of quinupristin/dalfopristin: administration guidelines. J Antimicrob Chemother 1999;44(Suppl A):37–46.

[40] Product information: Tygacil, tigecycline. Philadelphia: Wyeth Pharmaceuticals; 2005.

[41] Betino JS Jr, Booker LA, Franck PA, et al. Incidence of and significant risk factors for aminoglycoside-associated nephrotoxicity in patients dosed by using individualized pharmacokinetic monitoring. J Infect Dis 1993;167(1):173–9.

[42] Butkus DE, de Torrente A, Terman DS. Renal failure following gentamicin in combination with clindamycin. Nephron 1976;17(4):307–13.

[43] Harris KA, Garey KW, Rodvold KA. Drug–food interactions. In: Piscitelli SC, Rodvold KA, editors. Drug interactions in infectious diseases. 2nd edition. Totowa (NJ): Humana Press; 2005. p. 383–430.

[44] Park JY, Kim KA, Kim SL. Chloramphenicol is a potent inhibitor of cytochrome P450 isoforms CYP2C19 and CYP3A4 in human liver microsomes. Antimicrob Agents Chemother 2003;47(11):3464–9.

[45] Wen X, Wang J-S, Backman JT, et al. Trimethoprim and sulfamethoxazole are selective inhibitors of CYP2C8 and CYP2C9, respectively. Drug Metab Dispos 2002;30(6):631–5.

[46] Tseng A. Drugs for HIV-related opportunistic infections. In: Piscitelli SC, Rodvold KA, editors. Drug interactions in infectious diseases. 2nd edition. Totowa (NJ): Humana Press; 2005. p. 137–89.

[47] Hill G, Cihlar T, Oo C, et al. The anti-influenza drug oseltamivir exhibits low potential to induce pharmacokinetic drug interactions via renal secretion: correlation of in vivo and in vitro studies. Drug Metab Dispos 2002;30(1):13–9.

[48] Daniel MJ, Barnett JM, Pearson BA. The low potential for drug interactions with zanamivir. Clin Pharmacokinet 1999;36(Suppl 1):41–50.

[49] Yew WW. Clinically significant interactions with drugs used in the treatment of tuberculosis. Drug Saf 2002;25(2):111–33.

[50] Niemi M, Backman JT, Fromm MF, et al. Pharmacokinetic interactions with rifampicin: clinical relevance. Clin Pharmacokinet 2003;42(9):819–50.

[51] Namdar R, Ebert SC, Peloquin CA. Drugs for tuberculosis. In: Piscitelli SC, Rodvold KA, editors. Drug interactions in infectious diseases. 2nd edition. Totowa (NJ): Humana Press; 2005. p. 191–213.

[52] Yu MC, Skipper PL, Taghizadeh K, et al. Acetylator phenotype, aminobiphenyl-hemoglobin adduct levels, and bladder cancer risk in white, black, and Asian men in Los Angeles, California. J Natl Cancer Inst 1994;86(9):712–6.

ELSEVIER
SAUNDERS

Med Clin N Am 90 (2006) 1257–1264

THE MEDICAL
CLINICS
OF NORTH AMERICA

Antibiotic Selection in the Penicillin-Allergic Patient

Burke A. Cunha, MD[a,b,*]

[a]State University of New York School of Medicine, Stony Brook, NY, USA
[b]Infectious Disease Division, Winthrop-University Hospital, Mineola, NY 11501, USA

Many individuals with an infectious disease have a history of penicillin allergy. When a patient says that he or she is allergic to penicillin, the physician should clarify the nature of the penicillin allergy. Many patients do not, in fact, have a true penicillin allergy but rather an adverse effect to the medication, such as gastrointestinal intolerance, which is not related to drug allergy. The spectrum of penicillin allergy ranges from drug fever to anaphylactic reactions. After the nature of the penicillin allergy is determined, the clinician then selects an antimicrobial appropriate for the infectious disease being treated, while taking into account the patient's allergy history. In clinical practice, it is rarely if ever necessary to do skin testing for a penicillin allergy. Because so many antibiotics have no cross-allergenicity to penicillin, clinicians can almost always select an appropriate and safe antimicrobial for the penicillin-allergic patient. Skin testing for penicillin allergy and desensitization are rarely necessary in the hospital or outpatient setting [1–6].

Multiple drug hypersensitivity reactions are stereotyped in nature. In penicillin-allergic patients who develop a maculopapular rash to penicillins, the penicillin allergy has the same clinical manifestation on rechallenge. Re-exposure to penicillin will not result in a rash, hives, or anaphylaxis. This principle is important in selecting antimicrobial therapy in the penicillin-allergic patient. Clinicians can take comfort in being able to predict the type of penicillin reaction if a patient, upon re-exposure to the drug, has a hypersensitivity reaction. Physicians unaware of this fact usually are concerned that patients with a rash may develop hives or anaphylaxis. This is not the case. Hypersensitivity drug reactions are stereotyped and there is no progression of severity with repeated exposure. If the nature of the

---

* Infectious Disease Division, Winthrop-University Hospital, 222 Station Plaza North, Suite 432, Mineola, NY 11501.

0025-7125/06/$ - see front matter © 2006 Elsevier Inc. All rights reserved.
doi:10.1016/j.mcna.2006.07.005   *medical.theclinics.com*

penicillin allergy is known, the nature of potential subsequent exposures can be accurately predicted [3,7–10].

Determining the nature of the penicillin allergy

Many patients report a history in childhood to penicillin allergy in a way that is difficult to interpret. Others report that relatives have a penicillin allergy and therefore they think that they may be allergic to penicillin as well. In both of these situations, the probability of penicillin allergy is low and certainly is not anaphylactoid in nature. In clinical practice, the three main categories of clinical expression of penicillin allergy are drug fever, drug rash, and anaphylactic reactions [1,3,5,6,8–10].

Drug fever

Drug fever refers to hypersensitivity reaction to any medication, including antimicrobials, which is manifested clinically only by an increase in temperature. Many nonantibiotic drugs are more common causes of allergic reactions than most antibiotics, some antibiotics cause drug fevers. Drug fevers due to other medications or antibiotics are manifested clinically by increases in temperature from 100°F to over 106°F. Most drug fevers occur in the 102°F–104°F range. A clinical clue to the presence of drug fever is the "relatively good" appearance of the patient. That is, the patient does not appear to be toxemic from a bacterial infection. Drug fevers are regularly accompanied by a pulse–temperature deficit (ie, relative bradycardia). Physiologically, there is an increase in 10 beats per minute in the heart rate for every degree of temperature elevation above 98°F. This physiological relationship is an appropriate pulse–temperature response. For example, for a patient with 103°F fever, an appropriate pulse response would be a pulse of about 120 beats per minute. Alternatively, a patient with a 103°F temperature and a pulse rate of 88 beats per minute, has a pulse–temperature deficit and relative bradycardia. Relative bradycardia is an important clue to the presence of drug fever in a patient with an otherwise unexplained obscure fever. Relative bradycardia cannot be used as a diagnostic clue to the presence of drug fever if the patient is receiving β-blockers, verapamil, or diltiazem. These drugs in febrile patients do not allow an appropriate increase in pulse, and these patients have a blunted pulse response to fever. In trying to determine if relative bradycardia is present, patients on these medications, those with pacemaker-induced rhythms, and those with certain conduction abnormalities, such as Lev's disease and Lenegre's disease, should be excluded from consideration. In these patients, drug fever has to be diagnosed using other means [10,11].

Drug fever is a diagnosis of exclusion. It assumes that blood cultures, excluding skin contaminants obtained during venipuncture, are sterile. Patients may be ill with drug fevers, but look "inappropriately well" in terms of infection for the degree of fever. Laboratory tests also provide clues to the possibility of a drug fever. The presence of eosinophils in the peripheral smear in a patient with otherwise unexplained fever, should suggest the possibility of a drug hypersensitivity reaction. When the patient has eosinophilia, the relationship to the fever is likely to be realized. Unfortunately, eosinophils in the peripheral smear are more common than frank eosinophilia in patients with drug fever. Another difficulty in identifying eosinophils is that they are not routinely reported in complete blood cell counts (CBCs) obtained by automatic cell counters in the laboratory. Automated CBCs are relatively insensitive to eosinophils and atypical lymphocytes. If the clinician suspects drug fever, then a manual CBC should be ordered. A manual CBC identifies low numbers of eosinophils in the peripheral smear that would be missed in an automated differential white blood cell count (WBC). Atypical lymphocytes, even if present in low numbers (ie, without atypical lymphocytosis) are also clues to a drug hypersensitivity reaction in a patient with an otherwise unexplained fever. Physicians often associate atypical lymphocytes with viral infections. Indeed, most, but not all, viral infections contain atypical lymphocytes, which are also present in certain parasitic disorders, and importantly, in drug fevers. With drug fever, the number of atypical lymphocytes present in the peripheral smear is low, as in the case of eosinophils, and uncommonly reaches levels out of the normal range that would be reported. As with the eosinophils, atypical lymphocytes are best detected by manually performed WBC differential counts, which should be specifically requested when drug fever is a potential diagnosis [10–12].

Drug fevers often cause an increase in the WBC count with or without a left shift, which can mimic an infectious process. Less commonly, drug hypersensitivity reactions may also result in mild leukopenia or thrombocytopenia. Drug-induced leukopenia and thrombocytopenia are readily reversible when the drug causing a hypersensitivity reaction is discontinued. Other indirect tests indicating potential drug fever are an early and mild increase in the serum transaminases. Elevations of the aspartate aminotransferase are most common. Less common are mild elevations of the alanine aminotransferase. Serum transaminase elevations occur early and may reach levels of up to twice normal. The erythrocyte sedimentation rate (ESR) is also elevated in drug hypersensitivity reactions with fever. Few patients with drug fever have all of the laboratory abnormalities mentioned, but all patients have sufficient clues in the proper clinical setting to suggest the possibility of drug fever [10–12].

Maculopapular drug rashes

Drug rashes are drug hypersensitivity reactions manifested with cutaneous manifestations. Unless otherwise stated, drug rash implies a maculopapular eruption, not hives. Drug rashes are usually distributed about the body and are not localized. That is, they are not limited to the anterior trunk or the extremities, for example. Drug rashes may also involve the palms and soles, particularly if part of a total body maculopapular eruption. Early in the drug eruption process, maculopapular rashes are usually not pruritic but may become pruritic over time. Rarely are drug rashes pustular or vesiculopustular. Drug rashes may or may not be accompanied by fever. The diagnosis of drug rash is straightforward, unlike that of drug fever, because of the obvious presence of a rash. The most common diagnostic error made with drug fevers is to ascribe a localized rash, almost always representing contact dermatitis, as an allergic drug rash. Therefore, to be diagnosed with drug rash, a patient must be on a sensitizing medication and have a generalized maculopapular rash or an otherwise unexplained pruritic maculopapular rash [13–16].

Hives are cutaneous manifestations of a hypersensitivity reaction. Hives are discrete raised lesions, in contrast to the generalized exanthem of a maculopapular rash. As with other hypersensitivity drug reactions, patients with a history of hives to a given agent will, when re-exposed, again manifest a hypersensitivity reaction with hives. Hives are more serious manifestations of a hypersensitivity reaction than a maculopapular rash.

Anaphylactic reactions

The most severe clinical manifestations of a drug hypersensitivity reaction are anaphylactic reactions. Anaphylaxis may be clinically manifested by laryngospasm, bronchospasm, or hypotension, and shock. Anaphylactic reactions are life threatening and occur immediately after drug exposure. Patients with drug-induced hives usually do not have any of the laboratory abnormalities associated with drug fever or maculopapular drug eruptions [3,17–18].

Penicillin cross-reactivity with β-lactams

Penicillins as a group consist of penicillin G as well as extended spectrum penicillins, which are the antipseudomonal penicillins (carbenicillin, ticarcillin, mezlocillin, azlocillin, and piperacillin) and the antistaphylococcal penicillins (dicloxacillin, oxacillin, and nafcillin). Penicillin derivatives also include ampicillin and ampicillin derivatives (amoxicillin and bacampicillin). In the general category of penicillins are also β-lactamase–inhibitor combinations, which include a penicillin derivative. Among these combinations are ampicillin–sulbactam and piperacillin–tazobactam. β-lactamase inhibitors are hypoallergenic and if a drug hypersensitivity reaction occurs with β-lactam–β-lactamase–inhibitor combinations, the offending agent is always the β-lactam component. β-lactam antibiotics are structurally similar to the penicillins. For this reason, the cross-allergenicity rate between penicillins and β-lactams are 3% to 5%. Thus, earlier studies indicated much higher cross-reactivity rates between penicillins and β-lactams, such as cephalosporins. But the cross-reactions were not on the basis of cross-allergenicity but rather were reflective of individuals with multiple drug allergies [8–10,19–23].

Monobactams and carbapenems resemble β-lactam antibiotics but, from an allergy perspective, are unrelated. The only carbapenem with minimal potential for cross-reactivity with penicillins or β-lactams is imipenem [24,25]. Unlike other carbapenems, imipenem is combined with cilastatin and it probably is the cilastatin rather than the imipenem that is responsible for the rare cases of cross-reactivity between imipenem and β-lactams. There is no data suggesting cross-reactivity between meropenem and β-lactams, although ertapenem has been used for a shorter duration than the other carbapenems. To date, there are no reports of cross-allergenicity between β-lactams and ertapenem either. The only monobactam available for clinical use is aztreonam. As with carbapenems, there is no cross-allergenicity between monobactams and β-lactams [10,26,27].

Clinical approach to the penicillin-allergic patient

Penicillin allergy with drug fever or rash

For patients with penicillin allergy manifested by a drug fever or a maculopapular rash, the cross-reactivity with β-lactams is 3% to 5%, which is so low that β-lactams may be safely given in penicillin-allergic patients with either a drug fever or a maculopapular rash. β-lactams should not be given to patients with a history of penicillin allergy manifested by hives or anaphylaxis [10,18,28–30].

Penicillin allergy with hives or anaphylaxis

Antibiotics that have no cross-reactivity with penicillins or β-lactams should be used to treat infections in penicillin-allergic patients with serious systemic manifestations of drug allergenicity. Antibiotics that have no cross-allergenicity to either penicillin or β-lactams include aminoglycosides, tetracyclines, macrolides, clindamycin, chloramphenicol, metronidazole, vancomycin, quinupristin–dalfopristin, linezolid, daptomycin, tigecycline, quinolones, nitrofurantoin, monobactams, and carbapenems (eg, meropenem and ertapenem) (Table 1). Antibiotic selection depends on the severity of infection, route of administration, and a spectrum appropriate for the presumed pathogen, which is determined by the site of infection. In a group of patients with penicillin allergy, meropenem was given as appropriate therapy for the infection in those with a stated but unknown history of penicillin allergy and those with known anaphylactic reactions to penicillins or β-lactams. No patient receiving meropenem for 1 to 4 weeks had any allergic reaction. Significantly, no cross-allergenicity occurred in the penicillin anaphylactic group when treated with meropenem [31].

Table 1
Antibiotic alternatives in penicillin-allergic patients

Type of penicillin allergy	Alternative non–β-lactam antibiotics
Anaphylactic reaction or hives (hives, laryngospasm, bronchospasm, hypotension, shock)	Aminoglycosides (IV) Clindamycin (IV, PO) Macrolides (PO) Linezolid (IV, PO) TMP-SMX (IV, PO) Vancomycin (IV) Quinupristin–dalfopristin (IV) Colistin (IV) Polymyxin B (IV) Quinolones (IV, PO) Chloramphenicol (IV) Minocycline (IV, PO) Doxycycline (IV, PO) Aztreonam (IV) Meropenem (IV) Ertapenem (IV) Tigecycline (IV) Daptomycin (IV)
Drug fever (fever without rash) or drug rash (maculopapular rash, generalized)	β-Lactam antibiotic therapy or any of the non–β-lactam antibiotics listed

Abbreviations: IV, intravenous; PO, oral; TMP-SMX, trimethoprim-sulfamethoxazole.

Summary

Because of the numerous oral and parenteral antibiotics now available, clinicians can almost always find a suitable antibiotic that does not cross-react with penicillins or penicillin derivatives. Skin testing for penicillin allergy is rarely necessary because of the many therapeutic alternatives available [10,31]. In the rare instance of the need for penicillin desensitization, such as in the case of a pregnant patient with neurosyphilis and an anaphylactic reaction to penicillin, such desensitization should be done by an allergist or immunologist [32–34]. After 30 years of infectious disease practice, the author has never found it necessary to desensitize a patient because of a lack of an alternative medication for the clinical situation [10,31]. Most patients who give a history of penicillin allergy do not in fact have an allergy to penicillin, and skin testing is not always predictive of penicillin allergy [5,6,34]. To determine the nature of the penicillin allergy, if indeed it is present, the clinician must inquire for details regarding the nature of the penicillin allergy. This determination is important because patients with penicillin allergies manifested by drug fever or rash may safely be given β-lactam antibiotics, such as cephalosporins. In the worst-case scenario, if there is a reaction in 3% to 5% of patients that exhibit true cross-allergenicity to penicillin, then the patient will experience the same reaction (eg, drug fever or rash) that was experienced previously. Both drug fevers and drug rashes are recognizable clinical entities and readily reversible upon early discontinuation of the antibiotic. For patients with hives or an anaphylactic reaction to penicillin, then neither penicillins nor β-lactams should be used. An antibiotic with no cross-allergenicity with penicillins or β-lactams should be selected. That is, aminoglycosides, tetracyclines, fluoroquinolones, vancomycin, tigecycline linezolid, daptomycin, and carbapenems, particularly meropenem, may be given safely in penicillin allergies, including anaphylactic reactions, with virtually no potential for an allergic reaction [10,27,31].

Clinicians should be familiar with which antibiotics are safe to use for different types of penicillin-allergic reactions. Clinically, it is convenient to divide patients with penicillin reactions into three categories: those with unknown or possible reactions to penicillin, those with a drug fever or rash, and those with hives or anaphylactic reactions. B-lactam antibiotics may be used safely for patients with drug fever or rash. Penicillins or β-lactams should not be used for patients with hives or anaphylactic reactions. For such patients, clinicians should employ antimicrobial therapy with an antibiotic that does not cross-react with penicillins or β-lactams.

References

[1] Lin RY. A perspective on penicillin allergy. Arch Intern Med 1992;152:930–7.
[2] Lee CE, Zembower TR, Fotis MA, et al. The incidence of antimicrobial allergies in hospitalized patients. Arch Intern Med 2000;160:2819–22.
[3] Adkinson NF Jr. Drug allergy. In: Adkinson NR Jr, Yunginger J, Busse WW, et al, editors. Middleton's allergy: principles and practice. Philadelphia: Mosby; 2003. p. 1679–94.
[4] Pirmohamed M, James S, Meakin S, et al. Adverse drug reactions as a cause of admission to hospital: prospective analysis of 18,820 patients. BMJ 2004;329:15–9.
[5] Salkind AR, Cuddy PG, Foxworth JW. Is this patient allergic to penicillin? JAMA 2001;285:2498–505.
[6] Surtees SJ, Stockton MG, Gietzen TW. Allergy to penicillin: fable or fact? BMJ 1991;302:1051–2.
[7] Shepherd GM. Allergy to β-lactam antibiotics. Immunol Allergy Clin North Am 1991;11:611–33.
[8] Kelkar PS, Li JT. Cephalosporin allergy. N Engl J Med 2001;345:804–9.
[9] Gruchalla RS, Pirmohamed M. Antibiotic allergy. N Engl J Med 2006;354:601–9.
[10] Cunha BA, editor. Antibiotic essentials. 5th edition. Royal Oak (MI): Physicians' Press; 2006.
[11] Johnson DH, Cunha BA. Drug fever. Infect Dis Clin North Am 1996;10:85–91.
[12] Cunha BA. Laboratory tests in infectious disease. In: Cunha BA, editor. Educational review manual in infectious diseases. 2nd edition. New York: Castle Connolly Medical Publishing; 2005.
[13] Cunha BA. The diagnostic approach to rash and fever in the CCU. Crit Care Clin 1998;8:35–54.
[14] Cunha BA. Antibiotic side effects. Med Clin North Am 2001;85:149–85.
[15] Mendelson LM. Adverse reactions to β-lactam antibiotics. Immunol Allergy Clin North Am 1998;18:745–57.

[16] Pichler WJ. Delayed drug hypersensitivity reactions. Ann Intern Med 2003;139:683–93.

[17] Saxon A, Beall GN, Rohr AS, et al. Immediate hypersensitivity reactions to beta-lactam antibiotics. Ann Intern Med 1987;107:204–15.

[18] Segreti J, Trenholme GM, Levin S. Antibiotic therapy in the allergic patient. Med Clin North Am 1995;79:935–42.

[19] Kim S, Warrington RJ. Clinical cross-reactivity between penicillins and cephalosporins. Can J Allergy Clin Immunol 1998;3:12–5.

[20] Blanca M, Fernandez J, Miranda A, et al. Cross-reactivity between penicillins and cephalosporins: clinical and immunological studies. J Allergy Clin Immunol 1989;83:381–5.

[21] Blanca M, Vega JM, Garcia J, et al. New aspects of allergic reactions to beta-lactams: cross reactions and unique specificities. Clin Exp Allergy 1994;24:407–15.

[22] Anne S, Reisman RE. Risk of administering cephalosporin antibiotics to patients with histories of penicillin allergy. Ann Allergy Asthma Immunol 1995;74:167–70.

[23] Petz LD. Immunologic cross-reactivity between penicillins and cephalosporins: a review. J Infect Dis 1978;137(Suppl):74–9.

[24] Saxon A, Adelman DC, Patel A, et al. Imipenem cross-reactivity with penicillin in humans. J Allergy Clin Immunol 1988;82:213–7.

[25] McConnell SA, Penzak SR, Warmack TS, et al. Incidence of imipenem hypersensitivity reactions in febrile neutropenic bone marrow transplant patients with a history of penicillin allergy. Clin Infect Dis 2000;31:1512–4.

[26] Sullivan TJ. Allergic reactions to antimicrobial agents: a review of reactions to drugs not in the β-lactam antibiotic class. J Allergy Clin Immunol 1984;74:594–9.

[27] Cunha BA. Cross allergenicity of penicillin with carbapenems and monobactams. J Crit Illn 1998;13:344.

[28] Wickern GM, Nish WA, Bitner AS, et al. Allergy to beta-lactams: a survey of current practices. J Allergy Clin Immunol 1994;94:725–31.

[29] Robinson JL, Hameed T, Carr S. Practical aspects of choosing an antibiotic for patients with a reported allergy to an antibiotic. Clin Infect Dis 2002;35:26–30.

[30] Cunha BA. Antimicrobial selection in the penicillin-allergic patient. Drugs for Today 2001; 37:337–83.

[31] Cunha BA. Unpublished data. Mineola (NY): 2006.

[32] Fonacier L, David-Lorton M. Antibiotic adverse effects: penicillin allergy and desensitization. Antibiotics for Clinicians 1989;2:109–13.

[33] Sogn DD, Evans R, Shepherd GM, et al. Results of the National Institute of Allergy and Infectious Diseases collaborative clinical trial to test the predictive value of skin testing with major and minor penicillin derivatives in hospitalized adults. Arch Intern Med 1992;152: 1025–32.

[34] Levine BB, Zolov DM. Prediction of penicillin allergy by immunological tests. J Allergy 1969;43:231–44.

ELSEVIER
SAUNDERS

THE MEDICAL
CLINICS
OF NORTH AMERICA

Med Clin N Am 90 (2006) 1265–1277

Clinical Approach to Antibiotic Failure

David Schlossberg, MD, FACP[a,b,*]

[a]Temple University School of Medicine, 3401 North Broad Street, Philadelphia,
PA 19140, USA
[b]Tuberculosis Control Program, Department of Health, 500 South Broad Street,
Philadelphia, PA 19146, USA

Sometimes antibiotics fail or appear to fail, and the clinician must determine the reasons for a suboptimal response. However, before concluding that an antibiotic has failed, it is important to remember that, even when antibiotics have their desired effect, the patient's response may not be immediate. Most immunocompetent patients will show some clinical response to appropriate antibiotic therapy within 24 to 48 hours, although various objective parameters of the infectious process may lag behind the overall clinical response. For example, patients with Rocky Mountain spotted fever often feel better within 24 to 48 hours, but their fever may not begin to respond for an additional 2 to 3 days. Similarly, patients with pneumonia frequently experience a diminution in fever and toxicity in the first few days after institution of antibiotics, but the chest radiograph does not immediately reflect the patient's improvement and may actually appear to worsen before it ultimately improves. A similar observation describes cerebrospinal fluid during therapy for bacterial meningitis, which may temporarily worsen (ie, manifest a greater leukocytosis) even as the patient improves. Some classic parameters of infection are atypical on presentation. For example, patients with severe infection may develop leukopenia instead of leukocytosis, while others present with hypothermia instead of fever. Such patients will "respond" to treatment of their infection by an actual rise in white blood cell count or temperature.

Thus, in evaluating the response to antibiotic therapy, the clinician should consider primarily the patient's overall sense of well-being and symptoms, such as headache, generalized myalgias, and weakness. Objective signs of infection may lag and should not be misinterpreted as indicating a failed response. In this regard, it is crucial to assess the patient, not the laboratory parameters.

* 320 Orchard Way, Merion, PA 19066.
E-mail address: dschloss@ix.netcom.com

0025-7125/06/$ - see front matter © 2006 Elsevier Inc. All rights reserved.
doi:10.1016/j.mcna.2006.07.004

Nevertheless, some patients fail antibiotic therapy, and this review will discuss the approach to such real or perceived failure, as indicated in the algorithm (Fig. 1).

Noninfectious mimics of infection

The body's tissues have a limited repertoire of response to injury, and a multitude of noninfectious illnesses may mimic infection and fail to respond to antibiotic therapy until the correct diagnosis is made. Systemic inflammatory response syndrome, a response to tissue injury, is defined as a derangement in two of the four parameters of temperature, heart rate, respiratory rate, and white blood cell count. Sepsis, defined as systemic inflammatory response syndrome resulting from infection, is effectively mimicked by many diseases that produce fever with generalized manifestations, including vasculitis, drug hypersensitivity, malignant hyperthermia, neuroleptic malignant syndrome, thyroid storm, and adrenal insufficiency [1].

Localized syndromes also resemble a variety of infectious processes. For example, cellulitis is mimicked by contact dermatitis, drug reactions, eosinophilic cellulitis, arthritis, malignant infiltration, familial Mediterranean fever, panniculitis, insect stings, phlebitis, and infected Baker's cysts [2]; pulmonary infiltrate and fever imitating pneumonia are seen with pulmonary embolism, aspiration, hemorrhage, pulmonary hypersensitivity, tumor, vasculitis, and sickle cell pneumopathy; a variety of central nervous system processes can resemble meningitis, including medication reactions, vasculitis, malignancy, hemorrhage, sarcoidosis, and seizures; pancreatitis and ischemic bowel masquerade as abdominal infections; gastroenteritis is suggested by toxins, inflammatory bowel disease, and hyperthyroidism; and pyogenic arthritis is part of the differential diagnosis of rheumatoid arthritis, synovial tumors, and gout. The above lists are only partial but illustrate the capacity of many sterile illnesses to resemble infection.

Infectious processes not specifically treatable with antibiotics

Some infections will fail antibiotic therapy because they are not specifically treatable. These infections include most viral infections, especially upper respiratory infections and viral meningitis, and toxin-induced illness such as staphylococcal toxic shock. Some infections may appear to respond to antimicrobial therapy because of the anti-inflammatory activity of agents such as azithromycin.

Treatable infection with incomplete response

Frequently, after being treated for infection, a patient will appear to respond but remain febrile (Box 1). Such patients often feel and look better

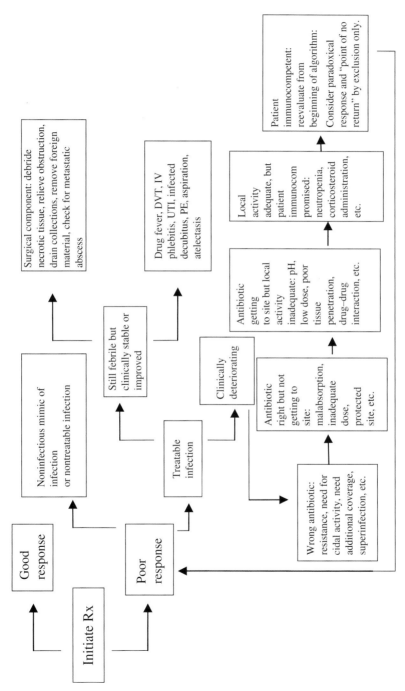

Fig. 1. Algorithm for antibiotic failure. DVT, deep venous thrombosis; IV, intravenous; PE, pulmonary embolism; Rx, antibiotic; UTI, urinary tract infection.

Box 1. Treatable infections with incomplete responses

Surgical component
Drain abscess
Relieve obstruction
Debride devitalized tissue
Identify intravascular sites
Remove prosthetic material

Miscellaneous complications
Drug fever
Intravenous site infection
Deep vein thrombosis
Pulmonary Embolism
Urinary tract infection
Atelectasis
Aspiration
Infected decubitus ulcer
Adrenal insufficiency
Myocardial infarction
Unsuspected concomitant infection
Exacerbation of underlying disease by the infection

---

and remain stable clinically, but some parameters of their infection, such as fever or leukocytosis, remain abnormal. The clinical approach to such patients should include (1) a search for a surgical component to their illness, and (2) exclusion of a group of miscellaneous complications of the underlying infection. Such complications are unrelated to the basic infection pathophysiologically and therefore represent a separate process (Box 1).

Surgical components

The possible surgical components include abscess drainage, relief of obstruction, debridement of devitalized tissue, removal of foreign material, and exclusion of persistent intravascular foci of infection. Abscess may complicate many infections, either at the outset or with subsequent tissue necrosis. Most abscesses require surgical drainage, which increasingly is accomplished percutaneously. Some abscesses, such as lung abscesses, normally drain themselves and do not require surgery. Others are exceptions to the general rule and usually resolve with medical therapy alone. These include tubo-ovarian abscesses, hepatic abscesses, and cerebritis (the early, pre-collection stage of brain abscess). But the general rule remains that pus should be drained, and the search for abscess should be repeated in patients with infections that may be accompanied by abscess but who are not resolving satisfactorily. Sometimes an early bacteremia may result in metastatic abscess formation that was not apparent at the onset of illness. Classic hiding sites for such abscesses are the spleen, liver, subdiaphragmatic locations, and skeletal muscle, especially the psoas and thigh and especially in immunocompromised patients. Although such patients are usually stable clinically, an occasional patient may develop bacteremia from the abscess or appear septic with negative blood cultures because of components of the bacterial cell wall that are released into the bloodstream.

Obstruction requiring relief is seen in cholecystitis, cholangitis, pyelonephritis, and pneumonia. Depending on the degree of obstruction, among other factors, some of these patients may stabilize yet remain febrile. Others continue to be ill until the obstruction is relieved on an emergency basis. In this regard, it is often distressing to see surgical reluctance to operate on a patient who is "too sick" to withstand surgery; on the contrary, such patients may not respond further until the obstruction is relieved. Temporizing procedures in such patients may be life saving. For example, nephrostomy can divert urinary flow in patients with infection proximal to a ureteral stone. Similarly, cholecystostomy can be performed under local anesthesia at the bedside to relieve cystic duct obstruction in cholecystitis, and percutaneous drainage or endoscopic retrograde cholangiopancreatography can decompress the biliary system in patients with cholangitis.

Debridement of devitalized tissue is crucial to recovery from soft tissue infections and should not be delayed pending the patient's improvement. Similarly, some infections involving foreign material, such as intravenous lines, pacemakers, urinary catheters, contact lenses, orthopedic hardware, prosthetic joints, artificial heart valves, intrauterine devices, vascular prostheses, and dialysis shunts, may require removal of the prosthetic material for the infection to resolve. Such prostheses allow organisms to adhere and, in some cases, to produce a biofilm, an extracellular polysaccharide matrix that protects the bacteria via physiologic as well as mechanical factors [3]. Usually such patients respond to therapy but require removal of the prosthetic material for ultimate eradication of infection and to prevent relapse. However, if the foreign material is in the bloodstream (eg, a central line or prosthetic heart valve) such patients can remain acutely ill and require immediate removal of the prosthesis.

A final category of surgical components of infection comprises persistent intravascular infection. This may result from refractory endocarditis or complications of endocarditis, such as valve ring abscess or septal abscess. Other endovascular infections include mycotic aneurysms complicating bacteremia and infection of a preexisting aneurysm. The classic example of the latter is persistent salmonella bacteremia in a patient with a known aortic aneurysm, with the clot in the aneurysm having become infected with salmonella. Salmonella may also infect atherosclerotic plaques and sites of venous thrombosis. As with the other intravascular infections described above, such patients may remain acutely ill and necessitate urgent surgical removal of their bloodstream focus of infection.

Miscellaneous complications

Miscellaneous indirect complications of the underlying infection include drug fever, intravenous site infection, deep venous thrombosis, pulmonary embolism, urinary tract infection, atelectasis, aspiration, decubiti, adrenal insufficiency, myocardial infarction, unsuspected concomitant infection, and exacerbation of underlying disease by the infection. Drug fever is easy to overlook because patients frequently lack a rash or eosinophilia, occasionally develop an extremely high temperature, or have been taking the causative medication for a long time. Helpful clues to fever resulting from drug allergy are relative bradycardia and atypical lymphocytosis. Although some drugs are relatively common causes of drug fever, such as sulfonamides and β-lactam antibiotics, it should be assumed that any drug can cause fever, with the possible exception of digoxin.

The site of an intravenous line, whether central or peripheral, may be a source of fever. When the site is reddened, with purulent drainage, the diagnosis is obvious. The line must be removed immediately and surgery consulted for consideration of resection or incision and drainage of the infected vein segment. However, some patients develop infection at the site of an indwelling line without evident inflammation, and these loci can be a cause of fever and bacteremia. Furthermore, even after a line is removed, prior sites should not be forgotten. If no erythema or drainage is visible, a sonogram can detect an area of phlebitis that might require resection. Deep venous phlebitis may complicate the course of a hospitalized, bedridden patient. This phlebitis may cause fever by itself or via a complicating pulmonary embolism. If the phlebitis is in the calf, sonography is relatively insensitive in the absence of physical signs of phlebitis. Also, phlebitis can be pelvic in location and even harder to detect clinically; this is most likely to occur in women who are postpartum or who have had pelvic surgery or infection, or in men with prostatic infection or surgery. Women with septic pelvic thrombophlebitis often defervesce when heparin is added to their antibiotic regimen.

Many pulmonary complications cause fever. Pulmonary embolism, aspiration, and atelectasis are all risks for the sick, hospitalized patient; decubitus ulcers may develop during a hospitalization or already be present in the patient admitted from a nursing home. It is easy to underestimate a decubitus ulcer. Relatively benign-looking decubiti may be a source of bacteremia, and unroofing the eschar overlying a decubitus ulcer sometimes, to everyone's surprise, reveals a purulent collection. Another indirect complication of infection is a myocardial infarction, often accompanied by fever, complicating the stress of infection in a predisposed patient.

Adrenal insufficiency may result in fever and hypotension in a patient maintained on corticosteroids but whose dose of corticosteroids is not increased following the stress of surgery or admission for pneumonia. In addition, adrenal involvement with varying degrees of adrenal hypofunction can complicate disseminated infection with *Neisseria meningitidis*, *Mycobacterium tuberculosis*, histoplasma, and cytomegalovirus (particularly in advanced AIDS). A different type of apparent antibiotic failure is a dual process, as seen in the patient with simultaneous pyogenic arthritis and acute gout; the antibiotics directed at the pyogenic arthritis will not quell the symptoms of the accompanying crystal-induced inflammation. Finally, infection can exacerbate an underlying illness, as in the patient with sickle cell disease whose pneumonia triggers an acute pulmonary syndrome.

Treatable infection clinically failing to respond

As seen in the algorithm (see Fig. 1), the category of treatable infections clinically failing to respond may result from prescribing the wrong antibiotic, from the antibiotic not reaching the site of infection, inadequate local activity of the antibiotic, immunosuppression, a paradoxical response, or a point of no return (Box 2).

Box 2. Treatable infection failing to respond

Wrong antibiotic
Need cidal therapy
Need additional coverage
Primary resistance
Secondary resistance
Superinfection

Antibiotic not reaching site of infection
Malabsorption
Intramuscular administration in diabetic or hypotensive patients
Protected sites (central nervous system, eye, prostate)

Inadequate local activity
Inadequate dose
Local pH effect
Drug–drug interaction
Organisms in stationary phase
Pregnancy
Concentration-dependent versus time-dependent activity

Immunosuppression
Paradoxical responses
Point of no return

The wrong antibiotic

The wrong antibiotic may be prescribed for a patient who needs bactericidal therapy. Most clinicians believe bactericidal activity is necessary to treat endocarditis—especially enterococcal endocarditis—and central nervous system infection, and many also prefer bactericidal therapy for osteomyelitis and patients with neutropenia. All of these clinical states represent inadequate local defenses. However, these rules have many exceptions, and the in vitro basis for the bactericidal–bacteriostatic distinction is not always clear-cut, with some classically bacteriostatic drugs exhibiting bactericidal activity under certain circumstances [4].

Another type of wrong antibiotic coverage occurs when additional pathogens in a polymicrobial infection are left untreated. For example, an intra-abdominal process requires coverage for anaerobes as well as for gram-negative aerobes and streptococci; fastidious organisms, such as anaerobes, may fail to grow on culture, and their presence must be inferred by organisms seen on Gram stain but not grown, or by clinical situations where their presence would be expected. A related issue is the requirement for combination coverage. For example, to eradicate enterococci from a heart valve, vancomycin or a penicillin must be added to an aminoglycoside; single antibiotic treatment of such infections ultimately fail.

Antibiotic therapy can also be wrong if the laboratory errs in identifying an organism or in susceptibility testing, or if the laboratory does not point out the in-vitro–in-vivo disparity known to occur for some organisms. For example, salmonella may appear susceptible to aminoglycosides in vitro, but clinical experience has taught us not to use these agents to treat salmonella infection. Similarly, methicillin-resistant *Staphylococcus aureus* may appear susceptible to cephalosporins in vitro, but methicillin-resistant strains will not respond to cephalosporins, regardless of the in vitro susceptibility studies. Resistance may also develop during therapy, especially if subinhibitory doses of antibiotics are used, or if an inducible resistance is encountered. An example of the latter is clindamycin resistance to staphylococci induced during therapy, which can be predicted by the D-zone test in erythromycin-resistant, clindamycin-susceptible straphylococci. It has been suggested that laboratories perform this testing routinely for staphylococci and for group A, B and G β-hemolytic streptococci [5]. Such resistance developing during therapy can result in failure of the primary infection or in relapse from a resistant strain after initial improvement. A related phenomenon is superinfection from resistant organisms that flourish under the selection pressure of the prescribed antibiotic.

Finally, certain bacteria that were once reliably susceptible to traditional empiric therapy have become resistant; the prevalence and degree of such emerging resistance varies geographically, so that local patterns must be constantly updated. In many instances, resistance must be assumed until susceptibility is known. Notorious examples of this change include

Streptococccus pneumoniae, whose resistance to penicillin is of greatest significance in meningitis; community-acquired staphylococcal infection, which may now be due to methicillin-resistant *S aureus*; *Neisseria gonorrhoeae,* which is increasingly resistant to fluoroquinolones; and campylobacter isolates that are increasingly resistant to fluoroquinolones in traveler's diarrhea acquired in southeast Asia.

Antibiotics not reaching site of infection

Antibiotics may fail to reach the site of infection. Malabsorption of the antibiotic can result from primary intestinal pathology or from superimposed ileus, bowel ischemia, or edema, or it may follow interaction with food or medication. Thus, fluoroquinolones are poorly absorbed with antacids containing magnesium or aluminum; products containing iron, calcium, or zinc; or sucralfate. Tetracyclines are poorly absorbed with antacids or dairy products; ketoconazole is better absorbed at a low pH, explaining its poor absorption with antacids and food. Antituberculosis drugs, especially rifampin (perhaps because it exhibits concentration-dependent killing, discussed below) but also isoniazid and ethambutol, may be absorbed late or incompletely, resulting in low serum concentrations with treatment failures and resistance. Such failures and resistance have been documented with HIV patients in the United States, and in both HIV-positive and HIV-negative patients from other countries, regardless of food or other factors, and indicates the importance of monitoring serum concentrations in selected patients [6,7]. A different type of malabsorption, with inadequate serum levels, occurs after intramuscular administration in patients who are diabetic or hypotensive.

An antibiotic can fail to reach the site of infection because of protected anatomic locations, especially the central nervous system, eye, and prostate. As opposed to the rest of the body, these three areas have nonfenestrated capillaries, so that antibiotics cannot pass between endothelial cells to reach extravascular locations but must pass directly through the cells. This is possible if the antibiotic is lipid-soluble, such as chloramphenicol, rifampin, metronidazole, quinolones, doxycycline, and trimethoprim. However, antibiotics that are weakly lipid-soluble (eg, β-lactams, aminoglycosides, and vancomycin) penetrate these protected sites poorly [8]. The presence of acute inflammation may facilitate entry of weakly lipid-soluble agents, so that most antibiotics treat acute prostatitis effectively. However, fluoroquinolones and trimethoprim–sulfamethoxazole are still preferred for chronic prostatitis because the β-lactams penetrate poorly in the absence of inflammation. For infections of the central nervous system, penicillins and third-generation cephalosporins given in high dosage can overcome the poor penetration of these agents when there is central nervous system inflammation. However, high doses should be maintained as the patient improves because decreasing inflammation reduces penetration of these drugs. Also, in view of the adjunctive use of dexamethasone in adult patients with pneumococcal meningitis, the desired reduction in inflammation might also reduce penetration of the antibiotic, with the potential for therapeutic failure. In such patients, a poor response or the presence of a highly resistant organism should prompt a repeat lumbar puncture to check adequacy of response [9]. Because of the poor central nervous system penetration of aminoglycosides and vancomycin, these agents have been administered intrathecally or intraventricularly for the treatment of meningitis and ventriculitis, respectively. In the treatment of endophthalmitis, intravitreal injection of antibiotics is the cornerstone of therapy, with the additional modalities of subconjunctival, topical, or systemic administration of antibiotics more controversial.

Protein binding, which renders a drug inactive, is another proposed reason for an antibiotic's failure to reach an infected site. However, protein binding is reversible and the importance of this factor is difficult to predict. Protein binding may also be a factor in extravascular sites if there is significant leakage of albumin. Similarly, vascular insufficiency may prevent antibiotic from reaching an infected area, a situation sometimes ameliorated by revascularization. Such vascular insufficiency may occur, for example, in an extremity infected with chronic osteomyelitis. Some protected sites are specific for individual drugs, such as the inadequate activity of daptomycin in pulmonary infection because of inhibition by surfactant [10,11], and the poor levels of aminoglycosides in bronchial secretions, which has resulted in the use of antipseudomonas aerosol therapy in cystic fibrosis.

On the other hand, antibiotics have little difficulty in reaching most body cavities, so that systemic administration is sufficient for infections involving pleura, peritoneum, pericardium, and joints, rendering unnecessary the direct instillation of antibiotics for these infections.

Inadequate local activity

Once the antibiotic reaches the site of infection, it can still fail if local activity is inadequate. This may result from insufficient dosage. It may also result from inactivation of antibiotics by low pH, as happens with aminoglycosides in abscesses or infected bone. Alkalinization appears to increase the activity of erythromycin, azithromycin, clarithromycin, clindamycin, and aminoglycosides. Drug–drug interactions may also render the local concentration of an antibiotic inadequate. For example, rifampin's effect on cytochrome P450 metabolism may reduce the levels of many drugs, including antibiotics, and this remains an important consideration in the interaction of rifampin and protease inhibitors for therapy of HIV infection.

Another local phenomenon that affects antibiotic effectiveness is the Eagle phenomenon, the tendency of some organisms that attain large populations to reach a stationary growth phase, during which penicillin-binding proteins are not expressed; this makes them less susceptible to cell-wall active antibiotics. This is one of the reasons that clindamycin has become an important adjunct to penicillin in the treatment of necrotizing fasciitis, in which massive numbers of organisms may accumulate [4]. Pregnancy promotes rapid clearance of many agents and an increased volume of distribution, which may dilute the concentration of some antimicrobial agents. In general, the concentration of an antibiotic at the site of infections should be 8 to 10 times the minimum inhibitory concentration to prevent the overgrowth of resistant populations and to avoid the selective pressure for emergence of resistance.

Pharmacodynamic principles may also determine activity at the site of infection [12–15]. One group of antibiotics has bactericidal activity that depends on the height of the serum concentration and a prolonged postantibiotic effect. Antibiotics in this group include the aminoglycosides, fluoroquinolones, metronidazole, azithromycin, and ketolides. Theoretically, the best results with these agents are obtained when the 24-hour ratio of the area under the curve to the minimal inhibitory concentration (AUC:MIC) equals 100 to 125 in the case of aminoglycosides and fluoroquinolones against gram-negative bacilli, and an AUC:MIC >25 to 35 for azithromycin and fluoroquinolones against S pneumoniae. Alternatively, a ratio of the maximum serum concentration to the MIC >10 is also considered a good predictor of success with these drugs. A second category of antibiotics comprises the β-lactams and vancomycin. These agents have time-dependent bactericidal action, and have a minimal or short postantibiotic effect. The goal of therapy with these drugs is maintenance of a serum concentration greater than the MIC for 40% to 50% of the dosing interval. As opposed to the concentration-dependent antibiotics, killing is maximized at four to five times the MIC with time-dependent drugs, and concentrations above that level do not kill bacteria more efficiently. A third category includes bacteriostatic agents whose efficacy depends on the AUC; they have moderate or prolonged postantibiotic effects but little concentration-dependent killing, with resultant effectiveness when their concentration exceeds the MIC for less than 50% of the dosing interval. Examples are the macrolides (erythromycin, clarithromycin), clindamycin, linezolid, and the tetracyclines.

However, these pharmacodynamic principles have limitations, as it is not always possible to extrapolate from in vitro observations. Some experimental conditions are not easily met in vivo, such as inoculum size, local pH, time of exposure to the antibiotic, effects of protein binding, and effects of drug concentration in urine or bile. Furthermore, the above considerations are based on expected serum concentrations, whereas the amount of drug at the site of infection may not reflect the serum level. The investigative technique of microdialysis attempts to address this disparity [16]. Also, a measured serum level does not predict intracellular concentrations of antibiotic, which may be crucial in treating intracellular pathogens, such as M tuberculosis, salmonella, listeria, and legionella. The fluoroquinolones, clindamycin, azithromycin, clarithromycin, and other macrolides all reach concentrations in cells sometimes exceeding extracellular fluid levels.

However, even this may not always be advantageous, since the antibiotic frequently localizes in lysosomes, which are acidic, so that macrolides and aminoglycosides will have reduced activity [17]. Pharmacodynamic properties of some antibiotics vary with different organisms, whereas others exhibit both time-dependent and concentration-dependent activity. Finally, in spite of the perceived importance of the MIC, subinhibitory concentrations often have desirable effects on phagocytosis, adherence, and intracellular killing. Therefore, in vitro observations do not always predict in vivo effects, and the ultimate gauge of an antibiotic's effectiveness remains the patient's clinical response [8,12].

Immunosuppression

Even if all the above factors are favorable—that is, the correct antibiotic concentration reaches the infected site and the antibiotic retains its activity—therapy may still fail. In some patients, this occurs because of immunosuppression, either iatrogenic (eg, corticosteroid administration, chemotherapy-induced leucopenia) or in disease states, such as AIDS or malignancy.

Paradoxical responses and the Jarisch–Herxheimer reaction

An apparent failure of antibiotic therapy may also indicate a paradoxical response to therapy, which is really not a failure. Such paradoxical responses are seen as an immune reconstitution phenomenon in the treatment of tuberculosis and are manifested by apparent exacerbation of a tuberculous focus (eg, an expanding lymph node or pulmonary infiltrate). However this paradox reflects an improving immunologic responsiveness, not therapeutic failure, and the temporary exacerbation can be treated with anti-inflammatory medication. Similarly, highly active antiretroviral therapy may be associated with paradoxical worsening of a variety of latent infections due to such opportunists as *Myobacterium avium*, cytomegalovirus, varicella-zoster, hepatitis C, cryptococcus, pneumocystis, and JC virus, the virus that causes progressive multifocal leukoencephalopathy. A similar worsening during therapy occurs with the Jarisch–Herxheimer reaction seen with syphilis and other spirochetal diseases (Lyme disease, leptospirosis, rat bite fever, relapsing fever), bacillary angiomatosis, and brucellosis. In this latter group, worsening stems from release of endotoxin or other pyrogens, which cause fever, rigors, myalgias, and sometime focal tissue damage. Sometimes this reaction is a diagnostic clue to the presence of an unsuspected infection. Such a reaction, for example, might suggest concomitant syphilis in a patient being treated for gonorrhea.

Point of no return

Finally, antibiotic treatment may fail because it is too late. Some infections are treatable initially, such as leptospirosis, which may respond to penicillin or tetracycline in the first few days of illness, or Rocky Mountain spotted fever, which responds poorly after 5 days. Other typically fulminant diseases, such as meningococcemia, must be treated extremely early to affect outcome.

If the evaluation of the apparent antibiotic failure still yields no answer, the clinician should repeat the steps in the algorithm (see Fig. 1). Some explanations may evolve over time and become apparent only later in the patient's course, so that review of the possible causes should be an ongoing process. Diagnosis of a paradoxical response, immunologic unresponsiveness, or a point of no return should be by exclusion only. In other words, don't give up.

References

[1] Cunha BA, editor. Infectious diseases in critical care medicine. New York: Marcel Dekker; 1998.
[2] Falagas ME, Vergidis PI. Narrative review: diseases that masquerade as infectious cellulitis. Ann Intern Med 2005;142(1):47–55.
[3] Donlan RM. Biofilm formation: a clinically relevant microbiological process. Clin Infect Dis 2001;33:1387–92.
[4] Pankey GA, Sabath LD. Clinical relevance of bacteriostatic versus bactericidal mechanisms of action in the treatment of gram-positive bacterial infections. CID 2004;38:864–70.
[5] Lewis JS II, Jorgensen JH. Inducible clindamycin resistance in staphylococci: should clinicians and microbiologists be concerned? CID 2005;40:280–5.
[6] Perlman DC, Segal Y, Rosenkranz S, et al. The clinical pharmacokinetics of rifampin and etahmbutol in HIV-infected persons with tuberculosis. CID 2005;41:1638–47.
[7] Tappero JW, Bradford WZ, Agerton TB, et al. Serum concentrations of antimycobacterial drugs in patients with pulmonary tuberculosis in Botswana. CID 2005;41:461–9.
[8] Hessen TH, Kaye D. Principles of use of antibacterial agents. Infect Dis Clin N Am 2004;18: 435–50.
[9] Tunkel AR. Acute meningitis. In: Mandell GL, Bennett JE, Dolin R, editors. Principles and practice of infectious disease. 6th edition. Philadelphia: Elsevier; 2005.
[10] Silverman JA, Mortin LI, Vanpraagh AD, et al. Inhibition of daptomycin by pulmonary surfactant: in vitro modeling and clinical impact. J Infect Dis 2005;191:2149–52.
[11] Schmidt-Ioanas M, de Roux A, Lode H. New antibiotics for the treatment of severe staphylococcal infection in the critically ill patient. Curr Opin Crit Care 2005;11:481–6.
[12] Levison ME. Pharmacodynamics of antimicrobial drugs. Infect Dis Clin N Am 2004;18: 451–65.
[13] Schentag JJ, Gilliland KK, Paladino JA. What have we learned from pharmacokinetic and pharmacodynamic theories? CID 2001;32:S39–46.
[14] Craig WA. Does the dose matter? CID 2001;33:S233–7.
[15] Craig WA. Pharmacokinetic/pharmacodynamic parameters: rationale for antibacterial dosing of mice and men. CID 1998;26:1–12.
[16] Liu P, Derendorf H. Antimicrobial tissue concentrations. Infect Dis Clin N Am 2003;17: 599–613.
[17] Barza M. Pharmacologic principles. In: Gorbach SL, Bartlett JG, Blacklow NR, editors. Infectious diseases. 3rd edition. Philadelphia: Lippincott Williams & Williams; 2004.

ELSEVIER
SAUNDERS

Med Clin N Am 90 (2006) 1279–1289

THE MEDICAL
CLINICS
OF NORTH AMERICA

Index

Note: Page numbers of article titles are in **boldface** type.

Sulfanilamide, discovery of, 1050

Sulfonamides, resistance to, 1063

Superantigens, 1079

Surgery, with antibiotic therapy,
1268–1270

Susceptibility testing, versus in vivo
effectiveness, **1077–1088,** 1167–1168
antibiotic intrinsic factors in,
1081–1084
host factors and, 1078–1081
methods for, 1084–1085
pathogen factors and, 1078–1081
pharmacodynamics and
pharmacokinetics effects on,
1081–1084
resistance impact on, 1084–1085

Synsorb 90 oligosaccharide, for *Clostridium
difficile*-associated diarrhea, 1149

Systemic infections, serious. *See* Serious
systemic infections.

T

Teicoplanin, 1057, 1148, 1150

Telithromycin
chemical structure of, 1109–1110, 1113
drug interactions with, 1229–1232
for pneumonia, 1192
for serious systemic infections, 1204
for *Streptococcus pneumoniae*
infections, 1171
resistance to, 1113–1114, 1118–1119,
1169

Tetracyclines, 1054–1055. *See also specific
agents.*
drug interactions with, 1238–1240
for *Helicobacter pylori* infections,
1131, 1134
for serious systemic infections, 1207
resistance to, 1063

Tiacumicins, for *Clostridium difficile*-
associated diarrhea, 1148

Ticarcillin, for serious systemic infections,
1206

Tigecycline, 1059
drug interactions with, 1239, 1241
for cellulitis, 1185
for endocarditis, 1191
for serious systemic infections, 1206
for *Staphylococcus aureus* infections,
1175
for *Streptococcus pneumoniae*
infections, 1171

Tinidazole, for *Helicobacter pylori*
infections, 1133

Tobramycin
drug interactions with, 1235–1236
for serious systemic infections, 1204

Tolevamer, for *Clostridium difficile*-
associated diarrhea, 1149

Toxic shock syndrome, 1079

Toxin-B cytotoxicity test, in *Clostridium
difficile*-associated diarrhea,
1144–1145

Toxins, *Clostridium difficile,* 1141–1142,
1151–1152

Transduction, in resistance transfer, 1060

Transformation, in resistance transfer,
1060

Transposition, in resistance transfer,
1060–1061

Trimethoprim-sulfamethoxazole,
1055–1056
Clostridium difficile-associated
diarrhea due to, 1143
drug interactions with, 1244, 1246
for endocarditis, 1191
for osteomyelitis, 1185–1186
for serious systemic infections, 1205,
1207
for *Staphylococcus aureus* infections,
1176–1177
resistance to, 1063, 1167, 1169

Tuberculosis, drugs for, drug interactions
with, 1250–1253

U

Ulcer(s)
decubitus, antibiotic failure in,
1270
peptic, *Helicobacter pylori* in, 1126,
1129

Urea breath tests, in *Helicobacter pylori*
infections, 1128

Urinary tract infections, nitrofurantoin for,
1092–1093

V

Vacuolizing cytotoxins, *Helicobacter pylori,*
1125–1126

Vancomycin, 1056
drug interactions with, 1236–1237
for cellulitis, 1185

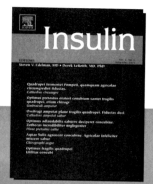

United States Postal Service
Statement of Ownership, Management, and Circulation

1. Publication Title	2. Publication Number		3. Filing Date
Medical Clinics of North America	3 3 7 - 3 3 4 0		9/15/06

4. Issue Frequency	5. Number of Issues Published Annually	6. Annual Subscription Price
Jan, Mar, May, Jul, Sep, Nov	6	$145.00

7. Complete Mailing Address of Known Office of Publication (*Not printer*) (*Street, city, county, state, and ZIP+4*)

Elsevier, Inc.
360 Park Avenue South
New York, NY 10010-1710

Contact Person
Sarah Carmichael
Telephone
(215) 239-3681

8. Complete Mailing Address of Headquarters or General Business Office of Publisher (*Not printer*)

Elsevier, Inc., 360 Park Avenue South, New York, NY 10010-1710

9. Full Names and Complete Mailing Addresses of Publisher, Editor, and Managing Editor (*Do not leave blank*)

Publisher (*Name and complete mailing address*)

John Schrefer, Elsevier, Inc., 1600 John F. Kennedy Blvd., Suite 1800, Philadelphia, PA 19103-2899

Editor (*Name and complete mailing address*)

Rachel Glover, Elsevier, Inc., 1600 John F. Kennedy Blvd., Suite 1800, Philadelphia, PA 19103-2899

Managing Editor (*Name and complete mailing address*)

Catherine Bewick, Elsevier, Inc., 1600 John F. Kennedy Blvd., Suite 1800, Philadelphia, PA 19103-2899

10. Owner (*Do not leave blank. If the publication is owned by a corporation, give the name and address of the corporation immediately followed by the names and addresses of all stockholders owning or holding 1 percent or more of the total amount of stock. If not owned by a corporation, give the names and addresses of the individual owners. If owned by a partnership or other unincorporated firm, give its name and address as well as those of each individual owner. If the publication is published by a nonprofit organization, give its name and address.*)

Full Name	Complete Mailing Address
Wholly owned subsidiary of	4520 East-West Highway
Reed/Elsevier, US Holdings	Bethesda, MD 20814

11. Known Bondholders, Mortgagees, and Other Security Holders Owning or Holding 1 Percent or More of Total Amount of Bonds, Mortgages, or Other Securities. If none, check box ▶ None

Full Name	Complete Mailing Address
N/A	

12. Tax Status (*For completion by nonprofit organizations authorized to mail at nonprofit rates*) (*Check one*)
The purpose, function, and nonprofit status of this organization and the exempt status for federal income tax purposes:
☐ Has Not Changed During Preceding 12 Months
☐ Has Changed During Preceding 12 Months (*Publisher must submit explanation of change with this statement*)

(*See Instructions on Reverse*)

PS Form **3526**, October 1999

---

13. Publication Title	14. Issue Date for Circulation Data Below
Medical Clinics of North America	July, 2006

15. Extent and Nature of Circulation			Average No. Copies Each Issue During Preceding 12 Months	No. Copies of Single Issue Published Nearest to Filing Date
a. Total Number of Copies (*Net press run*)			5,883	5,700
b. Paid and/or Requested Circulation	(1)	Paid/Requested Outside-County Mail Subscriptions Stated on Form 3541. (*Include advertiser's proof and exchange copies*)	3,082	2,916
	(2)	Paid In-County Subscriptions Stated on Form 3541 (*Include advertiser's proof and exchange copies*)		
	(3)	Sales Through Dealers and Carriers, Street Vendors, Counter Sales, and Other Non-USPS Paid Distribution	1,369	1,548
	(4)	Other Classes Mailed Through the USPS		
c. Total Paid and/or Requested Circulation [*Sum of 15b. (1), (2), (3), and (4)*]		▶	4,451	4,464
d. Free Distribution by Mail (*Samples, complimentary, and other free*)	(1)	Outside-County as Stated on Form 3541	120	135
	(2)	In-County as Stated on Form 3541		
	(3)	Other Classes Mailed Through the USPS		
e. Free Distribution Outside the Mail (*Carriers or other means*)		▶		
f. Total Free Distribution (*Sum of 15d. and 15e.*)		▶	120	135
g. Total Distribution (*Sum of 15c. and 15f.*)		▶	4,571	4,599
h. Copies not Distributed			1,312	1,101
i. Total (*Sum of 15g. and h.*)		▶	5,883	5,700
j. Percent Paid and/or Requested Circulation (*15c. divided by 15g. times 100*)			97.37%	97.06%

16. Publication of Statement of Ownership
☐ Publication required. Will be printed in the November 2006 issue of this publication. ☐ Publication not required

17. Signature and Title of Editor, Publisher, Business Manager, or Owner

[signature] Paul Frances — Executive Director of Subscription Services

Date 9/15/06

I certify that all information furnished on this form is true and complete. I understand that anyone who furnishes false or misleading information on this form or who omits material or information requested on the form may be subject to criminal sanctions (including fines and imprisonment) and/or civil sanctions (including civil penalties).

Instructions to Publishers

1. Complete and file one copy of this form with your postmaster annually on or before October 1. Keep a copy of the completed form for your records.
2. In cases where the stockholder or security holder is a trustee, include in items 10 and 11 the name of the person or corporation for whom the trustee is acting. Also include the names and addresses of individuals who are stockholders who own or hold 1 percent or more of the total amount of bonds, mortgages, or other securities of the publishing corporation. In item 11, if none, check the box. Use blank sheets if more space is required.
3. Be sure to furnish all circulation information called for in item 15. Free circulation must be shown in items 15d, e, and f.
4. Item 15h., Copies not Distributed, must include (1) newsstand copies originally stated on Form 3541, and returned to the publisher, (2) estimated returns from news agents, and (3), copies for office use, leftovers, spoiled, and all other copies not distributed.
5. If the publication had Periodicals authorization as a general or requester publication, this Statement of Ownership, Management, and Circulation must be published; it must be printed in any issue in October or, if the publication is not published during October, the first issue printed after October.
6. In item 16, indicate the date of the issue in which this Statement of Ownership will be published.
7. Item 17 must be signed.
Failure to file or publish a statement of ownership may lead to suspension of Periodicals authorization.

PS Form **3526**, October 1999 (*Reverse*)